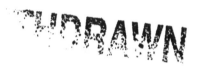

Dental Care
and Oral Health
SOURCEBOOK

Fifth Edition

Health Reference Series

Fifth Edition

Dental Care and Oral Health
SOURCEBOOK

Basic Consumer Health Information about Caring for the Mouth and Teeth, Including Facts about Dental Hygiene and Routine Care Guidelines, Fluoride, Sealants, Tooth Whitening Systems, Cavities, Root Canals, Extractions, Implants, Veneers, Dentures, and Orthodontic and Orofacial Procedures

Along with Information about Periodontal (Gum) Disease, Canker Sores, Dry Mouth, Temporomandibular Joint and Muscle Disorders (TMJ), Oral Cancer, and Other Conditions That Impact Oral Health, Suggestions for Finding and Financing Care, a Glossary of Related Terms, and Directories of Additional Resources

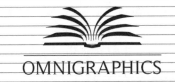

OMNIGRAPHICS

615 Griswold, Ste. 901, Detroit, MI 48226

Bibliographic Note
Because this page cannot legibly accommodate all the copyright notices, the Bibliographic
Note portion of the Preface constitutes an extension of the copyright notice.

* * *

Health Reference Series
Keith Jones, *Managing Editor*
***

OMNIGRAPHICS
A PART OF RELEVANT INFORMATION
***

Copyright © 2016 Omnigraphics
ISBN 978-0-7808-1530-8
E-ISBN 978-0-7808-1531-5

Library of Congress Cataloging-in-Publication Data

Names: Omnigraphics, Inc.

Title: Dental care and oral health sourcebook: basic consumer health information
about caring for the mouth and teeth, including facts about dental hygiene and
routine care guidelines, fluoride, sealants, tooth whitening systems, cavities, root
canals, extractions, implants, veneers, dentures, and orthodontic and orofacial
procedures; along with information about periodontal (gum) disease, canker sores,
dry mouth, temporomandibular joint and muscle disorders (tmj), oral cancer, and
other conditions that impact oral health, suggestions for finding and financing
care, a glossary of related terms, and directories of additional resources.

Description: Fifth edition. | Detroit, MI: Omnigraphics, [2016] | Series: Health
reference series | Includes bibliographical references and index.

Identifiers: LCCN 2016035617 (print) | LCCN 2016037005 (ebook) | ISBN
9780780815308 (hardcover: alk. paper) | ISBN 9780780815315 (ebook) | ISBN
9780780815315 (eBook)

Subjects: LCSH: Dentistry--Popular works. | Mouth--Diseases--Popular works. |
Mouth--Care and hygiene--Popular works.

Classification: LCC RK61 .O66 2016 (print) | LCC RK61 (ebook) | DDC 617.6--dc23

LC record available at https://lccn.loc.gov/2016035617

Table of Contents

Part II: Visiting Your Dentist's Office

Part III: Dental Care for Infants and Children

Part IV: Orthodontic, Endodontic, Periodontic, and Orofacial Procedures

Part V: Oral Diseases and Disorders

Part VII: Finding and Financing Oral Health in the United States

Part VIII: Additional Help and Information

Preface

About This Book

Oral health is essential to overall health. Good oral health includes more than maintaining healthy teeth and gums. Oral health also involves avoiding craniofacial conditions that can affect the face and mouth. When present these conditions can lead to systemic health conditions such as infections, immune disorders, cancer, or heart and lung disease. While there has been significant improvement in the oral health of Americans over the past 50 years due to increasingly effective prevention and treatment efforts, some challenges remain and new concerns have emerged. One important emerging oral health issue is the increase of tooth decay in preschool children. In addition, lack of access to dental care for all ages remains a public health challenge.

Dental Care and Oral Health Sourcebook, Fifth Edition, offers updated information about mouth and tooth care guidelines for effective hygiene, nutrition, and decay prevention. Facts about tooth pain, dental fillings, orthodontia, and other endodontic treatments, and dental implants are described. Facial trauma and cleft palate treatments are also discussed. Disorders such as bad breath, temporomandibular joint and muscle (TMJ) disorder, mouth sores, jaw disorders, and health conditions that impact oral health are addressed. The book concludes with guidelines for finding and financing dental care, a glossary of dental care terms, and directories with further information about dental care and oral health services.

How to Use This Book

This book is divided into parts and chapters. Parts focus on broad areas of interest. Chapters are devoted to single topics within a part.

Part I: Taking Care of Your Mouth and Teeth begins by outlining key steps for good dental health and provides an overview on the anatomy of the mouth. Information on home care products used to clean teeth and remove dental plaque is provided. The impact of nutrition and fluoride is described along with information about mouth injuries. Oral health for older adults is also discussed.

Part II: Visiting Your Dentist's Office explains common procedures, such as X-rays, fillings, sedation, air abrasion, and dental lasers for tooth pain. Details about types of dental restorations, having a tooth pulled, rebuilding and reshaping, and denture choices are also provided.

Part III: Dental Care for Infants and Children offers strategies for initiating and maintaining healthy primary teeth. Fluoride treatments and sealants with adequate calcium intake are addressed. Other specific concerns for children, such as teething, childhood bruxism, and the impact of sugar and snack foods on children's oral health, are detailed. It also discusses the importance of routine dental care visits and preventing tooth decay. The part ends with information on finding and visiting dental clinics for children.

Part IV: Orthodontic, Endodontic, Periodontic, and Orofacial Procedures offers details about braces and retainers, along with information about treatment for endodontic conditions, periodontal (gum) disease, and dental implants. Facial trauma and corrective jaw surgery are also discussed.

Part V: Oral Diseases and Disorders provides information about bad breath, burning mouth syndrome, cleft palate, dentinogenesis imperfecta, jaw problems, mouth sores, oral cancer, thrush, and tongue tie. Dry mouth disorders, such as sialadenitis and Sjögren's syndrome, are also explained.

Part VI: Health Conditions That Affect Oral Health describes specific medical conditions that cause—or result in—oral complications, including cancer treatment, celiac disease, diabetes, heart disease, immune system disorders, organ transplantation, osteoporosis, and the use of tobacco or illegal drugs.

Part VII: Finding and Financing Oral Health in the United States provides information on oral healthcare status and factors that impact access to oral healthcare. It reviews average dental expenses for dental care and includes suggestions for finding low-cost dental care. Specific information about school-based oral health services is also provided.

Part VIII: Additional Help and Information provides a glossary of terms related to dental care and oral health. Directories of local dental schools and other dental care and oral health resources are also included.

Bibliographic Note

This volume contains documents and excerpts from publications issued by the following U.S. government agencies: Agency for Healthcare Research and Quality (AHRQ); AIDS.gov; Centers for Disease Control and Prevention (CDC); Centers for Medicare and Medicaid Services (CMS); Early Childhood Learning and Knowledge Center (ECLKC); *Eunice Kennedy Shriver* National Institute of Child Health and Human Development (NICHD); Genetic and Rare Diseases (GARD) Information Center; Genetics Home Reference (GHR); National Institute of Arthritis and Musculoskeletal and Skin Diseases (NIAMS); National Institute of Dental and Craniofacial Research (NIDCR); National Institute of Diabetes and Digestive and Kidney Diseases (NIDDK); National Institute on Deafness and Other Communication Disorders (NIDCD); National Institute on Drug Abuse (NIDA); National Institutes of Health (NIH); NIDA for Teens; *NIH News in Health*; NIHSeniorHealth; Office of Disease Prevention and Health Promotion (ODPHP); Office on Women's Health (OWH); U.S. Environmental Protection Agency (EPA); U.S. Department of Health and Human Services (HHS); and U.S. Food and Drug Administration (FDA).

In addition, this volume contains copyrighted documents from the following organization: The Nemours Foundation

It may also contain original material produced by Omnigraphics and reviewed by medical consultants.

About the Health Reference Series

The *Health Reference Series* is designed to provide basic medical information for patients, families, caregivers, and the general public. Each volume takes a particular topic and provides comprehensive coverage. This is especially important for people who may be dealing with a newly diagnosed disease or a chronic disorder in themselves or in a family member. People looking for preventive guidance, information about disease warning signs, medical statistics, and risk factors for health problems will also find answers to their questions in the *Health Reference Series*. The *Series*, however, is not intended to serve as a tool for diagnosing illness, in prescribing treatments, or as a substitute for the physician/patient relationship. All people concerned about medical symptoms or the possibility of disease are encouraged to seek professional care from an appropriate health care provider.

A Note about Spelling and Style

Health Reference Series editors use *Stedman's Medical Dictionary* as an authority for questions related to the spelling of medical terms and the *Chicago Manual of Style* for questions related to grammatical structures, punctuation, and other editorial concerns. Consistent adherence is not always possible, however, because the individual volumes within the *Series* include many documents from a wide variety of different producers, and the editor's primary goal is to present material from each source as accurately as is possible. This sometimes means that information in different chapters or sections may follow other guidelines and alternate spelling authorities.

Medical Review

Omnigraphics contracts with a team of qualified, senior medical professionals who serve as medical consultants for the *Health Reference Series*. As necessary, medical consultants review reprinted and originally written material for currency and accuracy. Citations including the phrase, "Reviewed (month, year)" indicate material reviewed by this team. Medical consultation services are provided to the *Health Reference Series* editors by:

Dr. Senthil Selvan, MBBS, DCH, MD
Dr. K. Sivanandham, MBBS, DCH, MS (Research), PhD

Our Advisory Board

We would like to thank the following board members for providing initial guidance on the development of this series:

- Dr. Lynda Baker, Associate Professor of Library and Information Science, Wayne State University, Detroit, MI

- Nancy Bulgarelli, William Beaumont Hospital Library, Royal Oak, MI

- Karen Imarisio, Bloomfield Township Public Library, Bloomfield Township, MI

- Karen Morgan, Mardigian Library, University of Michigan-Dearborn, Dearborn, MI

- Rosemary Orlando, St. Clair Shores Public Library, St. Clair Shores, MI

Health Reference Series *Update Policy*

The inaugural book in the *Health Reference Series* was the first edition of *Cancer Sourcebook* published in 1989. Since then, the *Series* has been enthusiastically received by librarians and in the medical community. In order to maintain the standard of providing high-quality health information for the layperson the editorial staff at Omnigraphics felt it was necessary to implement a policy of updating volumes when warranted.

Medical researchers have been making tremendous strides, and it is the purpose of the *Health Reference Series* to stay current with the most recent advances. Each decision to update a volume is made on an individual basis. Some of the considerations include how much new information is available and the feedback we receive from people who use the books. If there is a topic you would like to see added to the update list, or an area of medical concern you feel has not been adequately addressed, please write to:

Managing Editor
Health Reference Series
Omnigraphics
615 Griswold, Ste. 901
Detroit, MI 48226

Part One

Taking Care of Your Mouth and Teeth

Chapter 1

Steps to Dental Health

Healthy teeth and gums make it easy for you to eat well and enjoy good food. Several problems can affect the health of your mouth, but good care should keep your teeth and gums strong as you age.

Tooth Decay

Teeth are covered in a hard, outer coating called enamel. Every day, a thin film of bacteria called dental plaque builds up on your teeth. The bacteria in plaque produce acids that can harm enamel and cause cavities. Brushing and flossing your teeth can prevent decay, but once a cavity forms, a dentist has to fix it.

Use fluoride toothpaste to protect your teeth from decay. If you are at a higher risk for tooth decay (for example, if you have a dry mouth because of a condition you have or medicines you take), you might need more fluoride. Your dentist or dental hygienist may give you a fluoride treatment during an office visit or may tell you to use a fluoride gel or mouth rinse at home.

Gum Disease

Gum disease begins when plaque builds up along and under your gum line. This plaque causes infections that hurt the gum and bone that hold your teeth in place. Gum disease may make your gums tender

This chapter includes text excerpted from "Taking Care of Your Teeth and Mouth," Centers for Disease Control and Prevention (CDC), June 2016.

and more likely to bleed. This problem, called gingivitis, can often be fixed by brushing and flossing every day.

A more severe form of gum disease, called periodontitis, must be treated by a dentist. If not treated, this infection can ruin the bones, gums, and other tissues that support your teeth. Over time, your teeth may have to be removed.

To prevent gum disease:

- Brush your teeth twice a day with fluoride toothpaste.

- Floss once a day.

- Visit your dentist regularly for a checkup and cleaning.

- Eat a well-balanced diet.

- Quit smoking. Smoking increases your risk for gum disease.

How to Clean Your Teeth and Gums

There is a right way to brush and floss your teeth. Every day:

- Gently brush your teeth on all sides with a soft-bristle brush and fluoride toothpaste.

- Use small circular motions and short back-and-forth strokes.

- Brush carefully and gently along your gum line.

- Lightly brush your tongue to help keep your mouth clean.

- Clean around your teeth with dental floss. Careful flossing removes plaque and leftover food that a toothbrush can't reach.

- Rinse after you floss.

People with arthritis or other conditions that limit hand motion may find it hard to hold and use a toothbrush. Some helpful tips are:

- Use an electric or battery-operated toothbrush.

- Slide a bicycle grip or foam tube over the handle of the toothbrush.

- Buy a toothbrush with a larger handle.

- Attach the toothbrush handle to your hand with a wide elastic band.

- See your dentist if brushing or flossing causes your gums to bleed or hurts your mouth. If you have trouble flossing, a floss holder may help. Ask your dentist to show you the right way to floss.

Dentures

Sometimes, false teeth (dentures) are needed to replace badly damaged teeth. Partial dentures may be used to fill in one or more missing teeth. Dentures may feel strange at first. In the beginning, your dentist may want to see you often to make sure the dentures fit. Over time, your gums will change shape, and your dentures may need to be adjusted or replaced. Be sure to let your dentist handle these adjustments.

Be careful when wearing dentures, because it may be harder for you to feel hot foods and drinks or notice bones in your food. When learning to eat with dentures, it may be easier if you:

- Start with soft, non-sticky food.

- Cut your food into small pieces.

- Chew slowly using both sides of your mouth.

Keep your dentures clean and free from food that can cause stains, bad breath, or swollen gums. Brush them every day with a denture-care product. Take your dentures out of your mouth at night, and soak them in water or a denture-cleansing liquid.

Dry Mouth

Dry mouth happens when you don't have enough saliva, or spit, to keep your mouth wet. It can make it hard to eat, swallow, taste, and even speak. Dry mouth can accelerate tooth decay and other infections of the mouth. Many common medicines can cause this problem.

There are things you can do that may help. Try sipping water or sugarless drinks. Don't smoke, and avoid alcohol and caffeine. Sugarless hard candy or sugarless gum that is a little tart may help. Your dentist or doctor might suggest using artificial saliva to keep your mouth wet.

Oral Cancer

Cancer of the mouth can grow in any part of the mouth or throat. It is more likely to happen in people over age 40. A dental checkup is a good time for your dentist to look for signs of oral cancer. Pain is not usually an early symptom of the disease. Treatment works best before the disease spreads. Even if you have lost all your natural teeth, you should still see your dentist for regular oral cancer exams.

You can lower your risk of getting oral cancer in a few ways:

- Do not use tobacco products, such as cigarettes, electronic cigarettes, chewing tobacco, snuff, pipes, or cigars.
- If you drink alcohol, do so only in moderation.
- Use lip balm with sunscreen.

Chapter 2

Anatomy of the Mouth

Basic Anatomy of the Mouth and Teeth

The entrance to the digestive tract, the mouth is lined with mucous membranes. The membrane-covered roof of the mouth is called the palate. The front part consists of a bony portion called the hard palate, with a fleshy rear part called the soft palate. The hard palate divides the mouth and the nasal passages above. The soft palate forms a curtain between the mouth and the throat or pharynx, to the rear. The soft palate contains the uvula, the dangling flesh at the back of the mouth. The tonsils are located on either side of the uvula and look like twin pillars holding up the opening to the pharynx.

A bundle of muscles extends from the floor of the mouth to form the tongue. The upper surface of the tongue is covered with tiny bumps called papillae. These contain tiny pores that are our taste buds. Four main kinds of taste buds are found on the tongue—those that sense sweet, salty, sour, and bitter tastes. Three pairs of salivary glands secrete saliva, which contains a digestive enzyme called amylase that starts the breakdown of carbohydrates even before food enters the stomach.

The lips are covered with skin on the outside and with slippery mucous membranes on the inside of the mouth. The major lip muscle, called the orbicularis oris, allows for the lips' mobility. The reddish tint

Text in this chapter is excerpted from "Mouth and Teeth," © 1995–2016. The Nemours Foundation/KidsHealth®. Reprinted with permission.

of the lips comes from underlying blood vessels. The inside portion of both lips is connected to the gums.

There are several types of teeth. Incisors are the squarish, sharp-edged teeth in the front of the mouth. There are four on the bottom and four on the top. On either side of the incisors are the sharp canines. The upper canines are sometimes called eyeteeth or cuspids. Behind the canines are the premolars, or bicuspids. There are two sets or four premolars, in each jaw.

The molars, situated behind the premolars, have points and grooves. There are 12 molars—three sets in each jaw called the first, second, and third molars. The third molars are the wisdom teeth, thought by some to have evolved thousands of years ago when human had larger jaws and ate mostly raw foods that required extra chewing power. But because they can crowd out the other teeth or cause problems like pain or infection, a dentist might need to remove them.

Human teeth are made up of four different types of tissue:

1. Pulp

2. Dentin

3. Enamel

4. Cementum.

The **pulp** is the innermost portion of the tooth and consists of connective tissue, nerves, and blood vessels, which nourish the tooth. The pulp has two parts—the pulp chamber, which lies in the crown, and the root canal, which is in the root of the tooth. Blood vessels and nerves enter the root through a small hole in its tip and extend through the canal into the pulp chamber.

Dentin surrounds the pulp. A hard yellow substance, it makes up most of the tooth and is as hard as bone. It's the dentin that gives teeth their yellowish tint.

Enamel, the hardest tissue in the body, covers the dentin and forms the outermost layer of the crown. It enables the tooth to withstand the pressure of chewing and protects it from harmful bacteria and changes in temperature from hot and cold foods. Both the dentin and pulp extend into the root.

A layer of **cementum** covers the outside of the root, under the gum line, and holds the tooth in place within the jawbone. Cementum is also as hard as bone.

Normal Development of the Mouth and Teeth

Humans are diphyodont, meaning that they develop two sets of teeth. The first set of 20 deciduous teeth are also called the milk, primary, temporary or baby teeth. They begin to develop before birth and begin to fall out when a child is around 6 years old. They're replaced by a set of 32 permanent teeth, which are also called secondary or adult teeth.

Around the eighth week after conception, oval-shaped tooth buds consisting of cells form in the embryo. These buds begin to harden about the 16th week. Although teeth aren't visible at birth, both the primary and permanent teeth are forming below the gums. The crown, or the hard enamel-covered part that's visible in the mouth, develops first. After the crown is formed, the root begins to develop.

Between the ages of 6 months and 1 year, the deciduous teeth begin to push through the gums. This process is called eruption or teething. At this point, the crown is complete and the root is almost fully formed. By the time a child is 3 years old, he or she has a set of 20 deciduous teeth, 10 in the lower and 10 in the upper jaw. Each jaw has four incisors, two canines, and four molars. The molars' purpose is to grind food, and the incisors and canine teeth are used to bite into and tear food.

The primary teeth help the permanent teeth erupt in their normal positions; most of the permanent teeth form close to the roots of the primary teeth. When a primary tooth is preparing to fall out, its root begins to dissolve. This root has completely dissolved by the time the permanent tooth below it is ready to erupt.

Kids start to lose their primary teeth, or baby teeth, at about 6 years old. This begins a phase of permanent tooth development that lasts over the next 15 years, as the jaw steadily grows into its adult form. From ages 6 to 9, the incisors and first molars start to come in. Between ages 10 and 12, the first and second premolars, as well as the canines, erupt. From 11 to 13, the second molars come in. The wisdom teeth (third molars) erupt between the ages of 17 and 21.

Sometimes there isn't room in a person's mouth for all the permanent teeth. If this happens, the wisdom teeth may get stuck, or impacted, beneath the gum and may need to be removed. Overcrowding of the teeth is one of the reasons kids get braces.

Problems of the Mouth and Teeth

Proper dental care—including a good diet, frequent cleaning of the teeth after eating, and regular dental checkups—is essential to maintaining healthy teeth and avoiding tooth decay and gum disease. Common mouth and dental diseases and conditions—some of which can be prevented, some of which cannot—are:

Disorders of the Mouth

- **Aphthous stomatitis (canker sores).** A common form of mouth ulcer, canker sores affect women more often than in men. Although their cause isn't completely understood, mouth injuries, stress, dietary deficiencies, hormonal changes (such as the menstrual cycle) or food allergies can trigger them. They usually appear on the inner surface of the cheeks or lips, under the tongue, on the soft palate, or at the base of the gums. They begin with a tingling or burning sensation followed by a painful sore called an ulcer. Pain subsides in 7 to 10 days, with complete healing usually occurring in 1 to 3 weeks.

- **Cleft lip and cleft palate.** These are birth defects in which the tissues of the lip and/or mouth don't form properly during fetal development. Children born with these disorders may have trouble feeding immediately after birth. Reconstructive surgery in infancy and sometimes later can repair the anatomical defects, and can prevent or lessen the severity of speech problems later on.

- **Enteroviral stomatitis.** This common childhood infection is caused by a family of viruses called enteroviruses. An important member of this family is coxsackievirus, which causes hand, foot, and mouth disease. Enteroviral stomatitis is marked by small, painful ulcers in the mouth that may decrease a child's desire to eat and drink and put him or her at risk for dehydration.

- **Herpetic stomatitis (oral herpes).** Kids can get a mouth infection with the herpes simplex virus from an adult or another child who has it. The infection can spread by direct contact, such as kissing, or by sharing utensils or a cup with someone with the virus. The resulting painful, clustered vesicles, or blisters, can make it difficult to drink or eat, which can lead to dehydration, especially in a young child.

- **Periodontal disease.** The gums and bones supporting the teeth are subject to disease. A common periodontal disease is gingivitis—inflammation of the gums characterized by redness, swelling, and sometimes bleeding. The accumulation of tartar (a hardened film of food particles and bacteria that builds up on teeth) usually causes this condition, and it's almost always the result of inadequate brushing and flossing. When gingivitis isn't treated, it can lead to periodontitis, in which the gums loosen around the teeth and pockets of bacteria and pus form, sometimes damaging the supporting bone and causing tooth loss.

Disorders of the Teeth

- **Cavities and tooth decay.** When bacteria and food particles stick to the teeth, plaque forms. The bacteria digest the carbohydrates in the food and produce acid, which dissolves the tooth's enamel and causes a cavity. If the cavity isn't treated, the decay process progresses to involve the dentin and pulp. Without treatment, serious infections can occur. The most common ways to treat cavities and more serious tooth decay problems are: filling the cavity; performing root canal therapy, involving the removal of the pulp of a tooth; crowning a tooth with a cap that looks like a tooth made of metal, porcelain or plastic; or removing and replacing the tooth. A common cause of tooth decay in toddlers is "baby bottle tooth decay," which occurs when a child goes to sleep with a milk or juice bottle in the mouth and the teeth are bathed in sugary liquid for an extended period of time. To avoid tooth decay and cavities, do not give your child a bottle when going to sleep. Also, teach your kids good dental habits—including proper tooth-brushing techniques—at an early age.

- **Impacted wisdom teeth.** In many people, the wisdom teeth are unable to erupt normally so they either remain below the jawline or don't grow in properly. Dentists call these teeth impacted. Wisdom teeth usually become impacted because the jaw isn't large enough to accommodate all the teeth that are growing in and the mouth becomes overcrowded. Impacted teeth can damage other teeth or become painful and infected. Dentists can check if a person has impacted wisdom teeth by taking X-rays of the teeth. If the X-rays show there's a chance that impacted teeth may cause problems, the dentist may recommend that the tooth or teeth be extracted.

- **Malocclusion** is the failure of the teeth in the upper and lower jaws to meet properly. Types of malocclusion include overbite, underbite, and crowding. Most conditions can be corrected with treatment such as braces, which are metal or clear ceramic brackets bonded to the front of each tooth. The wires connecting braces are tightened periodically to force the teeth to move into the correct position. There are also ways to correct the bite using removable clear appliances.

Chapter 3

Taking Care of Your Teeth

Chapter Contents

Section 3.1

Why Tooth Care Matters

This section contains text excerpted from the following sources:
Text in this chapter begins with excerpts from "Taking Care of
Your Teeth," © 1995–2016. The Nemours Foundation/KidsHealth®.
Reprinted with permission; Text under the heading "Everyday
Dental Care" is excerpted from "Take Care of Your Teeth and Gums,"
Office of Disease Prevention and Health Promotion (ODPHP), U.S.
Department of Health and Human Services (HHS), March 8, 2016.

When you get your picture taken, everyone says, "Say cheese! Smile!" So you do—you open your mouth and show your teeth. When you see the picture, you see a happy person looking back at you. The healthier those teeth are, the happier you look. Why is that?

It's because your teeth are important in many ways. If you take care of them, they'll help take care of you. Strong, healthy teeth help you chew the right foods to help you grow. They help you speak clearly. And yes, they help you look your best.

Why Healthy Teeth Are Important

How does taking care of your teeth help with all those things? Taking care of your teeth helps prevent plaque, which is a clear film of bacteria that sticks to your teeth.

After you eat, bacteria go crazy over the sugar on your teeth, like ants at a picnic. The bacteria break it down into acids that eat away tooth enamel, causing holes called cavities. Plaque also causes gingivitis, which is gum disease that can make your gums red, swollen, and sore. Your gums are those soft pink tissues in your mouth that hold your teeth in place.

If you don't take care of your teeth, cavities and unhealthy gums will make your mouth very, very sore. Eating meals will be difficult. And you won't feel like smiling so much.

Before Toothpaste Was Invented

We're lucky that we know so much now about taking care of our teeth. Long ago, as people got older, their teeth would rot away and be very painful. To get rid of a toothache, they had their teeth pulled out. Finally, people learned that cleaning their teeth was important, but they didn't have toothpaste right away. While you're swishing that minty-fresh paste around your mouth, think about what people used long ago to clean teeth:

- ground-up chalk or charcoal
- lemon juice
- ashes
- tobacco and honey mixed together

It was only about 100 years ago that someone finally created a minty cream to clean teeth. Not long after that, the toothpaste tube was invented, so people could squeeze the paste right onto the toothbrush! Tooth brushing became popular during World War II. The U.S. Army gave brushes and toothpaste to all soldiers, and they learned to brush twice a day. Back then, toothpaste tubes were made of metal; today they're made of soft plastic and are much easier to squeeze!

Today there are plenty of toothpaste choices: lots of colors and flavors to choose from, and some are made just for kids. When you're choosing a toothpaste, make sure it contains fluoride. Fluoride makes your teeth strong and protects them from cavities.

When you brush, you don't need a lot of toothpaste: just squeeze out a bit the size of a pea. It's not a good idea to swallow the toothpaste, either, so be sure to spit after brushing.

How You Can Keep Your Teeth Healthy

Kids can take charge of their teeth by taking these steps:

- Brush at least twice a day—after breakfast and before bedtime. If you can, brush after lunch or after sweet snacks. Brushing properly breaks down plaque.

- Brush all of your teeth, not just the front ones. Spend some time on the teeth along the sides and in the back. Have your dentist show you the best way to brush to get your teeth clean without damaging your gums.

- Take your time while brushing. Spend at least 2 or 3 minutes each time you brush. If you have trouble keeping track of the time, use a timer or play a recording of a song you like to help pass the time.

- Be sure your toothbrush has soft bristles (the package will tell you if they're soft). Ask your parent to help you get a new toothbrush every 3 months. Some toothbrushes come with bristles that change color when it's time to change them.

- Ask your dentist if an antibacterial mouth rinse is right for you.

- Learn how to floss your teeth, which is a very important way to keep them healthy. It feels weird the first few times you do it, but pretty soon you'll be a pro. Slip the dental floss between each tooth and along the gum line gently once a day. The floss gets rid of food that's hidden where your toothbrush can't get it, no matter how well you brush.

- You can also brush your tongue to help keep your breath fresh!

It's also important to visit the dentist twice a year. Besides checking for signs of cavities or gum disease, the dentist will help keep your teeth extra clean and can help you learn the best way to brush and floss.

It's not just brushing and flossing that keep your teeth healthy—you also need to be careful about what you eat and drink. Remember, the plaque on your teeth is just waiting for that sugar to arrive. Eat lots of fruits and vegetables and drink water instead of soda. And don't forget to smile!

Everyday Dental Care

The Basics

It's important to take care of your teeth and gums. You can prevent most problems with teeth and gums by taking these steps:

- Brush your teeth 2 times a day with fluoride toothpaste.
- Floss between your teeth every day.
- Visit a dentist regularly for a checkup and cleaning.
- Cut down on sugary foods and drinks.
- Don't smoke or chew tobacco.
- If you drink alcohol, drink only in moderation.

Why Do I Need to Take Care of My Teeth and Gums?

Healthy habits, including brushing and flossing, can prevent tooth decay (cavities) and gum disease. Tooth decay and gum disease can lead to pain and tooth loss.

What Causes Tooth Decay and Gum Disease?

Plaque is a sticky substance that forms on your teeth. When plaque stays on your teeth too long, it can lead to tooth decay and gum disease. Brushing and flossing help get plaque off your teeth so your mouth can stay healthy. Taking care of your teeth and gums is especially important if you:

- have diabetes
- have cancer
- are an older adult
- are pregnant

Take Action!

Follow these tips for a healthy, beautiful smile.

Brush Your Teeth

Brush your teeth 2 times every day. Use a toothbrush with soft bristles and toothpaste with fluoride. Fluoride is a mineral that helps protect teeth from decay.

- Brush in circles and use short, back-and-forth strokes.
- Take time to brush gently along the gum line.
- Brush your teeth for about 2 minutes each time.
- Don't forget to brush your tongue.
- Get a new toothbrush every 3 to 4 months. Replace your toothbrush sooner if it's wearing out.

Floss Every Day

Floss every day to remove plaque and any food between teeth that your toothbrush missed. Rinse your mouth with water after you floss. If you aren't sure how to floss, ask the dentist or dental assistant to show you at your next visit.

Get Regular Checkups at the Dentist

Visit a dentist once or twice a year for a checkup and cleaning. Get checkups even if you have no natural teeth and have dentures. If you have problems with your teeth or mouth, see a dentist right away.

What If I Don't Like Going to the Dentist?

Some people get nervous about going to the dentist. Try these tips to help make your visit to the dentist easier:

- Let your dentist know you are feeling nervous.
- Choose an appointment time when you won't feel rushed.
- Take headphones and a music player to your next visit.

What If I Don't Have Insurance?

Even if you don't have dental insurance, you can get dental care.

- Find a health center near you to learn more.
- Get tips for finding low-cost dental care.

Cut Down on Sugary Foods and Drinks

Choose low-sugar snacks like vegetables, fruits, and low-fat or fat-free cheese. Drink fewer sugary sodas and other drinks that can lead to tooth decay. Get ideas for eating healthy.

Quit Smoking

People who use tobacco in any form (cigarettes, cigars, pipe, smokeless tobacco) are at higher risk for gum disease and oral (mouth) cancer.

Drink Alcohol Only in Moderation

Drinking a lot of alcohol can increase your risk for oral cancer. If you choose to drink, have only a moderate amount. This means no more than 1 drink a day for women or 2 drinks a day for men.

Take Care of Your Children's Teeth

If you have kids, help them learn good habits for a healthy mouth. Start cleaning your child's teeth as soon as they come in.

Section 3.2

The Use and Handling of Toothbrushes

This section includes text excerpted from "The Use
and Handling of Toothbrushes," Centers for Disease
Control and Prevention (CDC), July 10, 2013.

Infection Control

Tooth brushing with a fluoride toothpaste is a simple, widely recommended and widely practiced method of caring for one's teeth. When done routinely and properly, tooth brushing can reduce the amount of plaque which contains the bacteria associated with gum disease and tooth decay, as well as provide the cavity-preventing benefits of fluoride.

To date, the Centers for Disease Control and Prevention (CDC) is unaware of any adverse health effects directly related to toothbrush use, although people with bleeding disorders and those severely immuno-depressed may suffer trauma from tooth brushing and may need to seek alternate means of oral hygiene. The mouth is home to millions of microorganisms (germs). In removing plaque and other soft debris from the teeth, toothbrushes become contaminated with bacteria, blood, saliva, oral debris, and toothpaste. Because of this contamination, a common recommendation is to rinse one's toothbrush thoroughly with tap water following brushing. Limited research has suggested that even after being rinsed visibly clean, toothbrushes can remain contaminated with potentially pathogenic organisms. In response to this, various means of cleaning, disinfecting or sterilizing toothbrushes between uses have been developed. To date, however, no published research data documents that brushing with a contaminated toothbrush has led to recontamination of a user's mouth, oral infections or other adverse health effects.

Recommended Toothbrush Care

- Do not share toothbrushes. The exchange of body fluids that such sharing would foster places toothbrush sharers at an increased risk for infections, a particularly important consideration for persons with compromised immune systems or infectious diseases.

• After brushing, rinse your toothbrush thoroughly with tap water to ensure the removal of toothpaste and debris, allow it to air-dry, and store it in an upright position. If multiple brushes are stored in the same holder, do not allow them to contact each other.

• It is not necessary to soak toothbrushes in disinfecting solutions or mouthwash. This practice actually may lead to cross-contamination of toothbrushes if the same disinfectant solution is used over a period of time or by multiple users.

• It is also unnecessary to use dishwashers, microwaves, or ultraviolet devices to disinfect toothbrushes. These measures may damage the toothbrush.

• Do not routinely cover toothbrushes or store them in closed containers. Such conditions (a humid environment) are more conducive to bacterial growth than the open air.

• Replace your toothbrush every 3–4 months, or sooner if the bristles appear worn or splayed. This recommendation of the American Dental Association (ADA) is based on the expected wear of the toothbrush and its subsequent loss of mechanical effectiveness, not on its bacterial contamination.

A decision to purchase or use products for toothbrush disinfection requires careful consideration, as the scientific literature does not support this practice at the present time.

Tooth Brushing Programs in Schools and Group Settings

Tooth brushing in group settings should always be supervised to ensure that toothbrushes are not shared and that they are handled properly. The likelihood of toothbrush cross-contamination in these environments is very high, either through children playing with them or toothbrushes being stored improperly. In addition a small chance exists that toothbrushes could become contaminated with blood during brushing. Although the risk for disease transmission through toothbrushes is still minimal, it is a potential cause for concern. Therefore, officials in charge of tooth brushing programs in these settings should evaluate their programs carefully.

Recommended measures for hygienic tooth brushing in schools:

- Ensure that each child has his or her own toothbrush, clearly marked with identification. Do not allow children to share or borrow toothbrushes.

- To prevent cross contamination of the toothpaste tube, ensure that a pea-sized amount of toothpaste is always dispensed onto a piece of wax paper before dispensing any onto the toothbrush.

- After the children finish brushing, ensure that they rinse their toothbrushes thoroughly with tap water, allow them to air-dry, and store them in an upright position so they cannot contact those of other children.

- Provide children with paper cups to use for rinsing after they finish brushing. Do not allow them to share cups, and ensure that they dispose of the cups properly after a single use.

Chapter 4

Nutrition Impacts Oral Health

Tooth development begins in the fetus as early as six weeks of age, when the basic material that makes up teeth starts to form. The impact of nutrition on oral health and dental development begins in the womb, with the mother's nutritional status and eating patterns playing a vital role in the process. Studies have shown that adequate nutrition is a key factor in defining the health of teeth and periodontal tissues and in maintaining salivary secretions at their optimum. Early nutritional imbalances can lead to developmental malformations of the dentition, while malnutrition can result in enamel hypoplasia (thin tooth enamel), poor periodontal health, increased risk of oral infectious disease, and the early onset of dental erosion.

Importance of Balanced Diet

Nutrition plays a vital role in boosting the body's immune system and preventing infections and inflammations. Malnutrition—deficiencies of essential nutrients, such as vitamins and minerals—can have a negative impact on general health and result in cavities and gum disease. Gum disease may start as gingivitis, an inflammation of the gums usually caused by bacterial infection which, if unchecked, may

"Nutrition Impacts Oral Health," © 2017 Omnigraphics. Reviewed September 2016.

progress to periodontal disease, a condition that affects the supporting tissues of the teeth.

Some Important Micronutrients

Studies show that nutrition and oral health are interrelated. Poor nutrition can cause oral and dental problems and, conversely, problems with oral health can trigger nutritional deficiencies. Food habits and eating patterns greatly impact the decay resistance of teeth in children and teens, and a well-balanced diet is an important factor in maintaining periodontal health in the adults and elderly.

A number of micronutrients (vitamins and minerals) are critical to the maintenance of healthy teeth and gums. These include:

Vitamin D (calciferol)

Vitamin D plays a vital role in maintaining musculoskeletal health by aiding in calcium absorption. Its direct effect on bone metabolism makes it an essential nutrient in preventing tooth loss and maintaining periodontal health. Vitamin D is also involved in certain immune regulatory pathways and reduces the risk of periodontitisor inflammation of periodontal tissues. Dietary sources of vitamin D include fish-liver oils, fatty fish, mushrooms, egg yolks, liver, and fortified foods, such as breakfast cereals, milk, and orange juice. The vitamin is also synthesized in the skin by the action of ultraviolet radiation of the sun on certain 7-dehydrocholesterol, a type of serum cholesterol that acts as a precursor to Vitamin D.

Vitamin C (ascorbic acid)

Vitamin C is essential for maintaining the integrity of the connective tissue and dentine, the hard material that makes up much of a tooth. It is also necessary for the proper functioning of the immune system. The deficiency ofvitamin C can lead to scurvy, a disease characterized by gingivitis (spongy, bleeding gums). Rich sources of vitamin C include citrus fruits—such as oranges, limes, and grapefruit—green leafy vegetables, tomatoes, and berries.

Choosing a Healthy Diet

- Fruits and vegetables are especially important in maintaining good oral health. Salads are ideal, as chewing raw vegetables stimulates the secretion of saliva, which helps to wash acid and food remnants from the mouth.

- Nuts are also good. Their low carbohydrate content reduces the risk of cavities. In addition to providing such benefits as minerals and vitamins, they also serve as rich sources of proteins that are important for maintaining overall health.

- Dairy products, such as milk, cheese, and yogurt, are excellent sources of proteins, as well as calcium, a mineral that is critical for the development and maintenance of healthy teeth and periodontal tissue.

- Lean meat, eggs, legumes, and green leafy vegetables, such as collards and spinach, are also rich sources of calcium and can help to build strong teeth and maintain good oral health.

Fluoridated Water and Oral Health

Drinking fluoridated water is highly beneficial for maintaining healthy teeth. Fluoride helps prevent tooth decay, and water washes away food debris in the mouth. The presence of food particles encourages the growth of bacteria that breakdown the sugars in food to release acids. These acids wear away the mineralized oral tissues, including enamel (the hard protective covering of the teeth), cementum (the exterior surface of the roots), and dentine. Water not only removes food residue in the mouth, but also dilutes the acid produced by cavity-causing bacteria.

Drinking water also prevents dehydration and xerostomia (dry mouth, or insufficient saliva). Saliva is an important factor in maintaining the integrity of oral structures. It helps lubricate, chew, and digest food; kill microorganisms in food; dilute sugars; and buffer acid in the mouth. Saliva also helps remineralize tooth enamel with calcium and phosphorous. Insufficient salivary secretions can increase therisk of gingivitis, dental cavities, and oral thrush, a fungal infection of the mouth.

Foods to Avoid for Better Oral Health

The connection between sugar and cavities has been studied for a long time, and it has been established that fermentable carbohydrates and sugars play a major role in the developmentof dental cavities. These cariogenic (cavity-causing) foods are acted upon by bacteria in the mouth, such as *streptococci* and *lactobacilli*, and are converted to acids. The acids demineralize teeth by dissolving calcium and phosphorus and causing tooth erosion. Normally, the demineralization of teeth is offset by remineralization with saliva, which is saturated with calcium and phosphorus. But if the acidic environment in the mouth persists, it interferes with the remineralization process, leading to tooth decay. Although cariogenic foods include a variety of sugars, such as glucose, lactose, fructose, and maltose—either naturally occurring or added to food—sucrose (table sugar) is by far the most cariogenic of all.

Avoiding high-sugar food, such as candies, confectionery, and sugar-sweetened drinks, is undoubtedly the most important prophylactic measure in controlling tooth decay and maintaining good oral health. While acids resulting from bacterial fermentation of sugars in the mouth are a major cause cavities, dietary acids can also, to some extent, contribute to decay by lowering pH below critical levels. Thus, foods and drinks with lower pH can cause teeth erosion. Vinegar-containing foods, as well as acids, naturally occurring in fruit or added to candies and sports drinks, can promote cavities and should be consumed in smaller amounts or eliminated from the diet entirely.

References

1. Touger-Decker, Riva, and Cor van Loveren. "Sugars and Dental Caries," American Journal of Clinical Nutrition, October 2003.

2. "The Best and Worst Foods for Your Teeth," Health Encyclopedia, University of Rochester Medical Center, 2016.

Chapter 5

Fluoride Prevents Tooth Decay

Chapter Contents

Section 5.1

Fluoridation Basics

This section includes text excerpted from
"Community Water Fluoridation," Centers for Disease
Control and Prevention (CDC), May 6, 2016.

What Is Water Fluoridation?

The mineral fluoride occurs naturally on earth and is released from rocks into the soil, water, and air. All water contains some fluoride. Usually, the fluoride level in water is not enough to prevent tooth decay; however, some groundwater and natural springs can have naturally high levels of fluoride.

Fluoride has been proven to protect teeth from decay. Bacteria in the mouth produce acid when a person eats sugary foods. This acid eats away minerals from the tooth's surface, making the tooth weaker and increasing the chance of developing cavities. Fluoride helps to rebuild and strengthen the tooth's surface, or enamel. Water fluoridation prevents tooth decay by providing frequent and consistent contact with low levels of fluoride. By keeping the tooth strong and solid, fluoride stops cavities from forming and can even rebuild the tooth's surface.

Community water fluoridation is the process of adjusting the amount of fluoride found in water to achieve optimal prevention of tooth decay.

Although other fluoride-containing products, such as toothpaste, mouth rinses, and dietary supplements are available and contribute to the prevention and control of tooth decay, community water fluoridation has been identified as the most cost-effective method of delivering fluoride to all, reducing tooth decay by 25% in children and adults.

Benefits: Strong Teeth

Fluoride benefits children and adults throughout their lives. For children younger than age 8, fluoride helps strengthen the adult (permanent) teeth that are developing under the gums. For adults, drinking water with fluoride supports tooth enamel, keeping teeth strong and healthy. The health benefits of fluoride include having:

- Fewer cavities.

- Less severe cavities.

- Less need for fillings and removing teeth.

- Less pain and suffering because of tooth decay.

History of Fluoride in Water

In the 1930s, scientists examined the relationship between tooth decay in children and naturally occurring fluoride in drinking water. The study found that children who drank water with naturally high levels of fluoride had less tooth decay. This discovery was important because during that time most children and adults in the United States were affected by tooth decay. Many suffered from toothaches and painful extractions—often losing permanent teeth, including molars, even as teenagers.

After much scientific research, in 1945, the city of Grand Rapids, Michigan, was the first to add fluoride to its city water system in order to provide residents with the benefits of fluoride. This process of testing the water supply for fluoride and adjusting it to the right amount to prevent cavities is called community water fluoridation.

Since 1945, hundreds of cities have started community water fluoridation and in 2012, nearly 75% of the United States served by community water systems had access to fluoridated water. Because of its contribution to the dramatic decline in tooth decay over the past 70 years, CDC named community water fluoridation as 1 of 10 great public health achievements of the 20th century.

Cost: Saves Money, Saves Teeth

Community water fluoridation has been shown to save money, both for families and the healthcare system. The return on investment for community water fluoridation varies with size of the community, increasing as the community size increases. Community water fluoridation is cost-saving, even for small communities. The estimated return on investment for community water fluoridation (including productivity losses) ranged from $4 in small communities of 5,000 people or less, to $27 in large communities of 200,000 people or more.

Fluoride in the Water Today

In 2012, more than 210 million people, or 75% of the U.S. population, were served by community water systems that contain enough fluoride to protect their teeth. However, approximately 100 million Americans still do not have access to water with fluoride. Because it is so beneficial, the United States has a national goal for 80% of Americans to have water with enough fluoride to prevent tooth decay by 2020.

Section 5.2

Questions about Community Water Fluoridation

This section contains text excerpted from the following sources: Text beginning with the heading "Fluoridated Water" is excerpted from "Community Water Fluoridation," Centers for Disease Control and Prevention (CDC), April 7, 2015; Text under the heading "What Is Community Water Fluoridation?" is excerpted from "FAQs," Centers for Disease Control and Prevention (CDC), April 20, 2015.

Fluoridated Water

The safety and benefits of fluoride are well documented. For 70 years, people in the United States have benefited from drinking water with fluoride, leading to better dental health.

Drinking fluoridated water keeps the teeth strong and reduced tooth decay by approximately 25% in children and adults. By preventing tooth decay, community water fluoridation has been shown to save money, both for families and the healthcare system.

Over the past several decades, there have been major improvements in the nation's oral health. Still, tooth decay remains one of the most common chronic diseases of childhood. Community water fluoridation has been identified as the most cost-effective method of delivering fluoride to all members of the community, regardless of age, educational attainment, or income level.

Nearly all water contains some fluoride, but usually not enough to help prevent tooth decay or cavities. Community water systems can add the right amount of fluoride to the local drinking water to prevent tooth decay.

Community water fluoridation is recommended by nearly all public health, medical, and dental organizations including the American Dental Association (ADA), American Academy of Pediatrics (AAP), U.S. Public Health Service (USPHS), and World Health Organization (WHO).

What Is Community Water Fluoridation?

Almost all water contains some naturally-occurring fluoride, but usually at levels too low to prevent tooth decay. Many communities adjust the fluoride concentration in the water supply to a level known to reduce tooth decay and promote good oral health (often called the optimal level). This practice is known as community water fluoridation, and reaches all people who drink that water. Given the dramatic decline in tooth decay during the past 70 years since community water fluoridation was initiated, the Centers for Disease Control and Prevention (CDC) named fluoridation of drinking water to prevent dental caries (tooth decay) as one of Ten Great Public Health Interventions of the 20th Century.

Why Did the U.S. Department of Health and Human Services (HHS) Make a New Recommendation for Community Water Fluoridation?

Sources of fluoride have increased since the early 1960s. At that time, nearly all fluoride intake came from drinking water and from food and from beverages prepared with fluoridated water. Today, water is one of several sources of fluoride. Other sources include dental products such as toothpaste and mouth rinses, prescription fluoride supplements, and professionally applied fluoride products such as varnish and gels. Because it is now possible to receive enough fluoride with slightly lower amounts of fluoride in water, U.S. Department of Health and Human Services (HHS) developed a new recommendation for the level of fluoride that is to be used in community water fluoridation.

Why Does HHS Recommend 0.7 Milligrams per Liter?

An optimal level of fluoride in drinking water provides enough fluoride to prevent tooth decay in children and adults while limiting the risk of dental fluorosis, which is the only unwanted health effect of community water fluoridation. Dental fluorosis is a change in the appearance of the dental enamel that occurs in children whose teeth are forming under the gums. The risk of dental fluorosis increases as children ingest higher levels of fluoride. The most common impact of fluorosis is faint white spots on teeth that usually only a dental professional would notice. National survey data show that prevention of tooth decay can be maintained at the recommended level of 0.7 milligrams of fluoride per liter of drinking water. This recommended level updates and replaces the previously recommended range of 0.7 to 1.2 milligrams per liter.

How Was the Updated Recommendation Developed?

In September 2010, the U.S. Department of Health and Human Services (HHS) convened a panel of scientists from across the U.S. government to review new information related to fluoride intake and to consider a new recommendation for community water fluoridation. The federal panel reviewed the best available information, including changes in the occurrence and severity of tooth decay and of dental fluorosis in U.S. children and adults. The panel also studied the U.S. Environmental Protection Agency's (EPA) scientific assessments of the major sources of fluoride intake and risk of severe dental fluorosis among children. Severe dental fluorosis is rare in the United States. Based on this review, the federal panel proposed changing the recommended level for community water systems to 0.7 milligrams per liter (the low end of the prior recommended range of 0.7 to 1.2 milligrams per liter). The proposed change was published in the Federal Register. Public comment on the proposed new level was sought—and considered carefully by the Panel—before finalizing the new recommendation. In addition, the proposed recommendation was submitted to a Peer Review Process, a step required by the federal government for influential scientific information.

How Does Fluoride Get into Tap Water?

Fluoride is a mineral that occurs naturally and is released from rocks into the soil, water, and air. Almost all water contains some fluoride, but usually not enough to prevent tooth decay. Fluoride can also be added to drinking water supplies as a public health measure for reducing cavities. Decisions about adding fluoride to drinking water are made at the state or local level.

Does My Public Water System Add Fluoride to the Water?

The best way to find the fluoride level of your local public water system is to contact your water utility provider. Consumers can find the name and contact information of the water utility on the water bill. The U.S. Environmental Protection Agency (EPA) requires that all community water systems provide each customer with an annual report on water quality, including the fluoride content.

Why Is the Drinking Water Standard from the U.S. Environmental Protection Agency (EPA)—Referred to as the MCL or MCLG—Different than the Optimal Fluoride Level Recommended for Community Water Systems by the Public Health Service (PHS)?

U.S. Environmental Protection Agency (EPA)'s drinking water standard differs from the Public Health Service (PHS) recommendation for fluoridation because the two have different purposes. EPA's enforceable standard for fluoride in public water supplies (4.0 milligrams per liter) is set to protect against exposure to high levels of naturally occurring fluoride. The PHS recommendation (0.7 milligrams per liter) identifies the optimal concentration of fluoride to prevent tooth decay while limiting the chance for dental fluorosis, which is a change in the appearance of the tooth enamel. The PHS recommendation only applies to those public water systems that add fluoride to reach the optimal concentration. Public water systems that contain naturally occurring fluoride at concentrations above 0.7 mg/L will not be affected by the new recommendation.

In Addition to Drinking Fluoridated "Tap" Water, How Else May Children Ingest Fluoride?

Young children often have trouble controlling their swallowing reflex and swallow toothpaste while toothbrushing. Commercial foods and beverages made with fluoridated water are an additional source of fluoride intake. Other fluoride-containing dental products, such as gels, varnishes, pastes, and dietary supplements are applied or prescribed by a healthcare professional. Most of these products are used only occasionally on the outside of the tooth and do not contribute much to a child's total intake of fluoride. Dietary fluoride supplements do contribute to the total amount of fluoride taken in.

Given That We Get Fluoride from Other Sources, Should Communities Still Fluoridate Water to Prevent Tooth Decay?

This optimal level recommendation is voluntary. If your local water system adds fluoride to the water, reducing the level is a simple process that can be completed almost immediately, although it may be several days before the entire water system is at the new level. If you want the most up-to-date information about the current fluoride level in your water, contact your local water system.

Are There Any Harmful Health Effects Due to Community Water Fluoridation?

The safety and effectiveness of community water fluoridation continues to be supported by scientific evidence produced by independent scientists and summarized by panels of experts. The independent, non-governmental Community Preventive Services Task Force has noted that the research evidence does not demonstrate that community water fluoridation results in any unwanted health effects other than dental fluorosis, a condition that causes primarily cosmetic changes in the appearance of tooth enamel.

Has the Safety of Community Water Fluoridation Been Evaluated?

The safety and effectiveness of fluoride at levels used in community water fluoridation have been thoroughly reviewed by multinational scientific and public health organizations (United States, Canada, Australia, New Zealand, Great Britain, and by the World Health Organization) using evidence-based reviews and expert panels. These panels include scientists with expertise in various health and scientific disciplines, including medicine, biophysics, chemistry, toxicological pathology, oral health, and epidemiology.

Experts have weighed the findings and quality of available evidence and concluded that there is no association between water fluoridation and any unwanted health effects other than dental fluorosis.

Are Children or Adults Exposed to Too Much Fluoride?

Since the 1962 Public Health Service recommendations were developed, there has been greater availability of fluoride products (fluoride toothpaste, mouth rinses, fluoride supplements, etc.), as well as an expansion in the number of persons in the U.S. receiving fluoridated tap water. Increased exposure to fluoride increases the risk of dental fluorosis in children, a condition that caused primarily cosmetic changes in the appearance of the enamel. The prevalence of dental fluorosis among 12- to 15-year-olds appears to have increased between 1986–1987 and 1999–2004, although the vast majority of cases were very mild or mild. Both the 1962 Public Health Service recommendation and the current updated recommendation for fluoride concentration in community drinking water were set to achieve a reduction in dental caries (tooth decay) while minimizing the risk of dental fluorosis. Implementation of the new recommendation is expected to lead to a reduction of approximately 25% (range: 12% to 42%) in fluoride intake from drinking water alone and a reduction of approximately 14% (range: 5% to 29%) in total fluoride intake.

Is My Child Getting the Right Amount of Fluoride to Prevent Tooth Decay from Drinking Water and Tooth Brushing?

If your child is among the more than 200 million Americans who receive their water from a community water system fluoridated at the optimal level and if you follow instructions for your child's tooth-brushing, your child is receiving the right amount of fluoride to prevent tooth decay. Centers for Disease Control and Prevention (CDC) recommends that children under 6 use a small, pea-sized amount of toothpaste, spit out the excess paste, and rinse well after brushing. Children should start using toothpaste with fluoride when they are 2 years old. Younger children should only use toothpaste with fluoride if your child's dentist or doctor recommends it.

If I Am Drinking Water with Fluoride, Why Do I Also Need to Brush with Toothpaste That Contains Fluoride?

Both drinking water and toothpaste with fluoride provide important and complementary benefits. Fluoridated water keeps a low level of fluoride in saliva and dental plaque all day. The much higher concentration of fluoride in toothpaste offers additional benefit. Fluoride slows the activity of bacteria that cause decay and combines with enamel on the tooth surface to make it stronger and better able to resist decay. Together, the two sources offer more protection than using either one alone.

Is It Safe to Mix Fluoridated Tap Water with Commercial Infant Formula?

All formulas, whether concentrates or ready-to-feed, have low levels of fluoride. A study by the American Dental Association (ADA) confirmed that fluoride concentrations in commercially available infant formulas are very low. In infant formula mixed from concentrate, whether liquid or powdered, the majority of fluoride comes from the water used. For this reason, some parents may choose to use low fluoride water to mix with the formula some of the time.

Will Using a Home Water Filtration System Remove the Fluoride from My Home's Water?

Removal of fluoride from water is a difficult water treatment action. Most point-of-use treatment systems for homes that are installed on single faucets use activated carbon filtration, which will not remove the fluoride ion. Other treatment systems (such as reverse osmosis, ion exchange, or distillation systems to reduce fluoride levels) vary in their effectiveness to reduce fluoride. Check with the manufacturer of the individual product.

Section 5.3

Bottled Water and Fluoride

This section includes text excerpted from "Community
Water Fluoridation," Centers for Disease Control and
Prevention (CDC), July 10, 2013.

Who Regulates Fluoride in Bottled Water?

The U.S. Environmental Protection Agency (EPA) regulates public drinking water (tap water), and the U.S. Food and Drug Administration (FDA) regulates bottled water products under the authority of the Federal Food, Drug, and Cosmetic Act.

Does Bottled Water Contain Fluoride?

Bottled water products may contain fluoride, depending on the source of the water. Fluoride can be naturally present in the original source of the water, and many public water systems add fluoride to their water. FDA sets limits for fluoride in bottled water, based on several factors, including the source of the water. Bottled water products labeled as de-ionized, purified, demineralized or distilled have been treated in such a way that they contain no or only trace amounts of fluoride, unless they specifically list fluoride as an added ingredient.

Is the Amount of Fluoride in Bottled Water Always Listed on the Label?

The FDA does not require bottled water manufacturers to list the amount of fluoride on the label unless the manufacturer has added fluoride within set limits.

How Can I Find out the Level of Fluoride in Bottled Water If It's Not on the Label?

Contact the bottled water's manufacturer to ask about the fluoride content of a particular brand.

What FDA Regulations for Bottled Water Relate to Fluoride?

As set forth in 21 CFR 165.110, FDA has established standards for the maximum amount of naturally occurring fluoride or added fluoride allowed in bottled drinking water.

If bottled water meets specific standards of identity and quality set forth by FDA, and the provisions of the authorized health claim, manufacturers may include the following health claim: "Drinking fluoridated water may reduce the risk of [dental caries or tooth decay]."

Can I Use Bottled Water for Mixing Infant Formula?

Yes, you can use bottled water to reconstitute (mix) powdered or liquid concentrate infant formulas, but be aware that the fluoride content in bottled water varies. If your child is exclusively consuming infant formula reconstituted with water that contains fluoride, there may be an increased chance for mild dental fluorosis (a change in the appearance of tooth enamel creating barely visible lacy white markings). To lessen this chance, parents may choose to use low-fluoride bottled water some of the time to mix infant formula. These bottled waters are labeled as de-ionized, purified, demineralized or distilled and are without any fluoride added after purification treatment (FDA requires the label to indicate when fluoride is added). Some water companies make available bottled waters marketed for infants and for the purpose of mixing with formula. When water is labeled as intended for infants, the water must meet tap water standards established by the EPA and indicate that the water is not sterile.

Section 5.4

Private Well Water and Fluoride

This section includes text excerpted from "Community Water Fluoridation," Centers for Disease Control and Prevention (CDC), July 10, 2013.

How Do I Know If My Water Is from a Public Water System or a Private Well?

The U.S. Environmental Protection Agency (EPA) defines a Public Water System as a system that serves 25 or more people per day. If you have water service from a well that has a limited delivery, such as to your house but not to your neighbor's house, then you likely have a private well.

What Are the Governmental Regulations for Private Wells?

Although most U.S. households are connected to a public water system, the U.S. Geological Survey report "Estimated Use of Water in the United States in 2005" estimates that 14% of United States residents rely on private wells that are not regulated by the EPA Safe Drinking Water Act. In most states, private wells are not regulated by governmental regulatory entities. Therefore, it is the responsibility of the homeowner to know and understand the quality of the water from their well. The U.S. Environmental Protection Agency (EPA) suggests that all wells be tested for quality once every three years since influences to well water quality can change over time. Contact your public health office for their advice on testing of private wells in your state or area.

My Home Gets Its Water from a Private Well. What Do I Need to Know about Fluoride and Groundwater from a Well?

Fluoride is present in virtually all waters at some level, and it is important to know the fluoride content of your water, particularly if you have children. A 2008 U.S. Geological Survey study found that 4% of sampled wells had natural fluoride levels above the EPA Secondary Maximum Contaminant Level (SMCL) of 2 mg/L. A smaller set of 1.2% of all wells exceeded the Maximum Contaminant Level (MCL) of 4 mg/L. If you have a home well, the EPA recommends having a sample of your water analyzed by a laboratory at least once every three years. Check with your dentist, physician, or public health department to learn how to have your home well water tested.

What Should I Do If the Water from My Well Has Less Fluoride than the Recommended Level of 0.7 Mg/L? Can I Add Fluoride?

The recommended fluoride level in drinking water for good oral health is 0.7 mg/L (milligrams per liter). If fluoride levels in your drinking water are lower than 0.7 mg/L, your child's dentist or pediatrician should evaluate whether your child could benefit from daily fluoride supplements. The prescription dosage of fluoride supplements should be consistent with the schedule established by the American Dental Association (ADA) Council on Scientific Affairs. Their recommendation will depend on your child's risk of developing tooth decay, as well as exposure to other sources of fluoride, such as drinking water at school or daycare, and fluoride toothpaste. It is not feasible to add fluoride to an individual residence's well.

What Should I Do If the Water from My Well Has Fluoride Levels That Are Higher than the Recommended Level of 0.7 Mg/L?

In some regions in the United States, community drinking water and home wells can contain levels of naturally occurring fluoride that are greater than the level recommended by the CDC for preventing tooth decay. The U.S. Environmental Protection Agency (EPA) currently has a non-enforceable recommended guideline for fluoride of 2.0 mg/L that is set to protect against dental fluorosis. If your home is served by a water system that has fluoride levels exceeding this recommended guideline, but lower than 4.0 mg/L, currently EPA recommends that children should be provided with alternative sources of drinking water. Continue to test your well water's quality every three years as recommended by EPA.

What Should I Do If My Well Water Was Measured as Having Too Much Fluoride (Level Greater than 4 Mg/L)?

It is unusual to have the fluoride content of water exceed 4 mg/L. If a laboratory report indicates that you have such excessive fluoride content, it is recommended that the water be retested. At least four samples should be collected, a minimum of one week apart, and the results compared. If one sample is above 4 mg/L and the other samples are less than 4 mg/L, then the high value may have been an erroneous measurement. If all samples register excessive levels greater than 4 mg/L, then you may want to consider investigating alternate sources of water for drinking and cooking or installing a device to remove the fluoride from your home water source. Physical contact with high fluoride content water, such as bathing or dishwashing, is safe since fluoride does not pass through the skin.

What Are the Health Risks of Consuming Water with Fluoride Levels Greater than 4 Mg/L?

Children aged 8 years and younger have an increased chance of developing severe tooth dental fluorosis. Consumption over a lifetime may increase the likelihood of bone fractures, and may result in skeletal fluorosis, a painful or even crippling disease. The U.S. Environmental Protection Agency (EPA) has determined that safe exposure of fluoride is below 4 mg/L in drinking water to avoid those effects.

Will Using a Home Water Filtration System Take the Fluoride out of My Home's Water?

Removal of fluoride from water is difficult. Most home point-of-use treatment systems that are installed at single faucets use activated carbon filtration, which does not remove the fluoride. Reverse osmosis point-of-use devices can effectively remove fluoride, although the amount may vary given individual circumstances. For a home point-of-use device to claim a reduction in fluoride, it must meet National Sanitation Foundation (NSF) Standard 58 criteria for fluoride removal. Standard 58 requires that a device must achieve a 1.5 milligrams per liter (mg/L) concentration in the product water if the original concentration was 8.0 mg/L, or approximately 80 percent removal. This percentage removal may not be consistent at lower concentrations of fluoride. Check with the manufacturer of the individual product for specific product information.

Fluoride is not released from water when it is boiled or frozen. One exception would be a water distillation system. These systems heat water to the boiling point and then collect water vapor as it evaporates. Water distillation systems are typically used in laboratories. For home use, these systems can be expensive and may present safety and maintenance concerns.

Can I Use Water with Fluoride for Preparing Infant Formula?

Yes, you can use well water for preparing infant formula. It is important, however, to ensure that the well water has been recently tested to verify safety. EPA suggests that well water should be tested a minimum of once every three years for micro-organisms and other substances. In addition, parents of young children should also have their well water tested for fluoride content.

For more information on private well testing, contact your local health department. Parents and caregivers should speak with their pediatrician to review the results of the private well testing and to determine if the well water should be boiled prior to mixing the formula. If you are advised to boil the water, be sure to boil the water only one time so that you don't concentrate substances by the boiling process itself.

If your child is exclusively consuming infant formula reconstituted with well water, and if that water contains fluoride, there is an increased chance for dental fluorosis. To lessen this chance, parents can use low-fluoride bottled water some of the time to mix infant formula; these bottled water are labeled as de-ionized, purified, demineralized or distilled.

Section 5.5

Fluoride Products for Dental Care

This section includes text excerpted from "Community
Water Fluoridation," Centers for Disease Control and
Prevention (CDC), July 10, 2013.

In the United States, water fluoridation is not the only form of fluoride delivery that is effective in preventing tooth decay in people of all ages. Use the information listed below to compare the other fluoride products that may lower the risk for tooth decay, especially for people who are at higher risk for decay. Although all of these products reduce tooth decay, combined use with fluoridated water offers protection greater than any of these products used alone.

Fluoride Products

Fluoride Toothpaste

Form. Concentrations of fluoride in toothpaste sold in the United States range from 1,000–1,500 ppm.

Use. Most people report brushing their teeth at least once per day, but more frequent use can offer additional protection. Fluoride in toothpaste is taken up directly by the dental plaque and demineralized enamel and also increases the concentration of fluoride in saliva.

Availability. Fluoride toothpaste is available over-the-counter and makes up more than 95% of toothpaste sales in the United States.

Recommendations. For most people (children, adolescents, and adults) brushing at least twice a day with a fluoride toothpaste—when you get up in the morning and before going to bed—is recommended.

Advice for Parents. For children aged 6 years and younger, some simple recommendations are advised to reduce the risk of dental fluorosis.

- Supervise brushing to discourage swallowing toothpaste.

- Place only a small pea-size amount of fluoride toothpaste on your child's toothbrush.

- Seek advice from a dentist or other healthcare professional before introducing fluoride toothpaste to children under 2 years of age.

Fluoride Mouth Rinse

Form. Fluoride mouth rinse is a concentrated solution intended for daily or weekly use. The most common fluoride compound used in mouth rinse is sodium fluoride. Over-the-counter solutions of 0.05% sodium fluoride (230 ppm fluoride) for daily rinsing are available for use by persons older than 6 years of age. Solutions of 0.20% sodium fluoride (920 ppm fluoride) are used in supervised, school-based weekly rinsing programs. Other concentrations also are available.

Use. Rinses are used daily or weekly for a prescribed amount of time. The fluoride from mouth rinse is retained in dental plaque and saliva to help prevent tooth decay.

Availability. Mouth rinses intended for home use can be purchased over-the-counter. Higher strength mouth rinses for those at high risk of tooth decay must be prescribed by a dentist or physician.

Recommendations. Children younger than 6 years of age should not use fluoride mouth rinse without consultation with a dentist or other healthcare provider because dental fluorosis could occur if such mouth rinses are repeatedly swallowed. Because fluoride mouth rinse has resulted in only limited reductions in tooth decay among school-children, especially as their exposure to other sources of fluoride has increased, its use should be targeted to individuals or groups at high risk for decay.

Fluoride Supplements

Form. Tablets, lozenges or liquids (including fluoride-vitamin preparations) are available. Most supplements contain sodium fluoride as the active ingredient. Tablets and lozenges are manufactured with 1.0, 0.5 or 0.25 mg fluoride.

Use. Fluoride supplements can be prescribed for children at high risk for tooth decay and whose primary drinking water has a low fluoride concentration. To maximize the topical effect of fluoride, tablets and lozenges are intended to be chewed or sucked for 1–2 minutes before being swallowed.

Availability. All fluoride supplements must be prescribed by a dentist or physician. The prescription should be consistent with the 2010 dosage schedule developed by American Dental Association (ADA).

Recommendations. For children aged less than 6 years, the dentist, physician, or other healthcare provider should weigh the risk for tooth decay without fluoride supplements, the decay prevention offered by supplements, and the potential for dental fluorosis. Consideration of the child's other sources of fluoride, especially drinking water, is essential in determining this balance. Parents and caregivers should be informed of both the benefit of protection against tooth decay and the possibility of dental fluorosis.

Fluoride Gel and Foam

Form. Fluoride gel is often formulated to be highly acidic (pH of approximately 3.0). Products available in the United States include gel of acidulated phosphate fluoride (1.23% [12,300 ppm] fluoride), gel or foam of sodium fluoride (0.9% [9,040 ppm] fluoride), and self-applied (i.e., home use) gel of sodium fluoride (0.5% [5,000 ppm] fluoride) or stannous fluoride (0.15% [1,000 ppm] fluoride).

Use. In a dental office, fluoride gel is applied for 1–4 minutes. Home use follows instructions provided on the prescription.

Availability. Most fluoride gel and foam applications are delivered in a dental office by a dental professional. These higher strength products, if used in the home, must be prescribed by a dentist or physician.

Recommendations. Because these applications are relatively infrequent, generally at 3 to 12–month intervals, fluoride gel poses little risk for dental fluorosis, even among patients younger than 6 years of age. Routine use of professionally applied fluoride gel or foam likely provides little benefit to persons not at high risk for tooth decay, especially those who drink fluoridated water and brush daily with fluoride toothpaste.

Fluoride Varnish

Form. Varnishes are available as sodium fluoride (2.26% [22,600 ppm] fluoride) or difluorsilane (0.1% [1,000 ppm] fluoride) preparations.

Use. High-concentration fluoride varnish is painted by dental or other healthcare professionals directly onto the teeth. Fluoride varnish is not intended to adhere permanently; this method holds a high concentration of fluoride in a small amount of material in close contact with the teeth for many hours. Varnishes must be reapplied at regular intervals with at least 2 applications per year required for effectiveness.

Availability. All fluoride varnish must be applied by a dentist or other healthcare provider.

Recommendations. No published evidence indicates that professionally applied fluoride varnish is a risk factor for dental fluorosis, even among children younger than 6 years of age. Proper application technique reduces the possibility that a patient will swallow varnish during its application and limits the total amount of fluoride swallowed as the varnish wears off the teeth over several hours.

Although it is not currently cleared for marketing by the U.S. Food and Drug Administration (FDA) as an anti-caries agent, fluoride varnish has been widely used for this purpose in Canada and Europe since the 1970s. Studies conducted in Canada and Europe have reported that fluoride varnish is as effective in preventing tooth decay as professionally applied fluoride gel.

Chapter 6

Dental Plaque

Dental Plaque and Its Causes

Plaque is a clear, sticky substance that builds up on and between teeth. Unlike other parts of the body, teeth do not have surfaces that follow a systemic cycle of shedding and renewal. This provides a rich area for micro-organisms to breed, creating a biofilm, an ecosystem of thousands of species of colonizing bacteria thatattach themselves to the enamel of the tooth. The biofilm or plaque is composed of a heterogeneous arrangement of bacterial cells, polysaccharides, proteins, and salt.

Plaque can form all over teeth, but it is found most often in the crevices of the molars. It tends to feel fuzzy or rough to the touch and is often difficult to see with the naked eye.

Problems Caused by Plaque

The bacteria in plaque live on sugars in the food that we eat. The fermentation of sugar produces acid byproducts that corrode teeth enamel and can subsequently result in a cavity. Unhindered, plaque may solidify into a hard substance called tartar or calculus. As the tartar and plaque progress further, the gums can become red and swollen and bleed when brushing. This is a condition known as gingivitis, an early-stage periodontal disease. If not treated properly,

---

"Dental Plaque," © 2017 Omnigraphics. Reviewed September 2016.

gingivitis may develop into periodontitis, a condition that is characterized by receding gums, infection, and damage to the bones supporting the teeth. Untreated, periodontitiscan eventually result in the loss of teeth.

Plaque Identification

Plaque is identified using two procedures:

1. A disclosing tablet is chewed for 30 seconds, and the mouth is rinsed with water. The tablet leaves a pink dye on the plaque that can easily be seen.

2. The mouth is rinsed with a special fluorescent solution and then rinsed gently with water. An ultraviolet light is shone on the teeth, revealing the existing plaque in a bright orange-yellow color. The advantage of this method is that it does not cause visible stains on teeth.

How to Deal with Dental Plaque

You cannot get rid of plaque completely on your own, but it can be prevented through proper dental hygiene:

- The best way to prevent dental plaque is to brush and floss daily. Brush your teeth once in the morning and again at night with fluoridated tooth paste. This dislodges the plaque and prevents the build-up of tartar.

- Use an interdental cleaner to remove plaque from hard to reach places where it is difficult to clean with a toothbrush.

- In addition to freshening breath, mouthwash can be useful in removing food debris, but do not depend on mouth rinses alone to keep plaque at bay. Brushing and flossing is essential.

- Eat healthy, balanced meals and limit snacks that may provide an environment for the bacteria in plaque.

- Make use of a sealant. If necessary, a dentist will cover teeth with a substance that forms a clear coating of plastic preventing the growth of bacteria and acids.

- Chewing sugar-free gum after meals can help prevent plaque by producing saliva, which washes away the acid present in the mouth after eating or drinking. Do not overuse chewing gum, though, because it may cause bruxism (tooth grinding) and problems in the joints of the jaw.

- Schedule regular visits to the dentist for a thorough oral examination and professional cleaning.

Failing to brush and floss is the single most common cause of plaque build-up that can lead to gingivitis and periodontitis later. Following a daily regimen of oral hygiene, combined with regular check-ups by a dentist, is the best way to prevent plaque and make sure teeth remain strong and healthy for a lifetime.

References

1. "Dental Plaque Identification at Home," A.D.A.M., Inc., August 23, 2016.

2. "What Is Plaque?" Delta Dental, March 2012.

3. Szalay, Jessie. "What Is Plaque?" LiveScience, August 26, 2014.

4. Laura, Manonelles. "What Is Tooth Plaque?" Propdental, May 16, 2014.

5. Hicks, Rob. "5 Bad Habits That Lead to Plaque on Your Teeth," WebMD, January 28, 2015.

Chapter 7

Mouth Injuries

What Are Mouth Injuries?

Mouth injuries are wounds or cuts on the lips, teeth, tongue, jaw, inner cheeks, and floor or roof of the mouth. These injuries often occur while playing sports or during other physical activity, and children tend to incur them more than adults. When mouth or dental injuries take place, there can be excessive bleeding, since a lot of blood vessels are concentrated in the mouth area. Though most of these types of injuries are minor and can be treated at home, severe cuts or bruises may call for professional medical attention.

Types of Mouth Injuries

Minor Injuries

Minor mouth injuries include cuts, bruises, and wounds that can be treated at home or that heal over time without treatment. Minor cuts are generally caused by playing, sports, or other daily activities. Even during routine activities like eating or sleeping a person may accidentally bite his or her tongue and cause minor injury, but these normally heal over time without treatment.

"Mouth Injuries," © 2017 Omnigraphics. Reviewed September 2016.

Major Injuries

Major injuries in the mouth require evaluation by a doctor, since they can affect the tonsils, soft palate (the fleshy area at the back of the roof of the mouth), or the throat. When a child falls with a pointed object in his or her mouth, it may lead to a major mouth injury, which can affect deeper tissues in the head or neck.

Upper and Lower Lip Cuts

Upper lip cuts usually occur when a person falls, which can cause a tear in the connective tissue between the upper lip and gum called frenulum. A suture is not always necessary, as this tear may heal on its own, although bleeding can recur during the healing process. A lower lip cut may take place during a fall when the lip is caught between the upper and lower teeth. In serious cases, sutures might be required.

Stitches may also be required for an injury to the mouth or lips that causes a loose flap of tissue, called a gaping wound. If the frenulum (the piece of skin between lips and gums) tears, it may require stitches or, if minor, it could heal on its own over time.

Dental Injuries

An injury to a tooth, which often occurs during a fall or sports activity, can cause it to crack, break off, lose color or be chipped. The tooth can also be displaced from its original position (dental luxation) or jammed into the gum (intruded). Other causes of dental injuries include grinding of the teeth, orthodontic procedures that cause mouth sores, and piercings in the mouth. A medical professional should evaluate all such injuries.

Symptoms of Mouth and Dental Injuries

Symptoms of mouth and dental injuries include bleeding, pain, laceration of tissue, tooth damage, swelling, bruising, tissue loss, and loose tissue flaps.

Treatment for Mouth and Dental Injuries

Most minor mouth injuries can be treated at home using some of the remedies listed below.

Stop the Bleeding

To stop bleeding from the inner lip or tissue that connects the inner lip with the gum, apply pressure to the bleeding site with sterile gauze or a clean cloth for ten minutes. Be careful reexamining the site, or bleeding may start again. Similarly, bleeding from the tongue can be stopped by pressing on the area with sterile gauze or a clean cloth. Applying a piece of ice or popsicle to the affected area may also help.

Reduce Pain in the Mouth

Pain in the mouth can be reduced with nonprescription medicines, such as:

- a topical medication like Orabase, Anbesol, or Ulcerease.
- pain relievers, such as acetaminophen (Tylenol).
- nonsteroidal anti-inflammatory drugs like ibuprofen (Advil or Motrin) or naproxen (Aleve or Naprosyn).

It is wise to read the instructions carefully before consuming nonprescription medicines, and only recommended doses are advisable. If a person is pregnant, allergic to certain medicines, or has been advised not to take certain medicines, a doctor should be consulted before treatment.

Promote Healing

Rinsing the mouth with warm salt water after every meal can promote the healing of many types of mouth wounds. Saltwater can be made by mixing 1 cup (250 ml) of warm water with 1 tsp (5g) of salt.

Recommended Diet

After a mouth or dental injury, a diet of soft foods is recommended in order to avoid disrupting the healing process.

Suggestions for soft foods include:

- dairy products like milk, yogurt, ice-cream, and cheese.
- fluids, such as milkshakes and sherbets, to avoid dehydration.
- eggs and tender or ground meats.
- fruits and vegetables that are well-ripened, or baked or mashed.

Things to be avoided include:

- citrus fruits and salty or spicy food that may cause stinging.
- alcoholic beverages.
- smoking or using other tobacco products.

When Must a Doctor Be Consulted for Mouth Injuries?

A doctor needs to be consulted if there is a major injury or if the following symptoms are observed:

- loose flaps of tissue or a gaping wound
- severe pain
- bleeding that won't stop
- swelling, redness, tenderness, or evidence of infection in the affected area
- severe toothache or one that persists for two weeks or interferes with daily activities
- fever
- cuts that are caused by a dirty or rusty object
- a tooth that is knocked out or torn out of its socket

Prevention of Mouth and Dental Injuries

Most mouth and dental injuries can be prevented by being careful and protecting oneself. Some suggestions:

- Get regular dental checkups to prevent tooth and gum problems.
- Wear a mouth guard to prevent injuries while playing sports.
- Follow instructions after an orthodontic procedure, and follow up with a medical professional if pain persists.

Children are particularly susceptible to mouth and dental injuries. Here are some steps parents can take to reduce the likelihood of such injuries:

- Make children aware of the dangers of playing or running with objects in their mouths.
- Teach children not to chew or suck on sharp or pointed objects.

- Be sure children wear mouth guards or face masks while playing sports.

- Teach children to sit while eating or drinking, especially while eating food on a stick.

- Discourage eating while riding in a car.

References

1. "Mouth and Dental Injuries: Topic Overview," WebMD, September 9, 2014.

2. "Cuts and Wounds of the Mouth and Lips," Stanford Children's Health, n.d.

3. Schmitt, Barton. "Should Your Child See a Doctor," Seattle Children's Hospital, n.d.

Chapter 8

Oral Health for Older Adults

Older Americans make up a growing percentage of the U.S. population; nearly 35 million are 65 years or older. By 2050, that number is expected to increase to 48 million. Oral diseases and conditions are common among these Americans who grew up without the benefit of community water fluoridation and other fluoride products.

Older Americans with the poorest oral health are those who are economically disadvantaged, lack insurance, and are members of racial and ethnic minorities. Being disabled, homebound, or institutionalized also increases the risk of poor oral health.

Many older Americans do not have dental insurance. Often these benefits are lost when they retire. The situation may be worse for older women, who generally have lower incomes and may never have had dental insurance.

Medicaid, the jointly-funded Federal-State health insurance program for certain low-income and needy people, funds dental care for

This chapter contains text excerpted from the following sources: Text in this chapter begins with excerpts from "Oral Health for Older Americans," Centers for Disease Control and Prevention (CDC), July 10, 2013; Text under the heading "Oral Health for Older Adults: Quick Tips" is excerpted from "Oral Health for Older Adults: Quick Tips," Office of Disease Prevention and Health Promotion (ODPHP), U.S. Department of Health and Human Services (HHS), December 17, 2015; Text under the heading "Myths and Facts about Oral Health" is excerpted from "Older Adults and Oral Health," National Institute of Dental and Craniofacial Research (NIDCR), June 10, 2015.

low income and disabled elderly in some states, but reimbursements for this care are low. Medicare, which provides health insurance for people over age 65 and people with certain illnesses and disabilities, was not designed to provide routine dental care.

About 25 percent of adults 60 years old and older no longer have any natural teeth. Interestingly, toothlessness varies greatly by state. Roughly 42 percent of Americans over age 65 living in West Virginia are toothless, compared to only 13 percent of those living in California. Having missing teeth can affect nutrition, since people without teeth often prefer soft, easily chewed foods. Because dentures are not as efficient for chewing food as natural teeth, denture wearers also may choose soft foods and avoid fresh fruits and vegetables.

Periodontal (gum) disease or tooth decay (cavities) are the most frequent causes of tooth loss. Older Americans continue to experience dental decay on the crowns of teeth (coronal caries) and on tooth roots (because of gum recession). In fact, older adults may have new tooth decay at higher rates than children.

Severity of periodontal (gum) disease increases with age. About 23 percent of 65- to 74-year-olds have severe disease, which is measured by 6mm loss of attachment of the tooth to the adjacent gum tissue. At all ages men are more likely than women to have more severe disease. At all ages, people at the lowest socioeconomic level have the most severe periodontal disease.

Oral and pharyngeal cancers, which are diagnosed in some 31,000 Americans each year, result in about 7,400 deaths each year. These cancers are primarily diagnosed in the elderly. Prognosis is poor. The five-year survival rate for white patients is 56 percent and for African American patients is only 34 percent.

Most older Americans take both prescription and over-the-counter drugs. Over 400 commonly used medications can be the cause of a dry mouth. Reduction of the flow of saliva increases the risk for oral disease, since saliva contains antimicrobial components as well as minerals that help rebuild tooth enamel attacked by decay-causing bacteria. Individuals in long-term care facilities—about 5 percent of the elderly—take an average of eight drugs each day.

Painful conditions that affect the facial nerves are more common among the elderly and can be severely debilitating. These conditions can affect mood, sleep, and oral-motor functions such as chewing and swallowing. Neurological diseases associated with age, such as Parkinson disease, Alzheimer disease, Huntington disease, and stroke also affect oral sensory and motor functions, in addition to limiting the ability to care for oneself.

What You Can Do to Maintain Your Oral Health

- Drink fluoridated water and use fluoride toothpaste; fluoride provides protection against dental decay at all ages.

- Practice good oral hygiene. Careful tooth brushing and flossing to reduce dental plaque can help prevent periodontal disease.

- It is important to see your dentist on a regular basis, even if you have no natural teeth and have dentures. Professional care helps to maintain the overall health of the teeth and mouth, and provides for early detection of pre-cancerous or cancerous lesions.

- Avoid tobacco. In addition to the general health risks posed by tobacco use, smokers have seven times the risk of developing periodontal disease compared to non-smokers. Tobacco used in any form—cigarettes, cigars, pipes, and smokeless (spit) tobacco—increases the risk for periodontal disease, oral and throat cancers, and oral fungal infection (candidiasis). Spit tobacco containing sugar also increases the risk of cavities.

- Limit alcohol. Drinking a high amount of alcoholic beverages is a risk factor for oral and throat cancers. Alcohol and tobacco used together are the primary risk factors for these cancers.

- Make sure that you or your loved one gets dental care prior to having cancer chemotherapy or radiation to the head or neck. These therapies can damage or destroy oral tissues and can result in severe irritation of the oral tissues and mouth ulcers, loss of salivary function, rampant tooth decay, and destruction of bone.

- Caregivers should reinforce the daily oral hygiene routines of elders who are unable to perform these activities independently.

- Sudden changes in taste and smell should not be considered signs of aging, but should be a sign to seek professional care.

- If medications produce a dry mouth, ask your doctor if there are other drugs that can be substituted. If dry mouth cannot be avoided, drink plenty of water, chew sugarless gum, and avoid tobacco and alcohol.

Oral Health for Older Adults: Quick Tips

Taking care of your teeth and gums as you get older can prevent problems like toothaches, cavities (tooth decay), and tooth loss. A healthy mouth also makes it easier for you to eat well and enjoy food.

It's especially important to take care of your teeth and gums if you have a health condition like diabetes or heart disease—or if you are taking medicines that can cause oral health problems.

Follow the steps below to keep your teeth and gums healthy as you get older.

Brush and Floss Your Teeth Every Day

Brushing and flossing helps remove dental plaque, a sticky film of bacteria (germs). If plaque builds up on your teeth, it can cause cavities or gum disease.

- Brush your teeth with fluoride toothpaste twice a day. Brush after breakfast and before bed.

- Floss between your teeth every day. If flossing is hard for you, ask a dentist about using a special brush or pick instead.

Watch for Changes in Your Mouth

Your risk of getting oral cancer increases as you get older. If you see any changes in your mouth, it's important to get them checked out.

See a doctor or dentist if you have any of these symptoms for more than 2 weeks:

- A spot in your mouth, lip, or throat that feels uncomfortable or sore

- A new lump or thick area in your mouth, lip, or throat

- A white or red patch in your mouth

- Difficulty chewing, swallowing, or moving your jaw or tongue

- Numbness or swelling in your mouth

- Pain in one ear without hearing loss

See the Dentist Regularly for a Checkup and Cleaning

- There's no single rule for how often people need to see the dentist—it varies from person to person. The next time you get a checkup and cleaning, ask your dentist how often you need to come in.

- Keep in mind that Medicare doesn't pay for routine dental care. You may want to get private dental insurance.

Talk to Your Doctor about Dry Mouth

Dry mouth means not having enough saliva (spit) to keep your mouth wet. Dry mouth can make it hard to eat, swallow, or talk. It can also lead to cavities or infection.

Dry mouth can be a side effect of some kinds of medicine. It can also happen if you have certain health problems (like diabetes) or if you are getting chemotherapy or radiation (treatment for cancer).

If you have dry mouth, you don't have to live with it. Talk with your doctor or dentist and ask what you can do.

Myths and Facts about Oral Health

Tooth Decay (Cavities)

Myth: Only school kids get cavities.

Fact: Tooth decay can develop at any age.

Tooth decay is not just a problem for children. It can happen as long as you have natural teeth. Dental plaque—a sticky film of bacteria—can build up on teeth. Plaque produces acids that, over time, eat away at the tooth's hard outer surface and create a cavity.

Even teeth that already have fillings are at risk. Plaque can build up underneath a chipped filling and cause new decay. And if your gums have pulled away from the teeth (called gum recession), the exposed tooth roots are also vulnerable to decay. But you can protect your teeth against decay. Here's how:

- Use toothpaste that contains fluoride. Fluoride can prevent tooth decay and also heal early decay. And it is just as helpful for adults as it is for children. Be sure to brush twice daily. This will help remove dental plaque that forms on teeth. Drinking fluoridated water also helps prevent tooth decay in adults.

- Floss regularly to remove plaque from between teeth. Or use a device such as a special brush or wooden or plastic pick recommended by a dental professional.

- See your dentist for routine check-ups. If you are at a higher risk for tooth decay (for example, if you have a dry mouth because of medicines you take), your dentist or dental hygienist may give you a fluoride treatment such as a varnish or foam during the office visit. Or, the dentist may tell you to use a fluoride gel or mouth rinse at home.

Gum Diseases

Myth: Gum disease is just a part of growing older.

Fact: You can prevent gum disease—it does not have to be a part of getting older.

Gum (periodontal) disease is an infection of the gums and surrounding tissues that hold teeth in place. Gum disease develops when plaque—a sticky film of bacteria—is allowed to build up along and under the gum line. The two forms of gum disease are:

1. **Gingivitis**, a mild form that is reversible with good oral hygiene. In gingivitis, the gums become red, swollen and can bleed easily.

2. **Periodontitis**, a more severe form that can damage the soft tissues and bone that support teeth. In periodontitis, gums pull away from the teeth and form spaces (called "pockets") that become infected. The body's immune system fights the bacteria as the plaque spreads and grows below the gum line. Bacterial toxins and the body's natural response to infection start to break down the bone and connective tissue that hold teeth in place. If not treated, the bones, gums, and tissue that support the teeth are destroyed. The teeth may eventually become loose and have to be removed.

The good news is that gum disease can be prevented. It does not have to be a part of growing older. With thorough brushing and flossing and regular professional cleanings by your dentist, you can reduce your risk of developing gum disease as you age.

And if you have been treated for gum disease, sticking to a proper oral hygiene routine and visiting your dentist for regular cleanings can minimize the chances it will come back. Here are some things you can do:

- Brush your teeth twice a day (with a fluoride toothpaste)

- Floss regularly to remove plaque from between teeth. Or use a device such as a special brush or wooden or plastic pick recommended by a dental professional.

- Visit the dentist regularly for a check-up and professional cleaning

- Don't smoke or use chewing tobacco or snuff

- Eat a well-balanced diet

If you smoke, you are at higher risk for developing periodontitis than a nonsmoker. In fact, smoking is one of the most significant risk factors for gum disease. Here's why:

- Smoking may impair blood flow to the gums, reducing the amount of oxygen and nutrients to the tissues and make them more vulnerable to infection

- Chemicals in tobacco smoke cause inflammation and cell damage, and can weaken the immune system

- Nicotine is toxic to cells that make new connective tissue, and also increases the production of an enzyme that breaks down tissue.

Smoking can also lower the chances that treatment for periodontitis will be successful and can lengthen the time it takes for treatments to work.

Dry Mouth

Myth: Dry mouth is a natural part of the aging process. You just have to learn to live with it.

Fact: Dry mouth is not a part of the aging process itself; it's important to find the cause of dry mouth so you can get relief.

Dry mouth is the condition of not having enough saliva, or spit, to keep the mouth wet. Without enough saliva, chewing, eating, swallowing and even talking can be difficult. Dry mouth also increases the risk for tooth decay because saliva helps keep harmful germs that cause tooth decay and other oral infections in check. Saliva also contains minerals (calcium and phosphate) that can help reverse early decay.

If you have dentures, dry mouth can make them uncomfortable and they may not fit as well. Without enough saliva, dentures can also rub against the gums and cause sore spots.

It's important to know that dry mouth is not part of the aging process itself. However, many older adults take medications that can dry out the mouth. And older adults are also more likely to have certain conditions that can lead to oral dryness. Here are some causes of dry mouth:

- Side effects of medicines. Hundreds of medicines can cause the salivary glands to make less saliva. Medicines for high blood pressure and depression often cause dry mouth.

- Disease. Some diseases affect the salivary glands. Sjögren's Syndrome and HIV/AIDS can cause dry mouth.

- Radiation therapy. The salivary glands can be damaged if they are exposed to radiation during cancer treatment.

- Chemotherapy. Drugs used to treat cancer can make saliva thicker, causing the mouth to feel dry.

- Nerve damage. Injury to the head or neck can damage the nerves that tell salivary glands to make saliva.

If you think you have dry mouth, see a dentist or physician. He or she can try to determine what is causing your dry mouth and what treatments might be helpful. For example, if dry mouth is caused by a medicine, your physician might change your medicine or adjust the dosage.

Your dentist or physician also might suggest that you keep your mouth wet by using artificial saliva, sold in most drug stores/pharmacies. Some people benefit from sucking sugarless hard candy or chewing sugarless gum.

Oral (Mouth) Cancer

Myth: If you don't use chewing tobacco, you don't need to worry about oral cancer.

Fact: It's not just smokeless tobacco ("dip" and "chew") that can increase your chances of getting oral cancer....

Tobacco use of any kind, including cigarette smoking, puts you at risk. Heavy alcohol use also increases your chances of developing the disease. And using tobacco plus alcohol poses a much greater risk than using either substance alone.

The likelihood of oral cancer increases with age. Most people with these cancers are older than 55 when the cancer is found.

Also, recent research has found that infection with the sexually transmitted human papillomavirus (HPV) has been linked to a subset of oral cancers.

It's important to catch oral cancer early–because treatment works best before the disease has spread. Pain is usually not an early symptom of the disease. So be on the lookout for any changes in your mouth, especially if you smoke or drink. If you have any of the following symptoms for more than two weeks, be sure to see a dentist or physician:

- A sore, irritation, lump or thick patch in the mouth, lip or throat
- A white or red patch in the mouth
- A feeling that something is caught in the throat
- Difficulty chewing or swallowing
- Difficulty moving the jaw or tongue
- Numbness in the tongue or other areas of the mouth
- Swelling of the jaw that causes dentures to fit poorly or become uncomfortable
- Pain in one ear without hearing loss

Most often, these symptoms do not mean cancer. An infection or other problem can cause the same symptoms. But it's important to get them checked out—because if it is cancer, it can be treated more successfully if it's caught early.

Part Two

Visiting Your Dentist's Office

Chapter 9

Routine Dental Visits and Overcoming Dental Phobia

Routine Dental Checkup

It is generally recommended that most people visit a dentist every six months for a routine dental checkup. Routine dental checkups usually include teeth cleaning, visual and physical exams, and sometimes dental X-rays.

Teeth Cleaning

A dental hygienist is a medical professional who specializes in teeth cleaning. This process involves removing tartar, a hard mineral that accumulates on teeth over time. The hygienist uses a small metal tool to scrape tartar off the tooth surface. The hygienist then flosses the teeth, and polishes teeth with a small rotating tool and tooth polishing compound. The hygienist may also apply a fluoride treatment to teeth. While cleaning the teeth, the hygienist also looks for evidence of tooth decay, cavities, gum disease, and other dental problems.

Dental X-rays

Sometimes a routine dental checkup includes the creation of dental X-rays. These special images allow dentists and other medical

"Routine Dental Visits and Overcoming Dental Phobia," © 2017 Omnigraphics. Reviewed September 2016.

professional to see inside the teeth and the bones of the face. X-rays are an important part of good dental health and are used for identifying, diagnosing, and monitoring dental problems.

Dental Exam

The dental exam is usually performed by a dentist. The exam typically includes a visual examination of the teeth and mouth as well as review of X-ray images. The dentist looks for possible problems with a person's bite and assesses any need for tooth restoration, removal, or replacement. For people who use dentures, the dentist and/or hygienist will check the fit of devices and discuss any problems or necessary adjustments. The dentist may provide recommendations on improving dental health, instructions on effective flossing and brushing, or other information. Dental exams sometimes also include a physical examination of the jaw, the area under the jaw, the soft tissue inside the mouth, the tongue, and the neck. These exams are done to check for signs of certain oral diseases and some types of cancer.

Dental Impressions

In some cases, dentists will order the creation of a dental impression. A bite impression is created by having the patient bite down on a special paper or other soft material that records the places where upper and lower teeth meet when the mouth is closed. This type of impression is useful in fitting tooth fillings, crowns, caps, and dentures.

Another type of dental impression is used to create a mold or model of a person's teeth and mouth tissue. These impressions are created by filling a U-shaped tray with special gelatin or paste, which is then placed over the arch of teeth and held for a few minutes. Once the impression material has partially hardened, the tray is removed. The resulting mold is used to create a cast of the teeth for the purpose of evaluating bite or making a custom mouth guard.

Dental Phobia

Although it is fairly safe to say that very few people enjoy dental visits, some people suffer from a severe form of anxiety known as dental phobia. For these people, a visit to the dentist can be a cause of extreme stress, fear, or panic. People who live with dental phobia generally avoid visiting a dentist, often for extended periods of time. The discomfort of tooth pain, broken teeth, or serious gum disease can seem more tolerable than seeking dental treatment for those with dental phobia. As a result, people with dental phobia are at a much higher risk for premature tooth loss and other health problems related to lack of dental care. Oral health has been linked to health conditions as diverse as diabetes, heart disease, and lung infections.

Causes of Dental Phobia

Phobias develop for a variety of reasons and it can be difficult to trace the origin of a fear that many people consider unreasonable. Among people with dental phobia, the reasons for fear can be different for each person. The most commonly expressed reason for avoiding dental care is a fear of pain. This fear is somewhat more common among older people whose early experiences with dental treatment occurred before modern advancements in dental sedation and pain management. Others express a fear of not being in control of a situation in which they are expected to remain still while someone works on their teeth and they are unable to anticipate what is happening. Some people are unable to tolerate the physical closeness with other people that is required as a hygienist or dentist works on their teeth.

Symptoms of Dental Phobia

Anyone might feel anxious before a visit to the dentist, but for some people, a pending dental visit produces feelings of terror and panic. People with dental phobia often describe their experiences during the time before a dental visit in similar terms: feeling tense, inability to sleep, feeling physically ill, trouble breathing, chest pains, vomiting, uncontrollable crying, and/or fear that builds as the time of the visit gets closer. During a dental procedure, people with dental phobia may also panic or have difficulty breathing. Sometimes the sight of dental instruments or dental staff can induce a panic attack.

Overcoming Dental Phobia

Dental phobia can be successfully treated and managed in a way that allows people to receive the dental care they need. Fear management begins with open communication to the dentist, hygienist, and other office staff. Modern dentistry offers many advancements and techniques that can be of great help to people with dental phobia. First among these techniques is the presentation and maintenance of the dental office environment, including the waiting room. A comfortable, soothing environment can help people with milder forms of dental anxiety feel more calm and confident. The use of artwork, background music, and color schemes can gently influence a person's first impression of the dental office as a safe place. Attention to details such as keeping dental instruments out of sight as much as possible and providing distractions such as headphones or personal television screens for patients can also help manage anxieties.

Dental phobia can also be alleviated somewhat through the use of continued communication. Dentists and hygienists may provide descriptions of procedures and outline what will be done before beginning, while responding to any questions or concerns that the patient may have. In some cases, alternative sedation may be offered to those with dental phobia. The dentist might prescribe an anti-anxiety medication to be taken earlier in the day of the dental visit. Inhalation sedation techniques (sometimes referred to as "laughing gas") can help people relax before any procedures are begun. Sedation via intravenous medication (IV sedation) is another option for people with dental phobia. IV sedation usually results in a deeper sedation that can be achieved through other means. Advances in dental equipment have produced tools engineered to be smaller and quieter than older equipment, and some modern dental drills include an emergency "stop" button that can be operated by the patient. This particular advancement has helped many with dental phobia to feel more in control of their experience during dental visits.

Some people with dental phobia find it helpful to bring a friend or relative with them to dental visits. This companion acts as an advocate, providing comfort and a feeling of safety for the person with dental phobia. In any case of dental phobia, communicating with the dental office staff is crucial to ensuring the needs of the patient are met.

References

1. "Oral Care," WebMD, November 14, 2014.

2. "Test and Procedures: Dental Exam," Mayo Clinic, February 14, 2015.

3. "What Is Dental Anxiety And Phobia?" Aetna, September 18, 2013.

4. "What Can Help?-Ways of Tackling Dental Fears," Dental Fear Central, 2016.

Chapter 10

Dental Caries (Cavities)

Chapter Contents

Section 10.1

What Is a Cavity?

Cavity

That's the word no one wants to hear at the dentist's office. A cavity develops when a tooth decays, or breaks down. A cavity is a hole that can grow bigger and deeper over time. Cavities are also called dental **caries**, and if you have a cavity, it's important to get it repaired.

But why would your tooth develop a hole? Blame plaque. That's a sticky, slimy substance made up mostly of the germs that cause tooth decay. The bacteria in your mouth make acids and when plaque clings to your teeth, the acids can eat away at the outermost layer of the tooth, called the **enamel**.

If you don't go to the dentist, the acids can continue to make their way through the enamel, and the inside parts of your tooth can begin to decay. If you've ever had a toothache or heard an adult complain about one, it may have been because there was a cavity that reached all the way inside a tooth, where the nerve endings are. Ouch!

Your dentist will carefully examine your teeth and may take X-rays. If your dentist discovers a cavity, he or she can repair it for you by first removing the rotted part of your tooth with a special drill. The dentist then fills the hole in your tooth with a special material. The result is called a filling.

Does it hurt? Sometimes it does, but your dentist can give you an anesthetic. That's a kind of medicine that will numb the area around the problem tooth while you're getting your new filling.

Cavity Prevention Tips

Though cavities can be repaired, try to avoid them by taking care of your teeth. Here's how:

- Brush your teeth with fluoride toothpaste after every meal or at least twice a day. Bedtime is an important time to brush.

- Brush up and down in a circular motion.

- Gently brush your gums as well to keep them healthy.

- Floss your teeth once a day to remove plaque and food that's stuck between your teeth.

- Limit sweets and sugary drinks, like soda or juice.

- See your dentist twice a year for regular checkups. We hope you'll hear those two wonderful words: "No cavities!"

Section 10.2

Dental Caries (Cavities) in Adults

This section includes text excerpted from "Dental Caries (Tooth Decay)," National Institute of Dental and Craniofacial Research (NIDCR), September 5, 2014.

Dental caries (tooth decay) remains the most prevalent chronic disease in both children and adults, even though it is largely preventable. Although caries has significantly decreased for most Americans over the past four decades, disparities remain among some population groups. In addition, this downward trend has recently reversed for young children.

Approximately 5% of adults age 20 to 64 have no teeth. This survey applies only to those adults who have teeth. Dental caries, both treated and untreated, in all adults age 20 to 64 declined from the early 1970s until 2004. The decrease was significant in all population subgroups. In spite of this decline, significant disparities are still found in some population groups.

Prevalence

- 92% of adults 20 to 64 have had dental caries in their permanent teeth.

- White adults and those living in families with higher incomes and more education have had more decay.

75

Unmet Needs

- 26% of adults 20 to 64 have untreated decay.

- Black and Hispanic adults, younger adults, and those with lower incomes and less education have more untreated decay.

Severity

- Adults 20 to 64 have an average of 3.28 decayed or missing permanent teeth and 13.65 decayed and missing permanent surfaces.

- Hispanic subgroups and those with lower incomes have more severe decay in permanent teeth.

- Black and Hispanic subgroups and those with lower incomes have more untreated permanent teeth.

Units of Measure

Dental caries is measured by a dentist examining a person's teeth, and recording the ones with untreated tooth decay and the ones with fillings. This provides three important numbers:

- **FT** (filled teeth): this is the number of decayed teeth that have been treated, which indicates access to dental care;

- **DMT** (decayed and missing teeth): this is the number decayed and missing teeth that have not been treated, which measures unmet need; and

- **DMFT** (decayed, missing, and filled teeth): this is the sum of DMT and FT, and is the measure of person's total lifetime tooth decay.

In addition to counting decayed and filled **teeth**, this same information can be gathered at the tooth surface level. Since every tooth has multiple surfaces, counting the decayed or filled surfaces provides a more accurate measure of the severity of decay.

Chapter 11

Dental Imaging

What Is Dental Imaging?

Dental imaging refers to the practice of creating pictures of a person's mouth and teeth using X-rays. X-rays, also known as radiographs, are electromagnetic waves of energy that can pass through many materials including bones and teeth. Because different materials absorb X-rays to varying degrees, X-rays are used to show the internal composition of things that are not normally visible. X-rays provide dentists with a way to see inside a person's teeth and jawbone without surgery or other invasive procedures. X-rays are an important part of good dental care and are the most commonly used form of radiograph technology.

Dentists use X-rays to identify, diagnose, and monitor dental health issues for their patients. Dental X-rays allow dentists and other medical professionals to see details of teeth, bones, and mouth tissue. X-rays are used to examine the roots of teeth and their position within the jaw, locate cavities, diagnose dental diseases and other problems, and monitor the development of teeth.

Dental Imaging Procedures

Dental X-rays are classified in two groups: intraoral and extraoral. To create intraoral X-rays, technicians place X-ray film inside a person's mouth. Extraoral X-rays are created using film that is located outside the mouth.

Intraoral X-rays result in a highly detailed images and are the most common form of dental imaging. There are four main types of intraoral dental X-ray that are used to examine different aspects of the teeth and mouth. Intraoral X-ray procedures are painless and quick, usually taking only a few seconds to complete.

- Bite-wing X-rays are used to see examine the crowns of teeth in the back of the mouth, including the molars and bicuspids. To create bite-wing X-ray images, the technician asks the patient to bite down on a device that holds the X-ray film while the image is created.

- Periapical X-rays are used to examine one or two teeth in full, including the entire length of the tooth from crown to root. The procedure for periapical X-rays is similar to that of bite-wing X-rays.

- A full-mouth radiographic survey, or FMX, is a set of intraoral X-rays that includes images of every tooth from crown to root, including supporting tissue. An FMX survey is created using both bite-wing and periapical X-rays.

- Occlusal X-rays are used to produce images that are larger than other types of dental imaging, including the full arch of teeth in either the upper or lower jaw. Occlusal X-rays are most often used to monitor the dental health of children.

Extraoral X-rays provide fewer details than intraoral X-rays, and are generally used to create images that provide a broad view of a person's teeth, jaw, and skull. Dentists use extraoral X-rays to monitor the growth of teeth, the position of teeth in relation to the bones of the jaw and face, and the position of teeth relative to each other within the jaw bone. There are five main types of extraoral X-rays.

- Panoramic X-rays allow dentists and other medical professionals to create a single image of the entire mouth, including all the teeth and upper and lower jaws. Panoramic X-rays are created using a machine that directs X-rays forward from behind the head, while the film is gradually moved from one side of the face to the other. The panoramic X-ray machine holds a fixed position and the film moves on a fixed path. The procedure requires people to be positioned with attachments that hold the head and jaw in place for the duration of the X-ray. The procedure is safe, painless, and typically takes only a few minutes to complete.

- Cephalometric projections are extraoral X-rays that provide a view of the entire side of a person's head. These images are used to examine a person's profile and the location of their teeth in relation to the jaw. These X-rays are most often used by orthodontists in planning treatment strategies.

- Cone-beam computed tomography (CT) is a type of extraoral X-ray that is used to create three-dimensional images of a person's entire head. During this procedure, a person stands or sits without moving while the X-ray machine moves around their head. These images are most often used to determine treatment strategies for people who need dental implants.

- Standard computed tomography (CT) is a type of dental imaging procedure that is usually conducted at a hospital or a radiologist's office. The procedure usually requires a person to lie down while the image is created. These images are similar to cone-beam computed tomography and are used for similar purposes.

- Digital radiography is a type of dental imaging that replaces standard X-ray film with a tablet computer or other type of sensor. Digital X-ray images are created and stored as computer files. These images can then be viewed on screen or printed.

Radiation and Radiation Dose

X-ray images are created through the use of emitted radiation (electromagnetic energy waves). Radiation dose is the measurement of the amount of energy that is absorbed when a person is exposed to X-rays. Dental and medical X-rays emit extremely small doses of radiation. Excessive absorption of radiation can cause health problems, and people working with X-rays or those who are exposed to many X-rays over time should take precautions to protect themselves.

Modern X-ray machines are built to limit the amount of emitted radiation to the smallest possible effective dose. Dental X-ray machines generally emit radiation in a narrow beam that is less than three inches in diameter. Very little radiation is emitted outside of this beam. Modern X-ray film has also been engineered to produce images using the smallest possible amount of radiation. Film holders keep X-ray films in place without the need for people to directly handle the film. Digital radiography further reduces the emitted radiation dose by as much as 80 percent. X-ray procedures commonly include the use of lead shields or aprons that cover patients from the neck to the knees. A lead collar is also sometimes used for further protection of people with thyroid disease or other specific health concerns. Lead blocks emitted radiation and therefore protects the body from harm. To limit exposure to X-ray radiation over time, X-ray technicians typically leave the procedure room and operate X-ray machines remotely.

Dental Radiology and Pregnancy

Pregnant women and their fetuses are considered to be at a higher risk of physical damage from excessive radiation exposure over time. Although dental X-rays expose people to extremely small doses of radiation, it is common practice to protect pregnant women with lead aprons when creating dental X-rays.

References

1. "Radiation Protection of Patients: Dental Radiology–X Rays," International Atomic Energy Agency, 2013.

2. "Treatments and Procedures: Types of Dental X-rays," Cleveland Clinic Foundation, 2015.

3. "Types of X-Rays," Aetna, 2013.

Chapter 12

Tooth Pain

What Are Toothaches?

Causes of Toothaches

Toothaches are primarily caused by tooth decay, which may initially result in pain when eating sweet, cold, or hot food. Decay can irritate the tooth's pulp—the inner core of teeth that contains nerves and connective tissue—stimulating the nerves and resulting in pain.

Other causes of toothache include infection, bleeding gums, tooth trauma, grinding teeth, abnormal bite, gum disease, and the emergence of new teeth (in babies and young children). Sinus problems, ear infections, temporomandibular joint disorders (TMJ/TMD), and tension in the facial muscles could also cause toothaches, generally accompanied by headaches. In some cases, pain surrounding the teeth and jaws could indicate an underlying heart disorder, such as angina.

Symptoms of a Toothache

Since toothache pain can be caused by a number of dental and medical conditions, the symptoms can only be diagnosed after a complete evaluation by a dentist. You may notice pus in the region of a toothache as a result of an abscess that is caused by an infection. An abscess could also be the result of gum disease, usually characterized

"Tooth Pain," © 2017 Omnigraphics. Reviewed September 2016.

by inflamed tissues and bleeding gums. Consult a dentist if you observe the following symptoms:

- fever
- difficulty breathing or swallowing
- swelling in the region of a tooth
- discharge of foul-tasting fluid
- continuous pain

Alleviating Pain in an Emergency

It is important to consult a dentist for a toothache, since leaving the condition untreated might lead to serious complications later.

If you are unable to consult a dentist right away, the self-care procedure below may help provide temporary relief:

- Use warm water to rinse your mouth.
- Floss gently to remove food particles that are stuck in your teeth.
- Take on over-the-counter medication, such as ibuprofen or acetaminophen, for pain relief.
- Do not apply aspirin directly to the affected tooth, since this may burn the gum tissue.
- Apply an over-the-counter antiseptic with benzocaine to the tooth or gums for pain relief. Clove oil (eugenol) applied to the gums may also help numb the pain. Rub the oil directly on the surface or soak a cotton swab with the oil and apply it to the tooth.
- Apply cold compresses to the cheek to reduce pain and swelling.

How a Dentist Helps

A dentist will determine the location and cause of the tooth pain with an oral examination. He or she will look for redness, swelling, and other visible indications of the cause. And an X-ray exam will help the dentist confirm an impacted tooth, decay, bone disorder, or other problems.

Depending on the underlying cause, antibiotics and pain relievers are typically prescribed to improve the healing of the toothache.

An advanced infection at the time of examination may require extraction of the tooth or root-canal surgery, which involves removal of the infected pulp from within the teeth.

Preventing Tooth Pain

The best way to prevent tooth pain is to practice regular oral hygiene. Failure to brush and floss after meals significantly increases the risk of developing cavities and the resulting toothaches.

Use the following tips to help prevent tooth pain:

- Brush at least twice a day, after meals and snacks.

- Floss daily to help prevent gum disease.

- Visit a dentist regularly for professional cleaning and an oral examination.

Hypersensitive Teeth

Causes of Sensitivity

If you experience a sharp, temporary pain on consuming hot coffee or ice cream, when breathing through the mouth, or when brushing or flossing, you may have a condition known as "sensitive teeth." Sensitive teeth can be caused by tooth decay, cracks in teeth, worn tooth enamel, exposed tooth roots, receding gums, periodontal disease, and overly aggressive brushing.

Symptoms of Sensitivity

The crowns of the teeth are covered by a strong protective layer of enamel. Below the gum line is a layer known as the cementum that covers the teeth and protects the root. Another layer called dentin covers the teeth underneath the enamel and the cementum. Dentin is less dense than enamel and cementum and has tubules that reach the core of the teeth. When the layers covering the dentin wear off, the tubules are exposed, allowing sensitivity to occur when hot or cold food stimulate the cells and nerves within the teeth.

Periodontal disease—disease of the gums—may also lead to hypersensitive teeth. If left untreated, periodontal disease can result in the separation of gum tissue from the tooth leaving pockets for bacteria to invade. The layers of the tooth can then erode leaving the root exposed. Regular dental checkups are highly recommended for the prevention, detection, and early treatment of periodontal disease and other problems.

Treatment of Sensitivity

An evaluation by a dentist is essential to diagnose hypersensitivity and rule out other causes of tooth pain. Based on circumstances, a dentist might recommend the following:

- **Desensitizing toothpaste:** Compounds present in desensitizing toothpaste block nerve impulses from causing pain. Several applications of the paste may be necessary for noticeable effects to be seen. Choose a tooth paste that carries the American Dental Association's Seal of Acceptance, which ensures compliance with the ADA's criteria for safety and effectiveness.

- **Fluoride:** Fluoride gel, possibly with a desensitizing agent, may be applied to sensitive areas of the teeth by the dentist as an in-office treatment. Fluoride may also be prescribed for use at home.

- **Bonding:** Sensitive and exposed root surfaces are sometimes treated by applying bonding resin under local anesthesia.

- **Surgical gum graft:** Healthy gum tissues extracted from elsewhere in the mouth are grafted onto exposed root surfaces to protect them and reduce sensitivity.

- **Root canal:** If other treatments do not work, and sensitivity is severe and persistent, root canal surgery may berecommended. This procedure involves replacing infected pulp in the teeth with inert material to eliminate sensitivity.

Preventing Teeth Sensitivity

Proper oral hygiene is essential to avoid teeth sensitivity. Brush twice per day using a soft-bristled toothbrush and fluoridated toothpaste. Floss on a daily basis. Do not use extremely abrasive toothpaste, and avoid aggressive and excessive brushing and flossing. Talk to your dentist about a mouth guard if you grind your teeth. Tooth-grinding can fracture teeth and lead to sensitivity.

Limit the intake of acidic foods and drinks, such as carbonated beverages, citrus fruits, yogurt, and wine. They can erode enamel over time and cause sensitivity. Use a straw to consume acidic liquids to prevent contact with teeth. After consuming acidic food and drinks, neutralize acidity levels in your mouth by drinking milk or water.

Do not brush immediately after consuming acidic substances because the acid softens the enamel, which could erode easily when brushing.

Cracked Teeth

Under the outer layer of enamel that surrounds the teeth, there is a hard layer of dentin. The dentin covers an inner core that is made of pulp. The pulp contains tissue, blood vessels, and nerves. When a tooth is cracked, chewing irritates the pulp and this causes pain. The pulp may become damaged to the extent that it does not heal completely. Extensive cracks may also lead to infection of the pulp, which can spread to the bone and gums.

It can sometimes be difficult to breathe cold air or consume hot or cold food with a cracked tooth. Bite on a clean piece of moist gauze to relieve the pain until you reach the dentist's office. Do not apply aspirin to tooth surfaces to relieve pain. It could cause burns.

Symptoms

Cracked teeth often cause erratic pain when chewing, when releasing pressure after biting, or when teeth are exposed to extremes in temperature. The pain may be intermittent, so a dentist may have difficulty determining which tooth is affected. It may be wise to consult an endodontist, a specialist in treating dental pulp, if you experience the symptoms of a cracked tooth.

Treatment

The treatment for cracked teeth depends on the location and the type of damage that has occurred. Do not delay seeing a dentist. With proper treatment cracked teeth can often be repaired to restore normal function.

Craze lines: Tiny cracks on the outer enamel of the teeth generally don't require treatment. They are very common and do not usually cause pain.

Chipped teeth: Chipped teeth are a common result of dental injuries. Chips can often be reattached or bonded with a tooth-colored filling. A crown can also be set over the tooth, if necessary.

Fractured cusp: The surface of a tooth may break off—often around a filling—and result in a fractured cusp. The fracture does not damage the pulp in most cases and does not usually cause pain. Treatments for the condition generally include fillings and crowns.

Vertical crack: In a vertically cracked tooth, the crack extends from the chewing surface down to the root. The tooth may not be broken, but the crack can eventually spread. Early diagnosis is necessary in order to save the tooth in such cases. If the crack does not extend to the pulp, root-canal surgery can save the tooth, but if the crack extends below the gum line, the tooth will likely need to be extracted.

Split tooth: A cracked tooth may progress in time into a split tooth, one that has separate segments that can divide into two portions. A split tooth generally cannot be saved fully, but proper endodontic treatment may be able to save part of it. An examination to evaluate the extent of damage will determine how much of the tooth can be saved.

Vertical root fracture: This is a fracture on the tooth that extends from the root upwards to the chewing surface. Symptoms and signs are usually minimal and might not be immediately noticeable. Such fractures are most often detected when the bone and gum near the site get infected. Treatment often involve extraction of the tooth, but endodontic treatment may help in retaining a portion of the tooth.

Healing

Broken teeth do not heal like broken bone. Cracked teeth may worsen and break off in spite of treatment, resulting in loss of teeth. A crown could provide maximum protection but is not appropriate in all cases. The specific kind of treatment you receive is important, because with proper intervention cracked teeth can be repaired to provide years of normal chewing function. Consult an endodontist to benefit from the best intervention in your case.

Prevention

You may not be able to prevent cracked teeth entirely, but here are some steps you can take to help make your teeth less vulnerable to cracks:

- Do not chew on very hard food substances, like ice or un-popped popcorn kernels. And don't make a habit of chewing on hard objects, such as pens.

- Try not to clench or grind your teeth.

- If you clench or grind your teeth while sleeping, talk to your dentist about a retainer or a mouth guard.

- When playing contact sports, wear a mouth guard or protective mask.

Tooth Abscess

A tooth abscess is a pus deposit caused by bacterial infection. Abscesses can occur in any region of the tooth for a number of different reasons. A periodontal abscess usually occurs in the gums next to a decayed root. Periapical abscesses form at the tip of a tooth's root, usually due to an untreated cavity or previous dental work. A dentist will drain the pus and treat the infection with medication. In order to save the tooth, a root-canal procedure might be necessary, but in some cases the tooth may need to be extracted. It is risky to leave a tooth abscess untreated, since it can lead to life-threatening complications.

Symptoms

Some of the symptoms of a tooth abscess include:

- severe and persistent throbbing pain radiating to the neck or ear.
- sensitivity to heat and cold.
- sensitivity to pressure when biting or chewing.
- fever, chills, nausea, or vomiting.
- swelling in the face or cheek.
- tender and swollen lymph nodes in the face or neck.
- foul smelling and tasting salty fluid in the mouth.

When to Consult a Dentist

When the above symptoms occur, you must consult a dentist immediately. If you have swelling in the face accompanied by fever and you cannot reach a dentist, go to an emergency room. Difficulty in breathing or swallowing indicates that the infection is advanced and has spread further into the jaws and other regions of the body.

Risk Factors

The risk of developing a tooth abscess is significantly increased with poor oral hygiene. Failing to brush and floss regularly can not only result in tooth decay and gum disease, but may also invite bacteria that could lead to abscesses and their serious complications. The risk of abscesses is also increased by a high-sugar diet. The regular consumption of sweets and sugary carbonated beverages can result in cavities that might later develop into abscesses.

Complications

Although a rupture in a tooth abscess may reduce pain significantly, it is essential to seek medical treatment. The pus may not drain completely, or the infection may spread to other areas of the body, like the neck or the head. Sepsis—a life-threatening condition—may develop if an abscess is left untreated and allowed to proliferate. And a weakened immune system could spread the infection from a tooth abscess even more quickly.

Diagnosis

- **Dental examination:** A dentist will first make a thorough oral examination to confirm a tooth abscess.

- **Tapping the teeth:** An abscess is usually present at the tip of the root, and a slight tap will induce pain.

- **X-ray:** An X-ray will confirm the presence of an abscess and allow the dentist to evaluate the spread of the infection.

- **CT scan:** If the abscess has spread, a CT scan will help the dentist determine the extent of infection.

Treatment

These are some of the procedures a dentist will likely follow to treat a tooth abscess:

- **Drain the abscess:** The dentist will make an incision in the abscess, drain the pus, then wash the area with saline.

- **Root canal:** A root canal can treat infection and help save a tooth. The dentist drills into the tooth and removes the pulp. The empty chamber is then filled inert material and sealed. Finally, a crown may be set on the tooth for protection.

- **Tooth extraction:** If the tooth cannot be saved, the dentist will extract the tooth and treat the abscess by draining it and treating the infection.

- **Prescribing antibiotics:** An infection that is limited to the area of the abscess may not require antibiotics, but a dentist will recommend antibiotics if the infection has spread to adjoining areas. Antibiotics will also be prescribed if you have a weakened immune system.

Phantom Tooth Pain

Phantom pain—also called atypical facial pain, neuropathic orofacial pain, or atypical odontalgia—presents as pain in a tooth or teeth without a specific cause. It usually begins after an extraction or following an endodontic procedure, and in time the pain can spread to other parts of the face.

The pain is termed atypical because it is dissimilar to normal tooth pain. Typical pain comes and goes and is aggravated by biting or chewing or by touch and pressure. It can be attributed to identifiable causes, such as decay, periodontal disease, or injury. Treatment usually relieves the pain.

Phantom pain, on the other hand, is a throbbing and constant pain at the site of an extraction or root canal that is not affected by hot or cold food substances or by biting or chewing. Local anesthetics and other pain treatments may or may not provide relief, and the intensity of pain may vary from mild to severe. This presents an inexplicable situation to the dentist who might attempt more treatment that provides no symptomatic improvement.

Causes

Since the causes of phantom tooth pain remain unclear, it is termed "idiopathic." It is more common in women than in men, and it tends to occur more often in middle-aged and older people. Research has found a link between anxiety and depression and phantom tooth pain, but the association remains unclear. Phantom tooth pain is a dysfunction or short-circuiting of the nerves that carry sensations from the teeth and jaw to the brain. Molecular or biochemical changes have been observed in areas of the brain that process pain, which could be the cause of the phantom pain.

Treatment

Dental treatment usually doesn't alleviate phantom tooth pain. It may lessen the severity, but it often returns. This is because the pain is a result of a dysfunction of the brain and nerves that process pain.

Phantom tooth pain is treated using a variety of medications, most commonly tricyclic antidepressants, such as amitriptyline, which in this case are prescribed for their pain-relieving properties, rather than their antidepressant benefits. Medicines prescribed for chronic pain conditions, such as gabapentin, baclofen, and duloxetine, are also often prescribed. This treatment reduces the pain but may not eliminate it completely.

Phantom tooth pain may or may not be a permanent condition, but in some cases the symptoms disappear after a length of time or with prolonged treatment. Sometimes the pain persists and may require lifelong medication.

Phantom tooth pain is a rare condition, and some dentists may not be familiar with its diagnosis and treatment. It is best to consult a dentist with an advanced specialization, such as oral medicine or orofacial pain.

References

1. "Sensitive Teeth: Causes and Treatment," American Dental Association, December 2003.

2. Carr, Alan. "What Causes Sensitive Teeth, and How Can I Treat Them?" Mayo Clinic, December 6, 2014.

3. "What Causes a Toothache?" Delta Dental, June 2010.

4. "Tooth Abscess," Mayo Clinic, February 16, 2016.

5. Falace, D. "Atypical Odontalgia," American Academy of Oral Medicine, January 22, 2015.

6. "Cracked Teeth," American Association of Endodontists, n.d.

Chapter 13

Medications Used in Dentistry

Dentists may prescribe several different types of medications as part of a patient's treatment plan. Medications are commonly used in oral care to help relieve pain and anxiety, prevent tooth decay, or control plaque and gingivitis, infections, and dry mouth. To ensure the effectiveness and reduce the risk of dental medications, it is important for patients to keep their dentist informed of any changes in symptoms, any health conditions they may have, and any other medications they may be taking.

Managing Pain and Anxiety

Many patients worry about the pain involved in dental procedures. As a result, pain management and anxiety control are important facets of dental care. At the dentist's office, patients may receive topical, local, or general anesthetics to help them deal with this common complication. They may also use prescription or over-the-counter analgesics at home to relieve discomfort following dental procedures.

- **Topical anesthetics**

    Many dentists apply topical anesthetics to numb the gums prior to injecting local anesthetics. In addition, they may prescribe

"Medications Used in Dentistry," © 2017 Omnigraphics. Reviewed September 2016.

topical anesthetics to provide patients with temporary relief from pain or irritation caused by cold sores, canker sores, fever blisters, teething, braces, or dentures. These medications are available in many forms, including gels, ointments, pastes, lozenges, and aerosol sprays. Some of the common brand name dental anesthetics include Anbesol, Chloraseptic, Orajel, and Xylocaine. It is important to note that topical anesthetics are generally intended to provide temporary pain relief, and patients should seek dental treatment if the discomfort lasts more than a few days.

- **Local anesthetics**

Dentists typically inject local anesthetics—such as lidocaine and mepivacaine—into the gum tissues of the mouth prior to dental procedures that involve drilling or cutting. These medications reduce pain by inhibiting the impulses from pain-sensing nerves.

- **General anesthetics**

Oral surgeons may administer intravenous anesthetic medications to enable patients to sleep through complex dental procedures.

- **Analgesics**

Analgesics are pain-relieving medications that are often recommended for patients who have undergone dental procedures. Narcotic analgesics such as codeine or hydrocodone (brand names Tylenol #3 or Vicodin) may be prescribed to manage severe pain conditions. To relieve minor pain and inflammation associated with toothaches or dental appliances, a number of non-narcotic analgesics are available over-the-counter, including ibuprofen (Advil, Nuprin, Motrin) and acetaminophen (Tylenol).

- **Anti-inflammatory medications**

Corticosteroids are anti-inflammatory medications that may help relieve discomfort from tooth and gum problems. They usually take the form of topical pastes and are sold under such brand names as Orabase-HCA, Oracort, and Oralone. It is important to note that corticosteroids should not be used for teething due to the potential for dangerous side effects in infants and young children.

- **Sedatives**

Dentists may also use medications to help patients relax during dental procedures. Inhaled anti-anxiety agents, such as nitrous

oxide, may be used along with local anesthetics. Benzodiazepines, such as diazepam (Valium), may also be prescribed to
help relieve the symptoms of anxiety. Finally, muscle relaxants
may be prescribed to reduce stress in patients who grind their
teeth or experience headaches or jaw pain from temporomandibular joint disorders (TMJ).

Controlling Plaque and Gingivitis

Plaque is a sticky, bacteria-containing film that coats the teeth
and other surfaces in the mouth. Gingivitis is a mild form of gum
disease that is caused by the buildup of plaque. Symptoms of gingivitis include redness, swelling, and irritation of the gums. Both
plaque and gingivitis can usually be controlled through good oral
hygiene, including brushing the teeth at least twice per day and
flossing between teeth regularly. In addition, many different antiseptic mouth rinses are available over-the-counter to help reduce
plaque and gingivitis and kill bacteria in the mouth that cause bad
breath.

Chlorhexidine is an antibiotic used to control plaque and gingivitis
in the mouth. Dentists may also prescribe chlorhexidine in conjunc-
tion with certain dental procedures, such as scaling or root planing,
or to reduce the depth of periodontal pockets (the space between
the teeth and gums). The medication is available as a mouth rinse
or in a chip form under the brand names Peridex, PerioChip, and
PerioGuard. Although chlorhexidine can help control bacteria in the
mouth, it may also cause unwanted side effects, such as an increase
in tartar on the teeth or staining of the teeth, dentures, or other
mouth appliances.

Tetracyclines are a category of antibiotics (including demeclocy-
cline, doxycycline, minocycline, oxytetracycline, and tetracyclineions)
that may be used to treat gingivitis and eliminate bacteria associated
with more advanced periodontal disease. Tetracyclines are available
as gels, mouth rinses, fibers, and particles for use as dental antibiotics.
Tetracyclines should not be used by pregnant women or children under
age eight, however, because they may cause permanent discoloration
of developing teeth.

Preventing Tooth Decay

Fluoride is a medication that helps prevent tooth decay by strengthening teeth and making them better able to resist damage from acids

and bacteria. Fluoride is added to many municipal water supplies, and it is also available in nonprescription form in many toothpastes and mouth rinses. Prescription-strength fluoride is also available in liquid, tablet, and chewable form for young children who do not have access to a fluoridated water supply.

Alleviating Dry Mouth

Dry mouth can occur as a complication of autoimmune disorders, certain medications, and some other conditions. The symptoms can often be alleviated through the use of saliva substitute medications, such as Moi-Stir, Mouth Kote, Optimoist, Salivar, Salix, and Xero-Lube. Most dry mouth treatments take the form of sprays that the patient can apply as needed. Pilocarpine, sold under the brand name Salagan, is a prescription medication that helps relieve dry mouth by stimulating saliva production.

Treating Dental Infections

In addition to helping control bacteria in the mouth that cause periodontal disease, antibiotics are also used in dentistry to prevent and treat infections and abscesses. Antibiotics are often used to treat infections that develop in the bone and soft tissue following dental procedures. In some cases, antibiotics are also prescribed prior to dental procedures to prevent bacteria in the mouth from entering the bloodstream. People with medical conditions that put them at high risk of infection—such as a compromised immune system, artificial heart valves, or liver disease—may need to take antibiotics both before and after undergoing dental procedures.

Penicillin and amoxicillin are among the antibiotics most commonly prescribed to treat infections that result from dental procedures. Patients who are allergic to penicillin are usually prescribed erythromycin instead. Clindamycin may be prescribed to treat infections that do not respond to other antibiotics. These medications may be administered orally, intramuscularly, or intravenously.

Antifungal medications such as nystatin are used to treat candidiasis (oral thrush), an infection caused by the *Candida albicans* fungus. Antifungal medications are available in lozenges or liquid suspensions that the patient holds in the mouth and swishes around before swallowing.

References

1. "Drugs Used in Dentistry," WebMD, 2016.

2. "Medications Used in Dentistry," Cleveland Clinic, 2010.

3. Ogbru, Annette. "Medications Used in Dentistry," WebMD, 2016.

Chapter 14

Sedation Techniques Used by Dentists

Sedation in dentistry involves administering medication to reduce patients' level of awareness and make them feel more relaxed and comfortable. Although sedation does not control pain, it can help decrease patients' level of anxiety about undergoing dental procedures. Studies have shown that up to 20% of people experience some form of anxiety or phobia with regard to dental treatment. Depending on its severity, dental anxiety can cause patients to postpone or avoid necessary dental care, resulting in poor oral health. People with poor oral health, in turn, generally require more extensive and complicated dental procedures, which serves to further increase their anxiety levels.

Fear and apprehension create physiological responses that can make dental treatment more difficult for patients and dentists alike. These emotions trigger the release of stress chemicals in the brain that put bodily systems on alert. Muscles become tense, nerves become hypersensitive to stimuli, and pain tolerance becomes lower. Management of patients' pain and anxiety is thus a major concern for successful dental practices. Various sedation techniques are available that suppress the central nervous system, allowing patients to feel relaxed, peaceful, and comfortable while still remaining conscious and in control. By helping patients overcome anxiety, sedation dentistry also enables the dental team to work more efficiently and confidently.

Levels of Sedation

There are several different levels of sedation available to meet patients' needs. The level of sedation is determined by the degree to which the medication suppresses the patient's central nervous system and awareness of their surroundings.

- Conscious or minimal sensation, also known as anxiolysis, induces a mildly depressed level of consciousness. The patient remains conscious and able to respond to verbal commands or physical stimuli. Although the patient's thought processes may be slightly impaired, this level of sedation should not affect breathing or heart function.

- Moderate sedation is similar to minimal sedation but involves a more depressed level of consciousness. Patients can generally respond to verbal commands, such as "open your mouth," that are accompanied by light tactile stimuli. Ventilation and cardiovascular function are usually unaffected.

- Deep sedation induces a loss of consciousness in the patient. Although the patient may respond to repeated stimulation, it may be difficult to arouse them. In addition, positive-pressure ventilation may be required and cardiovascular function may be impaired.

- General anesthesia is the deepest level of sedation. Patients cannot be aroused even by painful stimuli. Ventilation assistance is often required, and cardiovascular function may be impaired.

Sedation Techniques

Medications used for sedation in dentistry are typically administered orally, through inhalation, or intravenously. In some cases, different routes of drug administration are used in combination to induce the desired level of sedation.

- Oral (enteral) sedation is commonly used to help alleviate mild to moderate anxiety in dental patients. Patients take the medication by mouth, either by swallowing it or allowing it to dissolve under the tongue. Many people find the oral administration easy and convenient and appreciate the fact that injections are not required. Some of the oral sedatives often used in dentistry include benzodiazepines such as diazepam (Valium), lorazepam (Ativan), triazolam (Halcion), and midazolam (Versed), and non-benzodiazepines such as zolpidem (Ambien) and zaleplon (Sonata). These medications help patients relax and feel more comfortable during dental procedures. In some cases, they also produce an amnesia effect that dampens patients' memory of what happened in the dental chair. Even though the sedation effect is mild, patients should always be accompanied by a responsible person to drive them home from the dentist's office.

- Inhalation sedation involves the administration of nitrous oxide mixed with oxygen to the lungs. Patients inhale the gases through a nasal hood, which looks like a small plastic cup that fits over the nose. It produces a light-headed, euphoric feeling in patients that helps reduce pain and apprehension during dental treatment. Bodily functions remain unaffected, however, and the effects wear off quickly once the gas is turned off.

- Intravenous (IV) sedation involves the administration of sedatives directly into the bloodstream through the veins. The drugs most commonly used include a benzodiazepine in combination with an opioid, such as fentanyl or demerol. Since IV sedation requires specialized training, it is mainly used by oral surgeons and periodontists. Although IV sedation works quickly and allows the level of sedation to be adjusted easily, bodily functions like heart rate, blood pressure, and breathing must be monitored carefully. Due to the higher level of risk involved, IV sedation is typically considered when other sedation methods are ineffective.

Safety and Effectiveness

The sedative medications used in dentistry have been tested extensively and have proven safe and effective in most situations. To minimize the risk of adverse reactions, it is important for patients to provide their dentists with information about any underlying medical conditions they may have, such as diabetes; any prescription medications, over-the-counter drugs, or natural or herbal supplements they may be taking; and any lifestyle choices, such as smoking or excessive alcohol consumption, that may affect sedation. Patients should also follow the dentist's instructions about not eating or drinking for at least six hours before their appointment and bring a responsible person to drive them home following any dental procedure that involves sedation.

References

1. Assaf, Hussein M., and Marna L. Negrelli. "Sedation in the Dental Office: An Overview," DentalCare.com, January 5, 2015.

2. Silverman, Michael D. "Oral Sedation Dentistry," Dear Doctor: Dentistry and Oral Health, February 1, 2009.

Chapter 15

Alternatives to Dental Drills

Many patients dread going to the dentist because of the dental drill. Whether they object most to the noise, vibration, heat, or smell, many people find having their teeth drilled to be an unpleasant experience. In addition, procedures that require drilling usually involve the use of local anesthesia, which can entail several hours of discomfort due to numb lips, tongue, and cheeks. Recognizing the negative associations many patients have toward the dental drill, some dentists have adopted alternative methods of preparing and treating teeth, such as air abrasion and dental lasers.

Air Abrasion

Air abrasion, also known as micro-abrasion, is a technique that uses compressed air to propel a tiny stream of aluminum oxide particles onto the tooth. It has been compared to the process of sand blasting. Dentists can use air abrasion in place of a standard dental drill to fix minor cracks and discolorations or to remove decay from the tooth's surface and prepare it for fillings, sealants, or restoration placement.

Air abrasion offers several advantages over a traditional dental drill. It is very quiet and virtually painless, so patients do not require anesthetic. It also allows the dentist to operate with greater precision,

"Alternatives to Dental Drills," © 2017 Omnigraphics. Reviewed September 2016.

which helps to safeguard soft tissue, preserve more tooth structure, and reduce the risk of micro-fractures in tooth enamel. In addition, there is no odor or vibration associated with the air abrasion technique. Although patients may have some dust residue in their mouth, it can easily be removed by rinsing with water. The main disadvantage of air abrasion is that it cannot be used on restorations such as crowns and bridges.

Dental Lasers

Dental lasers offer another alternative to dental drills. Lasers use targeted pulses of infrared light energy to perform many of the typical functions of drills. Lasers can be used to remove decayed areas from a tooth to prepare it for filling and to strengthen the bond between the filling and the tooth. They can also be used in tooth-whitening procedures to enhance the action of bleaching chemicals applied to the tooth surface. Finally, lasers can be used to cut into gums and soft tissue during root canal procedures.

There are many different types of dental lasers available that use different wavelengths of light to vaporize water molecules or minerals like hydroxyapatite within teeth. A computer usually determines the pattern of laser pulses, although the dentist still controls the instrument. Most types of lasers do not produce heat or vibration, and many patients do not experience pain and thus avoid the need for anesthesia. In addition, dental lasers offer precision that can help preserve tooth structure and protect soft tissue from damage.

Dental lasers do have a few disadvantages, however. They cannot be used on teeth that already contain fillings, for instance, and they cannot be used to remove crowns or prepare teeth for bridgework. Even in situations when lasers can be used, traditional dental drills are sometimes needed to shape and polish fillings following laser treatment. Dental laser systems also tend to be an extremely costly investment for dental practices as compared to standard drills. Finally, although dental lasers have been approved for use by the U.S. Food and Drug Administration (FDA), as of 2015 they had not yet met the American Dental Association's (ADA) standards for safety and effectiveness. However, the ADA did express optimism about future applications of dental lasers as an alternative to more traditional treatment.

References

1. "Dental Alternative to the Drill: Drilless Dentistry," Drakeshire Dental, 2016.

2. Gwynne, Peter. "Laser Offers Alternative to the Dental Drill," Inside Science, June 4, 2014.

3. "Laser Use in Dentistry," WebMD, 2016.

Chapter 16

Dental Fillings

Chapter Contents

Section 16.1

Dental Amalgam Fillings

This section includes text excerpted from "About
Dental Amalgam Fillings," U.S. Food and Drug
Administration (FDA), February 10, 2015.

What Is Dental Amalgam?

Dental amalgam is a dental filling material used to fill cavities caused by tooth decay. It has been used for more than 150 years in hundreds of millions of patients around the world. Dental amalgam is a mixture of metals, consisting of liquid (elemental) mercury and a powdered alloy composed of silver, tin, and copper. Approximately 50% of dental amalgam is elemental mercury by weight. The chemical properties of elemental mercury allow it to react with and bind together the silver/copper/tin alloy particles to form an amalgam. Dental amalgam fillings are also known as "silver fillings" because of their silver-like appearance. Despite the name, "silver fillings" do contain elemental mercury.

Image of a capsule containing liquid mercury and amalgam putty. When placing dental amalgam, the dentist first drills the tooth to remove the decay and then shapes the tooth cavity for placement of the amalgam filling. Next, under appropriate safety conditions, the dentist mixes the powdered alloy with the liquid mercury to form an amalgam putty. (These components are provided to the dentist in a capsule as shown in the graphic.) This softened amalgam putty is placed and shaped in the prepared cavity, where it rapidly hardens into a solid filling.

What Should I Know Before Getting a Dental Amalgam Filling?

Deciding what filling material to use to treat dental decay is a choice that must be made by you and your dentist. U.S. Food and Drug Administration (FDA) continues to evaluate the available information on dental amalgam, and will update the information on this web page as necessary. As you consider your options, you should keep in mind the following information.

Benefits

Dental amalgam fillings are strong and long-lasting, so they are less likely to break than some other types of fillings. Dental amalgam is the least expensive type of filling material.

Potential Risks

Dental amalgam contains elemental mercury. It releases low levels of mercury in the form of a vapor that can be inhaled and absorbed by the lungs. High levels of mercury vapor exposure are associated with adverse effects in the brain and the kidneys.

FDA has reviewed the best available scientific evidence to determine whether the low levels of mercury vapor associated with dental amalgam fillings are a cause for concern. Based on this evidence, FDA considers dental amalgam fillings safe for adults and children ages 6 and above. The weight of credible scientific evidence reviewed by FDA does not establish an association between dental amalgam use and adverse health effects in the general population. Clinical studies in adults and children ages 6 and above have found no link between dental amalgam fillings and health problems.

The developing neurological systems in fetuses and young children may be more sensitive to the neurotoxic effects of mercury vapor. Very limited to no clinical data is available regarding long-term health outcomes in pregnant women and their developing fetuses, and children under the age of six, including infants who are breastfed. Pregnant women and parents with children under six who are concerned about the absence of clinical data as to long-term health outcomes should talk to their dentist.

However, the estimated amount of mercury in breast milk attributable to dental amalgam is low and falls well below general levels for oral intake that the Environmental Protection Agency (EPA) considers safe. Despite the limited clinical information, FDA concludes that the existing risk information supports a finding that infants are not at risk for adverse health effects from the mercury in breast milk of women exposed to mercury vapor from dental amalgam. Some individuals have an allergy or sensitivity to mercury or the other components of dental amalgam (such as silver, copper or tin). Dental amalgam might cause these individuals to develop oral lesions or other contact reactions. If you are allergic to any of the metals in dental amalgam, you should not get amalgam fillings. You can discuss other treatment options with your dentist.

Why Is Mercury Used in Dental Amalgam?

Approximately half of a dental amalgam filling is liquid mercury and the other half is a powdered alloy of silver, tin, and copper. Mercury is used to bind the alloy particles together into a strong, durable, and solid filling. Mercury's unique properties (it is a liquid at room temperature and that bonds well with the alloy powder) make it an important component of dental amalgam that contributes to its durability.

What Is Bioaccumulation?

Bioaccumulation refers to the build-up or steadily increasing concentration of a chemical in organs or tissues in the body. Mercury from dental amalgam and other sources (e.g., fish) is bioaccumulative. Studies of healthy subjects with amalgam fillings have shown that mercury from exposure to mercury vapor bioaccumulates in certain tissues of the body including kidneys and brain. Studies have not shown that bioaccumulation of mercury from dental amalgam results in damage to target organs.

Is the Mercury in Dental Amalgam the Same as the Mercury in Some Types of Fish?

No. There are several different chemical forms of mercury: elemental mercury, inorganic mercury, and methylmercury. The form of mercury associated with dental amalgam is elemental mercury, which releases mercury vapor. The form of mercury found in fish is methylmercury, a type of organic mercury. Mercury vapor is mainly absorbed by the lungs. Methylmercury is mainly absorbed through the digestive tract. The body processes these forms of mercury differently and has different levels of tolerance for mercury vapor and methylmercury.

If I Am Concerned About the Mercury in Dental Amalgam, Should I Have My Fillings Removed?

If your fillings are in good condition and there is no decay beneath the filling, FDA does not recommend that you have your amalgam fillings removed or replaced. Removing sound amalgam fillings results in unnecessary loss of healthy tooth structure, and exposes you to additional mercury vapor released during the removal process.

However, if you believe you have an allergy or sensitivity to mercury or any of the other metals in dental amalgam (such as silver, tin or copper), you should discuss treatment options with your dentist.

Section 16.2

Mercury in Dental Amalgam

This section includes text excerpted from "Mercury in Dental Amalgam," United States Environmental Protection Agency (EPA), March 3, 2016.

What Are Dental Amalgam Fillings?

Sometimes referred to as "silver filling," dental amalgam is a silver-colored material used to fill (restore) teeth that have cavities. Dental amalgam is made of two nearly equal parts:

1. liquid mercury and

2. a powder containing silver, tin, copper, zinc and other metals.

Amalgam is one of the most commonly used tooth fillings, and is considered a safe, sound, and effective treatment for tooth decay.

Are Dental Amalgam Fillings Safe?

When amalgam fillings are placed in or removed from teeth, they can release a small amount of mercury vapor. Amalgam can also release small amounts of mercury vapor during chewing. People can absorb these vapors by inhaling or ingesting them.

However, the U.S. Food and Drug Administration (FDA) considers dental amalgam fillings safe for adults and children over the age of six. FDA regulates dental amalgam as a medical device. FDA is responsible for ensuring that dental amalgam is reasonably safe and effective.

Among other things, FDA also makes sure the product labeling for dentists has adequate directions for use and includes applicable warnings.

Are There Alternatives to Using Dental Amalgam Fillings?

Presently, there are five other types of restorative materials for tooth decay:

- resin composite
- glass ionomer
- resin ionomer
- porcelain
- gold alloys

The choice of dental treatment rests with dental professionals and their patients, so talk with your dentist about available dental treatment options.

How Does Amalgam Waste Affect the Environment?

If improperly managed by dental offices, dental amalgam waste can be released into the environment. Although most dental offices currently use some type of basic filtration system to reduce the amount of mercury solids passing into the sewer system, dental offices are the single largest source of mercury at sewage treatment plants.

The installation of amalgam separators, which catch and hold the excess amalgam waste coming from office spittoons, can further reduce discharges to wastewater. Without these separators, the excess amalgam waste will be released to the sewers.

From sewers, amalgam waste goes to publicly-owned treatment works (POTWs) (sewage treatment plants). POTWs have around a 90% efficiency rate of removing amalgam from wastewaters. Once removed, the amalgam waste becomes part of the POTW's sewage sludge, which is then disposed:

- **in landfills.** If the amalgam waste is sent to a landfill, the mercury may be released into the ground water or air.

- **through incineration.** If the mercury is incinerated, mercury may be emitted to the air from the incinerator stacks.

- **by applying the sludge to agricultural land as fertilizer.** if mercury-contaminated sludge is used as an agricultural fertilizer, some of the mercury used as fertilizer may also evaporate to the atmosphere.

Through precipitation, this airborne mercury eventually gets deposited onto water bodies, land and vegetation. Some dentists throw their excess amalgam into special medical waste containers, believing this to be an environmentally safe disposal practice. If waste amalgam is improperly disposed in medical waste bags, however, the amalgam waste may be incinerated and mercury may be emitted to the air from the incinerator stacks. This airborne mercury is eventually deposited into water bodies and onto land.

Section 16.3

Amalgam Filling Alternatives

This section includes text excerpted from
"Alternatives to Dental Amalgam," U.S. Food and Drug
Administration (FDA), January 27, 2015.

Alternatives to Dental Amalgam

Other materials can also be used to fill cavities caused by dental decay. Like dental amalgam, these direct filling materials are used to restore the biting surface of a tooth that has been damaged by decay. Your dentist can discuss treatment options based on the location of cavities in your mouth and the amount of tooth decay. The primary alternatives to dental amalgam are as follows:

- Composite Resin Fillings

- Glass Ionomer Cement Fillings

Every restorative material has advantages and disadvantages.

Composite Resin Fillings

Picture of a tooth with a composite resin filling. Composite resin fillings are the most common alternative to dental amalgam. They are sometimes called "tooth-colored" or "white" fillings because of their color. Composite resin fillings are made of a type of plastic (an acrylic resin) reinforced with powdered glass filler. The color (shade) of composite resins can be customized to closely match surrounding teeth. Composite resin fillings are often light cured by a "blue-light" in layers to build up the final restoration.

Advantages of composite resin fillings include:

• Blend in with surrounding teeth

• High strength

• Require minimal removal of healthy tooth structure for placement

Disadvantages of composite resin fillings include:

• More difficult to place than dental amalgam

• May be less durable than dental amalgam and may need to be replaced more frequently

• Higher cost of placement

Glass Ionomer Cement Fillings

Glass ionomer cements contain organic acids, such as eugenol, and bases, such as zinc oxide, and may include acrylic resins. Like some composite resins, glass ionomer cements include a component of glass filler that releases fluoride over time. Also like composite fillings, glass ionomer cements are tooth-colored. The composition and properties of glass ionomer cements are best suited for very small restorations. Unlike composite resin fillings, glass ionomer cements are self-curing and usually do not need a "blue light" to set (harden). The advantages of glass ionomer cements are ease of use and appearance. Their chief disadvantage is that they are limited to use in small restorations.

Chapter 17

Rebuilding and Reshaping Teeth

Crowns and Bridges

What Is a Dental Crown?

A dental crown is a cap that covers a tooth that is cracked, broken, or discolored, or one in which fillings have deteriorated or been lost. The purpose of a dental crown is to restore the shape, size, and strength of the tooth, as well as to improve its appearance.

Numerous options are available for dental crown material. Depending on its location, the dentist may suggest permanent crowns made of resin, ceramic, stainless steel, metal (gold or other alloy), or porcelain that is fused to metal. A dental crown should last between five and 15 years, depending on how much wear and tear it receives and how good the oral hygiene is, as well as on other individual habits, such as grinding or clenching teeth, biting fingernails, and chewing ice.

When Is a Crown Needed?

A person could require a dental crown to:

- Prevent cracking or breaking of a weak tooth.

"Rebuilding and Reshaping Teeth," © 2017 Omnigraphics. Reviewed September 2016.

- hold together or restore an already broken tooth.
- act as an anchor for a dental bridge.
- cover worn out or discolored teeth.
- provide the tooth with cover and support for a large filling.
- cover a dental implant or a root canal.

A crown may be required for children on primary (baby) teeth to:

- save a tooth severely damaged by decay.
- protect teeth when the child is at high risk of tooth decay, especially when there is difficulty in maintaining proper dental hygiene.
- decrease use of general anesthesia in children unable to sit through proper dental care requirements (due to age, behavior, or medical history).

How Is a Tooth Prepared for a Crown?

Usually, two visits to the dentist are required to prepare the tooth for a crown. In the first visit, the dentist examines the tooth by taking X-rays to check its root and the surrounding bone. A root canal may be required if there is either extensive tooth decay or the risk of injury or infection to the pulp of the tooth. The tooth will then be reshaped to accommodate the crown, and a paste or putty impressions will be made of the tooth that will receive the crown, along with those above or below it.

These impressions will then be sent to a dental lab, and the crown will arrive at the dentist's office in about two or three weeks. In the interim, the patient will be fitted with a temporary crown made of acrylic, which will protect the prepared tooth. The dentist will usually suggest a few special precautions to take care of this temporary crown. In the second visit, the dentist will inspect the fit and color of the permanent crown, and if they are satisfactory, it will be cemented in place.

What Is a Dental Bridge?

A dental bridge is a ceramic structure that fills the gap created by a missing or extracted tooth. It is used for a number of purposes, including to restore the ability to speak or chew properly, to prevent teeth from moving out of position, to restore the person's smile, and to maintain the shape of the face.

To create a bridge, an artificial tooth (called a pontic), commonly made of ceramic, is fused with two or more crowns on the teeth on either side of the gap. These crowns become the anchors for the pontic, and are known as abutment teeth. Porcelain, gold, alloys, or a combination of these materials can be used to make a bridge, which can last from five to 15 years, depending on good oral hygiene and regular dental checkups.

How Is a Bridge Prepared?

Preparing a bridge generally requires at least two dental visits. In the first, the abutment teeth are reshaped to make room for the crowns to be placed over them. The impressions of these teeth are then made and will be used as the model in the dental lab to prepare the pontic, crowns, and bridge. The shape and color of both the crowns and the pontic will be made to match those of the patient's natural teeth. As with crowns, the dentist will make a temporary bridge to help protect the exposed teeth and gums between visits.

In the second visit, the fit and appearance of the bridge will be checked. Adjustments will be made if required, and when the bridge fits properly, it will be installed permanently. This fitting process sometimes requires more than one visit, and in some cases the dentist may cement it only temporarily for a few weeks to ensure that it fits properly before the final placement.

Is Special Care Required for Dental Crowns and Bridges?

Special care is not generally needed for a crowned tooth or a bridge, however, it is important to maintain good oral hygiene. In addition to brushing at least twice daily and flossing (especially where the gum meets the tooth), using an antibacterial mouthwash to rinse at least once per day is recommended. In the case of a bridge, strong and healthy adjoining teeth are needed to provide sturdy support, so practicing good oral hygiene is crucial to prevent tooth loss due to decay or gum disease. And a regular cleaning schedule and visits to the dentist will help identify complications at an early stage.

Dental Veneers

A dental veneer, sometimes called a porcelain veneer or a dental porcelain laminate, is a thin shell used to cover the front surface of a tooth. It is made from either porcelain or resin composite material to provide strength to the tooth and improve its appearance. The veneer is custom-made to match the person's natural teeth and is typically used to correct teeth that are slightly out of position, discolored, fractured or chipped, unevenly shaped, or have gaps between them. It functions as an intermediate option between bonding (the application of resin directly to the tooth) and a crown for individuals who want only a slight change in the appearance of the tooth. Veneers usually last from five to ten years, after which they need to be replaced.

How Is a Veneer Prepared?

Preparing a veneer might require multiple visits to the dentist's office. The first visit will be a consultation with the dentist to determine if a veneer is the right option for the patient. The dentist will examine the teeth, discuss the procedure, outline plusses and minuses, and suggest alternatives, if there are any.

To prepare for a veneer, the dentist will remove about half a millimeter of enamel from the surface of the tooth. This is roughly equal to the thickness of the veneer that will be bonded to that tooth's surface. An impression of the tooth will then be made and sent to the dental lab that will make the veneer. It can take up to two weeks for the dentist to receive the veneer from the lab, and in the interim the patient may opt for a temporary veneer, usually at additional cost.

In the next visit, the veneer will be placed temporarily on the tooth to test its fit and color. Small adjustments will be made to the fit if needed, and the color can be fine-tuned with different shades of cement. The tooth will then be prepared to receive the veneer by cleaning, polishing, and then etching the surface to roughen it for a stronger bond. Once the veneer is cemented into position, the excess cement is removed, the bite is evaluated, and final adjustments are made, if needed. A follow-up visit might be required after a couple of weeks for the dentist to see how the gums respond to the veneer and to examine its placement once again. Regular professional visits to the dentist will also be required to polish the veneer with a special non-abrasive paste.

Is Special Care Required for a Veneer?

Maintaining a porcelain veneer does not generally demand special care, other than normal oral hygiene, including brushing twice daily, flossing, and rinsing daily with an antiseptic mouthwash. But the dentist might recommend a nighttime bite guard if the patient grinds or clenches his or her teeth often. Though veneers are stain resistant, the dentist might also recommend avoiding food and beverages that stain teeth, like coffee, tea, and red wine.

References

1. "Crowns & Bridges," National Dental Care, n.d.

2. Wyatt Jr., Alfred D. "Dental Crowns," WebMD, September 29, 2014.

3. Friedman, Michael. "Dental Health and Bridges," WebMD, May 24, 2016.

4. Wyatt Jr., Alfred D. "Dental Health and Veneers," WebMD, January 30, 2015.

5. "Porcelain Veneers," American Academy of Cosmetic Dentistry, n.d.

Chapter 18

Having a Tooth Pulled

Tooth extraction, or having a tooth pulled, is a dental procedure that involves removing a tooth from its socket in the jawbone. Simple extractions are typically performed by a general dentist using a local anesthetic. Surgical extractions, on the other hand, are usually performed by an oral surgeon and often require an intravenous (IV) or general anesthetic.

Reasons for Tooth Extraction

People have teeth extracted for a number of different reasons. One or more teeth may need to be pulled in cases where they:

- become damaged by trauma or decay and cannot be repaired with a filling, crown, or other dental treatment;

- become loose due to periodontal (gum) disease affecting the bones and tissues of the mouth;

- are too crowded for permanent teeth to come in properly or for orthodontic treatment to align teeth properly;

- become impacted (stuck in the jaw), especially wisdom teeth;

- develop an infection that cannot be successfully treated with antibiotics or root canal therapy;

"Having a Tooth Pulled," © 2017 Omnigraphics. Reviewed September 2016.

- create a high risk of infection in people with weakened immune systems due to chemotherapy, organ transplant, or other medical conditions; or

- get in the way of radiation treatment to the head or neck.

Before Having a Tooth Pulled

When a dentist diagnoses a problem that requires the removal of a tooth, the first step in the process involves assessing the patient's medical condition and history. Although tooth extraction is generally considered to be a very safe procedure, it can allow bacteria from the mouth to enter the bloodstream. As a result, people with medical conditions that put them at high risk of infection—such as a compromised immune system, heart disease, or liver disease—may need to take antibiotics before and after having a tooth pulled.

Patients should also provide a list of all medications they take, including prescriptions, over-the-counter drugs, vitamins, and dietary supplements. Some medications, such as bisphosphonates (which are commonly prescribed to treat osteoporosis and other forms of bone loss), can increase the risk of complications from oral surgery.

After taking a medical history, the dentist or oral surgeon will usually take a series of X-rays or a panoramic X-ray to help them plan the extraction. X-rays can provide important information about the relationship between upper teeth and sinuses, or between lower teeth and the inferior alveolar nerve in the jawbone. In addition, X-rays can help identify infections, tumors, or bone diseases that may be affecting the teeth.

The Tooth Extraction Process

Prior to the tooth extraction, the patient usually receives some form of anesthesia. For a simple extraction where the tooth is fully exposed or already loose, the dentist may inject a local anesthetic to numb the area of the mouth near the tooth. For more complex procedures involving an impacted tooth or multiple teeth, an oral surgeon may administer a general anesthetic. Depending on the type of anesthetic used, the patient may remain conscious but feel very calm and sedated, or the patient may sleep through the entire procedure. It is important for patients to follow preoperative instructions and avoid eating, drinking, or smoking if they will receive general anesthesia.

For a simple extraction, the dentist will typically use an instrument called an elevator to loosen the tooth, then grasp it with forceps and wiggle it gently to remove it. In a surgical extraction, the oral surgeon will usually make a small incision in the gum to expose the tooth and then cut away the bone and tissue holding it in place. Finally, the oral surgeon will grasp the tooth with forceps and rock it gently to loosen and remove it. Teeth that are impacted or difficult to pull out sometimes must be broken and removed in pieces.

Once the extraction has been completed, the dentist will pack the tooth socket with gauze and ask the patient to bite down to put pressure on the wound for 20 to 30 minutes. Since cuts in the mouth cannot dry out and form a scab, they tend to bleed for a longer period of time than cuts on the skin. In some cases, minor bleeding may continue for 24 hours. Eventually, however, a blood clot should form in the socket. The dentist may use a few stitches to close the edges of the gum over the extraction site. The stitches may dissolve on their own, or they may need to be removed by the dentist at a follow-up appointment.

After Having a Tooth Pulled

Most people who have a tooth extracted are able to return home a few hours after the procedure is completed. In most cases, patients are encouraged to have a responsible person accompany them and drive them home. The initial recovery from a tooth extraction typically takes a few days. During that time, the following suggestions can help patients minimize pain and discomfort, reduce the risk of infection, and promote a quick and full recovery:

- Keep a gauze pad in place for three to four hours to control bleeding and allow a blood clot to form in the tooth socket. Change the pad whenever it becomes soaked with blood or saliva.

- Avoid spitting, rinsing, or drinking from a straw for 24 hours after the extraction to prevent the clot from being dislodged.

- Take nonsteroidal anti-inflammatory drugs (NSAIDs), such as ibuprofen, as directed by the dentist to help manage pain and reduce swelling. Stronger painkillers may be prescribed for the first few days following a surgical tooth extraction.

- Apply an icepack to the face in 15-minute increments to help control inflammation.

- Limit physical activity for one to two days after the procedure.

- When lying down, prop the head up on pillows to inhibit bleeding.

- Brush the teeth and tongue gently to reduce the risk of infection, being careful to avoid the extraction site.

- After 24 hours, rinse the mouth gently with a warm saltwater solution (1/2 teaspoon salt dissolved in 8 ounces of warm water) to keep the extraction area clean.

- Eat foods that are soft and cool—such as yogurt, pudding, or applesauce—for the first 24 hours, reintroducing solid foods gradually as the wound heals.

- Do not smoke, which can delay healing.

Risks of Tooth Extraction

Although tooth extraction is generally viewed as a very safe procedure, there are a few risks associated with it. Some of the complications the patient may experience after having a tooth pulled include the following:

- infection of the extraction site

- accidental damage to nearby teeth or fillings

- fracture of the jaw

- puncture of the sinus cavity

- injury to the inferior alveolar nerve in the jaw, causing temporary or permanent numbness of the chin and lower lip

- dry socket, a painful condition in which the blood clot in the socket breaks off, exposing the underlying bone to air and food

Some pain, discomfort, swelling, and soreness of the jaw is normal after a tooth extraction. Patients are advised to seek medical attention, however, if they experience the following symptoms:

- severe pain or bleeding that continues for more than 4 hours after the procedure

- redness, oozing, or excessive discharge that occurs after the first 24 hours

- swelling that becomes worse over time rather than better

- fever, chills, or other signs of infection

- trouble swallowing

- nausea or vomiting

- pain in the extraction site that begins 3 days after the procedure, which may indicate dry socket

Most people who have a tooth pulled will fully recover within one to two weeks, although it may take several months for new bone and gum tissue to fill the gap where the tooth used to be. In many cases, the dentist may recommend a second procedure to replace the missing tooth with an implant, bridge, or denture.

References

1. "Pulling a Tooth." WebMD, 2014.

2. "Tooth Extraction," Colgate Oral Care Center, May 2, 2014.

Chapter 19

Dentures

Chapter Contents

Section 19.1

What Are Dentures?

"What Are Dentures?" © 2017 Omnigraphics.
Reviewed September 2016.

Dentures, also called false teeth, are prosthetic devices that replace two or more natural teeth that have been lost as a result of decay, periodontal disease, or developmental defects. They are held in place by the hard and soft tissues of the mouth and can, to a large extent, take over the functions of natural teeth, such as chewing and speech. In addition to functional benefits, dentures also help maintain facial structure and improve appearance.

The Process

Dentures are made in commercial laboratories by technicians called denturists. Today, manydentures are made from acrylic resins and have better functionality and aesthetic appeal than their forerunners. They are very resilient and generally have a life of about eight years. Porcelain may also be used, but this material is not generally recommended for some applications, as it can wear away the natural teeth that comein contact with them. The teeth in dentures are mounted on a saddle-shaped plastic or metal frame whose form is designed to conform to the user's gums and palate. Plastic frames are becoming more common, because they are highly wear-resistant and can easily be reshaped at the dentist's office.

The manufacturing process begins with the creation of adiagnostic cast. This involves making a preliminary wax impression of the patient's maxillary and mandibular arches (upper and lower sets of dentition). The preliminary cast is adjusted by applying pressure to the soft tissues to simulate a biting effect. This helps ensure proper-alignment of the dentures and gums. The preliminary cast is used as a template for the permanent cast, which is made of gypsum. Acrylic resin is filled in the final mold to manufacture the denture. The packed mold is then heated to enable the resin to harden. Finally, the hardened acrylic denture is removed by breaking the mold.

Types of Dentures

Depending on whether they replace all or some of the teeth, dentures are classified as full or partial. A full denture replaces the complete set of teeth and requires the removal of any remaining natural teeth prior to its placement. The denture is typically not fixed immediately following tooth removal, as the gums and jawbones take a while to heal and reshape. The dentist may, in fact, wait several months after tooth removal to order a full denture. This helps avoid the need for alterations or relining of the denture to accommodate structural changes in the gums and bones, a process which inevitably follows tooth removal.

A partial denture, on the other hand, is designed to replace one, or a few, missing teeth. It is usually anchored to the natural teeth using metal clasps and can be easily removed. The clips may occasionally be made from material that closely resembles gum or tooth, although this type is generally not as strong as those made from metal.

Dentures, whether full or partial, may be permanent or removable. Removable dentures depend on the underlying bone for support and are low in cost and less invasive to fit. In many cases, however, removable dentures mightnot be the ideal solution, since bone loss may result in the lack of a suitable anchoring point. Permanent dentures may be the only option in such cases. This type of denture is permanently fixed in the mouth and is supported by dental implants. More invasive and more expensive than removable dentures, permanent dentures replace both visible structures and the root structures of the teeth.

Disadvantage of Dentures

Although dentures have helped many people regain the ability to eat normally, enunciate better, enhance their appearance, and boost their self-esteem, they are not without problems. While some of the issues associated with dentures may subside after a break-in period, during which the patient becomes accustomed to the prosthesis, others may persist and often require additional visits to the dentist or orthodontist.

Common Problems with Dentures

Before considering being fitted with dentures, it is important to be aware of some of the problems associated with them, including:

Awkwardness

One of the most common issues experienced by denture-wearers is getting used to having a foreign object in their mouths. And the dentures may slip out frequently. When this happens, especially with the lower denture, the user will in time learn to bite down softly and push the denture back into position. Pronunciation of certain sounds may also take some practice. But, usually, these issues tend to lessen after a brief period of adjustment.

Irritation

Pain, swelling, and increased salivation are other common problems following denture placement. However, these issues usually subside as healing takes place and the wearer adapts to the dentures. The dentist may recommend a special adhesive to help keep the denture in place, however it's best not to overuse denture adhesives and to avoid those containing zinc. If pain and irritation persist, the dentist may recommend pain-relieving gels, as well as antiseptics to prevent possible infection.

Difficulty Chewing

Chewing feels different with dentures, and this may take some getting used to. Unlike natural teeth, prostheses lack nerve sensations, and the wearer may not become aware of food textures and changes in temperature. While dentures help you eat most foods, there are some sticky or crunchy foods that pose problems for the denture wearer. For example, nut butters and crunchy fruits and vegetables may not be denture-friendly, and you may need to substitute these with non-sticky protein-rich spreads, cooked vegetables, stewed fruit, or smoothies.

Resorption

Bone resorption is a process that normally accompanies tooth removal. When there are no teeth to support, the bony ridges that once held the natural teeth begin to reduce in mass and density. As the body recognizes the loss of function in the supporting bones, the nutrients that normally aid bone growth are rerouted elsewhere. This resorption can be accelerated as the dentures exert pressure on the gums and underlying bony tissues. As a result, dentures may begin to lose their fit after some time and might need to be remodeled or relined on occasion.

Care and Hygiene

Caring for your dentures is as important as caring for your natural teeth. Your dentist or orthodontist will recommend how long you need to wear your dentures and how to care for them properly. Clean dentures contribute to good oral health and hygiene and can prevent problems such as gum disease, bad breath, and oral infections.

Some tips for denture care include:

- Soak dentures overnight in warm water and cleansing solution to prevent drying or warping.

- Brush dentures at least once per day, ideally after every meal, to remove food remnants and prevent the buildup of tartar.

- Brush with a soft-bristled brush and soapy water or a commercial denture cleaner.

- Never use house-cleaning liquids or abrasive chemicals.

- Massage and clean the roof of the mouth, tongue, and gums each day before putting on your dentures.

- Never sleep with your dentures in place.

References

1. "Dental Health and Dentures," WebMD, 2005–2016.

2. Horne, Steven B., DDS. "Dentures," MedicineNet, Inc., 2016.

3. "Denture," MadeHow.com, 2016.

Section 19.2

Denture Adhesives

This section includes text excerpted from "Denture Adhesives," U.S. Food and Drug Administration (FDA), June 4, 2014.

Denture adhesives are pastes, powders or adhesive pads that may be placed in/on dentures to help them stay in place. Sometimes denture adhesives contain zinc to enhance adhesion.

In most cases, properly fitted and maintained dentures should not require the use of denture adhesives. Over time, shrinkage in the bone structure in the mouth causes dentures to gradually become loose. When this occurs, the dentures should be relined or new dentures made that fit the mouth properly. Denture adhesives fill gaps caused by shrinking bone and give temporary relief from loosening dentures.

Zinc and Potential Risk

Zinc is a mineral that is an essential ingredient for good health. It is found in protein-rich foods such as shellfish, beef, chicken and nuts, as well as in some dietary supplements.

However, an excess of zinc in the body can lead to health problems such as nerve damage, especially in the hands and feet. This damage appears slowly, over an extended period of time. Overuse of zinc-containing denture adhesives, especially when combined with dietary supplements that contain zinc and other sources of zinc, can contribute to an excess of zinc in your body.

Advice for Denture Wearers

Denture wearers may have difficulty determining the proper amount of denture adhesive to use if the instructions are not clear. If a denture wearer is uncertain about how much to use, he or she should contact a dental health professional to help determine the correct amount.

Denture wearers should know that a large amount of denture adhesive will not necessarily address problems with ill-fitting dentures, and prolonged use of ill-fitting dentures may lead to an increase in bone loss.

The U.S. Food and Drug Administration (FDA) recommends that consumers of denture adhesive products:

- Follow the instructions provided with the denture adhesive. If the product does not come with instructions or the instructions are unclear, consult with a dental professional.

- **Do not use more adhesive than recommended.**

- Understand that some denture adhesives contain zinc, and that although they are safe to use in moderation as directed, if over-used, they could contribute to harmful effects if over-used.

- Know that manufacturers may not always list their product ingredients.

- Know that there are zinc-free denture adhesives products.

- Stop using the denture adhesive and consult your physician if you experience symptoms such as numbness or tingling sensations in the extremities.

- Start with a small amount of adhesive—if the adhesive oozes off the denture into your mouth, you are likely using too much adhesive.

- Know that a 2.4-ounce tube of denture adhesive used by a consumer with upper and lower dentures should last seven to eight weeks.

- Track how much denture adhesive you use by marking on a calendar when you started a new tube, and when the tube is empty.

- Consider speaking to your dentist to see that your dentures fit properly. Dentures can become ill-fitting as a person's gums change over time.

Reports of Problems

The U.S. Food and Drug Administration (FDA) is aware of case reports in the medical literature linking negative reactions such as nerve damage, numbness or tingling sensations from denture adhesives that contain zinc to chronic overuse of the products.

The FDA has not found conclusive evidence that these problems result from using zinc-containing denture adhesive as instructed in the product labeling.

To help address the potential risk that overuse of zinc-containing denture adhesives may pose, the FDA asked makers of zinc-containing denture adhesives to consider:

- Including directions that will prevent overuse if zinc is an ingredient. (Some companies include graphics of the amount of adhesive to use or the amount of time that a tube should last under correct usage.)

- Modifying the labeling to specify that the product contains zinc as an ingredient, if appropriate and consider replacing zinc with an ingredient that presents less health risks in situations of overuse.

Part Three

Dental Care for Infants and Children

Chapter 20

Oral Health for Infants

Chapter Contents

Section 20.1

A Healthy Mouth for Your Baby

This section includes text excerpted from "A Healthy Mouth for Your Baby," National Institute of Dental and Craniofacial Research (NIDCR), August 24, 2015.

Healthy teeth are important—even baby teeth. Children need healthy teeth to help them chew and to speak clearly. And baby teeth hold space for adult teeth. This section can help you keep your baby's mouth healthy and give him a healthy start!

Protect Your Baby's Teeth with Fluoride

Fluoride (said like floor-eyed) protects teeth from tooth decay. It can even heal early decay. Fluoride is in the drinking water of many towns and cities. Ask a dentist or doctor if your water has fluoride in it. If it doesn't, ask about other kinds of fluoride (such as fluoride varnish or drops) that can help keep your baby's teeth healthy.

Check and Clean Your Baby's Teeth

CHECK your baby's teeth.

Healthy teeth should be all one color. If you see spots or stains on the teeth, take your baby to a dentist.

CLEAN your baby's teeth.

Clean them as soon as they come in with a clean, soft cloth or a baby's toothbrush. Clean the teeth at least once a day. It's best to clean them right before bedtime.

At about age 2 (or sooner if a dentist or doctor suggests it) you should start putting fluoride toothpaste on your child's toothbrush. Use only a pea-sized drop of toothpaste.

Young children cannot get their teeth clean by themselves. Until they are 7 or 8 years old, you will need to help them brush. Try brushing their teeth first and then letting them finish.

Feed Your Baby Healthy Food

- Choose foods without a lot of sugar in them.

- Give your child fruits and vegetables for snacks.

- Save cookies and other treats for special occasions.

Don't Put Your Baby to Bed with a Bottle

Milk, formula, juice, and other drinks such as soda all have sugar in them. If sugary liquids stay on your baby's teeth too long, it can lead to tooth decay. (And decayed teeth can cause pain for your baby.)

What's one of the most important things you can do to keep your baby from getting cavities?

Avoid putting him to bed with a bottle—at night or at nap time. (If you do put your baby to bed with a bottle, fill it only with water.)

Here are some other things you can do:

- Between feedings, don't give your baby a bottle or sippy cup filled with sweet drinks to carry around.

- Near his first birthday, teach your child to drink from an open cup.

- If your baby uses a pacifier, don't dip it in anything sweet like sugar or honey.

Take Your Child to the Dentist

Your child should have a dental visit by his first birthday. At this visit, the dentist will:

- Check your child's teeth.

- Show you the best way to clean your child's teeth.

- Talk to you about other things such as a healthy diet and fluoride that can keep your child's mouth healthy.

Section 20.2

Teething

This section includes text excerpted from "Brush Up on Oral Health," Early Childhood Learning and Knowledge Center (ECLKC), U.S. Department of Health and Human Services (HHS), April 2014.

Did You Know?

- By the time a child is three years old, he or she will have 20 primary (baby) teeth.

- Typically, the two bottom front teeth come in first, followed by the two top front teeth a few weeks later.

Head Start and Babies Who Are Teething

Teething happens when a baby's primary teeth come into the mouth. For some babies, teething is uncomfortable. **Head Start** staff, including home visitors, classroom teachers, and family service coordinators, can give guidance and support to parents whose babies are teething.

Teething Basics

Teething can start any time between ages 3 and 12 months. Most babies begin teething around age 6 months. As the primary teeth come into the mouth, babies might become cranky, drool more, not want to eat solid foods, have sore or swollen gums, and chew on things to ease the pressure from the tooth pushing through the gum.

Strategies for Parents Whose Babies Are Teething

- **Keep it safe:** Choose safe teething toys. Here are some ideas:
- Make sure liquid-filled teething toys are made of durable material that the baby can't chew a hole into.
  - Find teething toys that don't have loose pieces that could break off in a baby's mouth and cause choking.

- Don't put a teething toy, including chewbeads, a chew necklace, or a pacifier on a cord and hang it around a baby's neck or attach it to clothes. It could get tangled around the baby's neck and cause choking.

- **Clean it:** Many strategies for comforting a teething baby include putting something in the baby's mouth. Everything that goes in the mouth should be cleaned first to keep the baby healthy. Read the pacifier's or teething toy's package for directions on how to clean it. Some items are dishwasher safe and some are not.

- **Massage it:** Gently rub the baby's gums with a clean finger for about 2 minutes. Many babies find the pressure soothing. For babies who already have some teeth, be careful the baby doesn't bite you!

- **Cool it:** Cold helps ease the pain of sore gums. Give the baby a cool clean wet washcloth, spoon, pacifier, or teething ring to chew on. Teething rings can be put in the refrigerator but not the freezer. Chewing frozen teething rings can make a baby's cheeks or chin become bumpy and turn reddish-purple. Note: To prevent mouth injuries, do not let a baby walk while holding a spoon.

- **Freeze it:** Some frozen foods can help ease teething pain.

- **Don't use it:** Oral health and medical providers don't recommend using teething gels and liquids on babies' gums because they can cause serious health problems, including death. If nothing works to ease a baby's teething pain, encourage parents to ask their baby's physician or dentist for directions on how to use pain medicine safely.

Foods to Ease Teething Pain

Here's a delicious healthy snack that can be given to babies who are teething.

Ingredients

1 banana or plain bagel

Directions

1. If using a banana, peel it and cut into 6 thick pieces. If using a bagel, cut bagel halves into quarters.

2. Place the banana or bagel pieces on a cookie sheet, making sure they don't touch each other.

3. Put the sheet in the freezer for 20–30 minutes, or until the banana or bagel pieces are frozen.

4. Place the frozen banana or bagel pieces in a plastic freezer bag or container.

5. Squeeze the air out of the freezer bag (if using), mark the date on the bag or container, and put it in the freezer. Frozen bananas and bagel pieces can be stored for up to 4 months.

6. Comfort the teething baby with one frozen banana or bagel piece.

Bananas and bagels contain sugar that can cause tooth decay. Give these foods to a teething baby once in a while and not throughout the day. Offer the food while the baby is sitting in a high chair.

Section 20.3

Medicines for Teething Babies

This section includes text excerpted from "Do Teething Babies Need Medicine on Their Gums?" U.S. Food and Drug Administration (FDA), July 25, 2015.

Do Teething Babies Need Medicines?

There are more theories about teething and "treating" a baby's sore gums than there are teeth in a child's mouth. One thing doctors and other healthcare professionals agree on is that teething is a normal part of childhood that can be treated without prescription or over-the-counter (OTC) medications. Too often well-meaning parents, grandparents, and caregivers want to soothe a teething baby by rubbing numbing medications on the tot's gums, using potentially harmful drugs instead of safer, non-toxic alternatives.

That's why the U.S. Food and Drug Administration (FDA) is warning parents that prescription drugs such as viscous lidocaine are not safe for treating teething in infants or young children, and that they have hurt some children who used those products. FDA has previously recommended that parents and caregivers not use benzocaine products for children younger than two years, except under the advice and supervision of a healthcare professional. Benzocaine—which, like viscous lidocaine, is a local anesthetic—can be found in such OTC products as Anbesol, Hurricaine, Orajel, Baby Orajel, and Orabase.

The use of benzocaine gels and liquids for mouth and gum pain can lead to a rare but serious—and sometimes fatal—condition called methemoglobinemia, a disorder in which the amount of oxygen carried through the blood stream is greatly reduced. And children under two years old appear to be at particular risk.

Parents Have Safer Alternatives

On average, children get one new tooth every month from 6 months of age to about age 3, for a total of 20 "baby teeth." According to the American Academy of Pediatrics (AAP), occasional symptoms of teething include mild irritability, a low-level fever, drooling and an urge to chew on something hard. Because teething happens during a time of much change in a baby's life, it is often wrongly blamed for sleep disturbances, decreased appetite, congestion, coughing, vomiting, and diarrhea.

If your child's gums are swollen and tender,

- gently rub or massage the gums with your finger, and

- give your child a cool teething ring or a clean, wet, cool washcloth to chew on.

Chill the teething ring or washcloth in the refrigerator for a short time, making sure it's cool—not cold like an ice cube. If the object is too cold, it can hurt the gums and your child. The coolness soothes the gums by dulling the nerves, which transmit pain.

"The cool object acts like a very mild local anesthetic," says Hari Cheryl Sachs, M.D., a pediatrician at FDA. "This is a great relief for children for a short time."

Parents should supervise their children so they don't accidentally choke on the teething ring or wash cloth.

Avoid Local Anesthetics

For teething, avoid local anesthetics such as viscous lidocaine or benzocaine-containing teething products except under the advice and supervision of a healthcare professional.

Viscous lidocaine is a prescription medication, a local anesthetic in a gel-like syrup. Doctors may prescribe it for chemotherapy patients (children and adults) who are unable to eat because of mouth ulcers that can occur with chemotherapy. Dentists may use it to reduce the gag reflex in children during dental X-rays and impressions.

Parents may have viscous lidocaine on hand if it has been prescribed to treat another family member for pain relief from conditions such as mouth or throat ulcers. But it should never be used to comfort a teething baby.

The Institute for Safe Medication Practices (ISMP)—a nonprofit organization dedicated to preventing medication errors—has received reports of teething babies suffering overdoses of viscous lidocaine. Symptoms include jitteriness, confusion, vision problems, vomiting, falling asleep too easily, shaking, and seizures.

The drug also "can make swallowing difficult and can increase the risk of choking or breathing in food. It can lead to drug toxicity and affect the heart and nervous system," says Michael R. Cohen, RPh, MS, ISMP president.

Parents have been known to repeatedly apply viscous lidocaine if a baby keeps fussing, says Cohen. They have also been known to put liquid gel forms of a topical anesthetic into a baby's formula or even soak a pacifier or a cloth in it, then put that in their baby's mouth. How much the baby gets is not measured, so it may be too much, he says. For all these reasons, FDA recommends viscous lidocaine not be used to treat the pain associated with teething.

"Teething is a normal phenomenon; all babies teethe," says Ethan Hausman, M.D., a pediatrician and pathologist at FDA. "FDA does not recommend any sort of drug, herbal or homeopathic medication or therapy for teething in children."

Section 20.4

Benzocaine and Teething

This section includes text excerpted from "Benzocaine and Babies: Not a Good Mix," U.S. Food and Drug Administration (FDA), April 7, 2016.

Reaching Out for Pain Remedies

When a baby is teething, many a mom or dad reaches for a pain remedy containing benzocaine to help soothe sore gums. Benzocaine is a local anesthetic and can be found in such over-the-counter (OTC) products as Anbesol, Hurricane, Orajel, Baby Orajel, and Orabase. But the use of benzocaine gels and liquids for mouth and gum pain can lead to a rare but serious—and sometimes fatal—condition called methemoglobinemia, a disorder in which the amount of oxygen carried through the blood stream is greatly reduced. In the most severe cases, says U.S. Food and Drug Administration (FDA) pharmacist Mary Ghods, R.Ph., methemoglobinemia can result in death. And children under 2 years old appear to be at particular risk.

Since the FDA first warned about potential dangers in 2006, the agency has received 29 reports of benzocaine gel-related cases of methemoglobinemia. Nineteen of those cases occurred in children, and 15 of the 19 cases occurred in children under 2 years of age, says FDA pharmacist Kellie Taylor, Pharm.D., MPH.

The agency repeated the warning in April 2011 and remains particularly concerned about the use of OTC benzocaine products in children for relief of pain from teething, says Taylor. This concern is fueled by the serious potential outcomes and the difficulty parents may have recognizing the signs and symptoms of methemoglobinemia when using these products at home. These symptoms may not always be evident or attributed to the condition.

For these reasons, U.S. Food and Drug Administration (FDA) recommends that parents and caregivers not use benzocaine products for children younger than 2 years, except under the advice and supervision of a healthcare professional.

Danger Signs

Symptoms of methemoglobinemia include:

- pale, gray, or blue-colored skin, lips and nail beds
- shortness of breath
- fatigue
- confusion
- headache
- light-headedness
- rapid heart rate

"Symptoms can occur within minutes to hours after benzocaine use," Ghods says. "They can occur after using the drug for the first time, as well as after several uses."

If your child has any of these symptoms after using benzocaine, she adds, stop using the product and seek medical help immediately by calling 911

Methemoglobinemia caused by benzocaine may require treatment with medications and admission to a hospital. Serious cases should be treated right away. If left untreated or if treatment is delayed, methemoglobinemia may cause permanent injury to the brain and body tissues, and even death, from the insufficient amount of oxygen in the blood.

Teething: What's a Parent to Do?

As for the crying baby, what's a mom or dad to do? The American Academy of Pediatrics (AAP) offers some alternatives for treating teething pain:

- Give the child a teething ring chilled in the refrigerator.
- Gently rub or massage the child's gums with your finger.

If these remedies don't provide relief, contact your healthcare professional for advice on other treatments.

Adults Can Be Affected Too

Benzocaine products—which are sold as gels, liquids, sprays, and lozenges—are also widely used by adults. Doctors and dentists often use sprays containing benzocaine to numb the mucous membranes of the mouth and throat during such procedures as transesophageal echocardiograms, endoscopy, intubation, and feeding tube replacements.

Even though children are more at risk, it's still a good idea to talk to your healthcare professional about using benzocaine, especially if you have heart disease; are a smoker; or have breathing problems such as asthma, bronchitis or emphysema.

FDA advises consumers to:

- store any products containing benzocaine out of the reach of children.

- use benzocaine gels and liquids sparingly and only when needed. Do not use them more than 4 times a day.

- read the label to see if benzocaine is an active ingredient when buying OTC products. Labels on OTC products containing benzocaine are not currently required to carry warnings about the risk of methemoglobinemia. If you have any concerns, talk to your healthcare professional before using them.

Chapter 21

Routine Care for Children's Teeth

Chapter Contents

Section 21.1

Primary Teeth

This section includes text excerpted from "Brush Up on Oral Health," Early Childhood Learning and Knowledge Center (ECLKC), U.S. Department of Health and Human Services (HHS), June 2015.

Did You Know?

- By the time a child is 2 to 3 years old, she or he usually has all 20 primary teeth.

- A child generally does not lose his or her last primary tooth until age 10 to 12.

Primary (Baby) Teeth

Many parents believe that primary (baby) teeth are less important than permanent teeth because primary teeth are going to "fall out anyway." However, primary teeth are key to a child's growth and development. **Head Start** staff play a vital role in helping parents better understand the importance primary teeth.

This issue talks about why primary teeth are important and offers information about primary teeth that **Head Start** staff can share with parents. A recipe for a healthy snack that can be made in the **Head Start** classroom or at home is also included.

Facts about Primary Teeth

- **Primary teeth are important.** Primary teeth are key to young children's health and development in five very important ways. These include:

  1. **Maintaining good health.** The health of primary teeth affects children's overall health and well-being. Untreated tooth decay in primary teeth can lead to infections that can cause fever and discomfort. Infection from an abscessed primary tooth can spread to other areas in the head and neck and lead to pain, severe swelling, and, in rare cases, death. Using

antibiotics to treat dental infections may work temporarily. However, the infection will always return if the decay is not treated.

2. **Maintaining good nutrition with proper chewing.** To grow and be strong, children need to eat healthy food every day. Children with decay in their primary teeth are less likely to eat crunchy foods, such as fresh fruits and vegetables, that promote good nutrition and a healthy weight. These children are also at risk for developing dietary deficiencies and becoming malnourished.

3. **Helping with development of speech.** Missing teeth can interfere with the development a young child's speech. Young children with missing teeth have difficulty making "th," "la," and other sounds. This can make it hard for others to understand the child. In some cases the child may need speech therapy to change speech patterns he or she developed because of missing teeth.

4. **Maintaining space for permanent teeth.** Primary teeth hold space for permanent teeth developing underneath them in the jaw. If primary teeth are lost too early, teeth in the mouth move into the space and block the space for the incoming permanent teeth. This can cause crowding of the permanent teeth.

5. **Promoting self-esteem and confidence.** Young children can be quick to point out other children with teeth that are decayed, chipped, or discolored. Children with tooth decay tend to avoid smiling, cover their mouth with their hands when they speak, or minimize interaction with others. A healthy smile gives children the self-confidence they need to have positive social experiences.

• **Tooth decay in primary teeth matters.** Children with pain from tooth decay do more poorly in school and have more behavior problems. Untreated tooth decay can also spread from one tooth to another. Children with severe tooth decay may need to be put to sleep and receive treatment in a hospital operating room.

• **Brushing primary teeth with fluoride toothpaste every day promotes good oral health.** Parents should begin brushing a baby's teeth with a smear (rice-sized amount) of fluoride toothpaste twice a day as soon as the first tooth appears in the mouth. Making this a daily habit lowers the amount of bacteria in the mouth, helps prevent tooth decay, and starts a lifetime of good oral health habits.

- **Having a dental visit by age one promotes good oral health.** The American Academy of Pediatric Dentistry (AAPD) recommends that a child have his or her first dental visit by age one. A young child's dental visit is simple and quick. The oral health professional examines the child's mouth, identifies potential problems, and explains what changes to expect in the child's mouth as he or she develops and grows. The oral health professional also shows parents how to take care of their child's teeth and applies fluoride varnish to the child's teeth.

Section 21.2

Keeping Children's Teeth Healthy

This section includes text excerpted from "Healthy Teeth for Baby and Beyond," *NIH News in Health*, National nstitutes of Health (NIH), February 2013.

Teeth help us bite, chew, speak clearly and smile. Even babies need healthy teeth. But teeth need proper care to stay healthy and strong. It's never too early to start kids on the path to good dental health.

Diet plays a role in tooth decay. When you eat or drink foods that contain sugar, germs in your mouth use the sugar to make acids. Over time, the acids can cause tooth decay, or **cavities.** Tooth decay is the most common chronic disease in children, yet it's mostly preventable.

Although baby teeth eventually fall out, it's still important to take care of them. They play an important role in the mouth. "Baby teeth of course are used to chew, but they also guide growth of the jaw bones and create room for permanent teeth to come in," says Dr. Tim Iafolla, a dental health expert at National Institutes of Health (NIH).

"Start cleaning your baby's mouth even before the first teeth come in, so your baby gets used to having his or her mouth cleaned. Wipe gums with a clean, soft cloth," says Iafolla. "When teeth come in, clean them twice a day with a cloth or soft brush, as they are immediately susceptible to tooth decay and **plaque.**"

One important way to protect baby teeth is not putting your baby to bed with a bottle. Milk, formula and juice all contain sugar. If sugary liquids stay on your baby's teeth too long, it can lead to tooth decay. If you give your baby a bottle to keep at bedtime or to carry around between feedings, fill it only with water.

"It's important to catch tooth decay early," Iafolla says. He recommends bringing your child to the dentist by age 1. The dentist can tell if teeth are coming in properly, detect early signs of decay, and give you tips on caring for your child's teeth.

The best defense against tooth decay is fluoride, a mineral found in most tap water. If your water doesn't have fluoride, ask a dentist about fluoride drops, gel or varnish.

Start using fluoride toothpaste at about age 2. Iafolla recommends using just a pea-sized drop of fluoridated toothpaste until kids have the ability to spit and rinse. Young kids need help brushing their teeth properly. Try brushing their teeth first and letting them finish. You might try using a timer or a favorite song so your child learns to brush for 2 minutes. Continue to supervise brushing until your child is 7 or 8 years old. Have kids brush their teeth at least twice daily in the morning, at bedtime, and preferably after meals. Offer healthy foods and snacks to children. If kids do eat sugary or sticky foods, they should brush their teeth afterward. Also ask your child's dentist about sealants—a simple, pain-free way to prevent tooth decay. These thin plastic coatings are painted on the chewing surfaces of permanent back teeth. They quickly harden to form a protective shield against germs and food. If a small cavity is accidentally covered by a sealant, the decay won't spread because germs trapped inside are sealed off from their food supply.

By following these tips, you can help your children develop healthy dental habits for life.

Section 21.3

Brushing Your Child's Teeth

This section includes text excerpted from "Brush Up on Oral Health,"
Early Childhood Learning and Knowledge Center (ECLKC), U.S.
Department of Health and Human Services (HHS), December 2013.

Did You Know?

Young children don't have the fine motor skills until around age
7 or 8 (when they can tie their shoelaces without help) to brush their
teeth well. But, to help young children form healthy habits, it's good
for them to brush their teeth with an adult supervising. An adult
should thoroughly brush the child's teeth at least once a day (in the
morning or before bed).

Helping Children Brush Their Teeth

Young children, including those with disabilities, often want to do
things "all by myself." This can make brushing a child's teeth challenging. To help children keep their mouths healthy, start brushing
as soon as the first tooth appears in the infant's mouth. It's important
for an adult to supervise brushing and help brush the child's teeth.

Toothbrushing Challenges for Children

Young children, especially those with a physical, emotional, behavioral, intellectual, or communication disability, don't have the fine
motor skills they need to clean their teeth well. Some things to watch
for when helping children brush:

- **Holding the toothbrush.** Can the child hold the toothbrush
  firmly and bring it to his or her mouth? Is the handle too thin? Is
  the child able to close his or her hand over the handle?

- **Brushing and having teeth brushed.** Can the child keep his
  or her mouth open during brushing? Does the child gag when a

toothbrush is in his or her mouth? Can the child hold still when an adult is helping brush the child's teeth? Can the child place and move the toothbrush over all of the tooth surfaces when brushing?

- **Using toothpaste.** Does the child dislike some toothpaste flavors? Does the child dislike how the toothpaste feels in his or her mouth? Is the child able to spit toothpaste out?

- **Brushing safely.** Can the child brush his or her teeth without hurting the mouth, tongue or gums?

It is important to know what is working and not working well in brushing a child's teeth. Then Head Start staff or parents can reinforce good habits and help address any problems.

Toothbrushing Tips: What Parents Can Do

Each child has different skills and needs that can guide Head Start staff and parents in helping him or her brush. Here are some tips to help young children practice brushing and to make it a good experience:

- **Choosing a toothbrush.** Use a soft-bristled toothbrush designed for brushing an infant's or child's teeth.

- **Holding a toothbrush.** If the child has trouble holding a toothbrush, try making the handle thicker by putting it inside a tennis ball. The toothbrush handle can also be strapped to the child's hand with a wide rubber band, a hair band, or Velcro. Toothbrushes with thick handles can also be found in retail and discount stores.

- **Teaching the child how to brush.** Break the process into small steps that the child can understand and practice. Ask a dentist, dental hygienist, occupational therapist, or early childhood specialist for help, if needed. Another way is to place a hand over the child's hand to guide the toothbrush as the child brushes. In Head Start programs, a staff person or volunteer can be assigned to a child who needs extra help.

- **Using toothpaste with fluoride.** Use toothpaste with fluoride that the child likes and that feels good in his or her mouth. An adult should always place toothpaste on the toothbrush. For children under age 2, use a small smear of toothpaste. For children ages 2–5, use a pea-size amount of toothpaste. If a child cannot spit, have the child tilt his or her mouth down so that the toothpaste can dribble out into the sink, a cup, or a washcloth.

• **Positioning the child.** There are many ways a child can be positioned to make the child feel comfortable and allow an adult to brush his or her teeth.

• **Keeping the child engaged in brushing.** Use a timer, a short song, or counting as a game to encourage brushing for 2 minutes.

Section 21.4

Calcium Is Critical for Tooth Development

This section includes text excerpted from "Healthy Teeth for Baby and Beyond," Eunice Kennedy Shriver National Institute of Child Health and Human Development (NICHD), September 2005. Reviewed September 2016.

Building Strong Bones in the Tween and Teen Years Makes a Lifelong Difference

Having a calcium-rich diet when you're young makes a big difference in health, now and later. By getting the calcium they need now, tweens and teens will:

• **Strengthen bones now.** Our bodies continually remove and replace small amounts of calcium from our bones. If more calcium is removed than is replaced, bones will become weaker and have a greater chance of breaking. Some researchers suspect that the rise in forearm fractures in children is due to decreased bone mass, which may result because children are drinking less milk and more soda and are getting less physical activity.

• **Help prevent osteoporosis later in life.** Osteoporosis is a condition that makes bones weak so they break more easily. Although the effects of osteoporosis might not show up until adulthood, tweens and teens can help prevent it by building strong bones when they are young.

Calcium Keeps Mouths Healthy Too

Calcium is important for a healthy mouth too. Even before they come in, baby teeth and adult teeth need calcium to develop fully. And after the teeth are in, calcium may also help protect them against decay. Calcium makes jawbones strong and healthy too! Besides making sure your children get enough calcium, there are other things you can do to keep their teeth healthy:

- Make sure your children brush with a fluoride toothpaste. Fluoride protects teeth from decay and helps heal early decay.

- Ask your child's dental care or healthcare provider if there is fluoride in your town or city's drinking water. If there is not, ask about fluoride tablets or drops for your child.

- Ask your child's dental care provider about proper brushing and flossing techniques and other ways your tween or teen can make sure teeth stay healthy.

Here's Where Tweens and Teens Can Get the Calcium They Need

These foods help tweens and teens reach the 1,300 mg of calcium they need every day.

Table 21.1. Calcium-Rich Foods

Calcium-Rich Foods			
Food	**Serving Size**	**Calories**	**Amount of Calcium**
Plain yogurt, fat-free	1 cup	127	452 mg
Orange juice with added calcium	8 fluid ounces (1 cup)	120	350 mg
Fruit yogurt, low-fat	1 cup	232	345 mg
Ricotta cheese, part skim	1/2 cup	170	334 mg
American cheese, low-fat and fat-free	2 ounces (about 3 slices)	(Calories vary)	312 mg
Milk (fat-free, low-fat, whole, or lactose-free)	8 fluid ounces (1 cup)	(Calories vary)	300 mg
Soybeans, cooked	1 cup	175	298 mg

Table 21.1. Continued

Calcium-Rich Foods			
Food	Serving Size	Calories	Amount of Calcium
Cheddar cheese, low-fat and fat-free	1/2 cup	(Calories vary)	204 mg
Tofu, firm, with added calcium sulfate	1/2 cup	97	204 mg
Soy beverage with added calcium	8 fluid ounces (1 cup)	100–130	200–300 mg
Cheese pizza	1 slice	240	200 mg

There are lots of different calcium-rich foods to choose from, making it easy for tweens and teens to get the calcium they need every day. For example, just 1 cup of yogurt gives young people 25 percent of their daily calcium requirement. Low-fat and fat-free milk and milk products, such as low-fat or fat-free cheese and yogurt, are also excellent sources of calcium. Remember: tweens and teens can get most of their daily calcium from 3 cups of low-fat or fat-free milk (900 mg of calcium), but they also need additional servings of calcium rich foods to get the 1,300 mg of calcium necessary. Food labels can tell you how much calcium is in one serving of food. Look at the % Daily Value (% DV) next to the calcium number on the food label.

Here are some other foods young people can eat to boost their calcium intake.

Table 21.2. Other Foods with Calcium

Other Foods with Calcium			
Food	Serving Size	Calories	Amount of Calcium
Broccoli, raw	1 medium stalk	106	180 mg
Broccoli, cooked	1 cup	52	94 mg
Bok choy, boiled	1 cup	20	158 mg
Spinach, cooked from frozen	1/2 cup	27	139 mg
Frozen yogurt, softserve vanilla	1/2 cup	114	103 mg
Macaroni and cheese	1 cup	230	100 mg
Almonds	1 ounce (22 nuts)	169	75 mg
Tortilla, flour (7–8 inches)	1 tortilla	150	58 mg
Tortilla, corn (6 inches)	1 tortilla	53	42 mg

"But My Child Doesn't Like the Taste of Milk!"

Even if your tweens or teens don't like the taste of plain milk, there are still plenty of ways to get calcium in the diet:

- Try a flavored low-fat or fat-free milk, such as chocolate, vanilla or strawberry. Flavored milk has just as much calcium as plain.

- Serve foods that go with milk, such as fruit bars and fig bars.

- Drink milk or yogurt smoothies for breakfast or a snack. You can make these at home or try one of the ready-made versions now available at many grocery stores.

- Keep portable, calcium-rich foods on hand for snacks on the run, such as low-fat or fat-free string cheese or individual pudding cups with calcium added.

- In moderation, low-fat or fat-free ice cream and frozen yogurt are calcium-rich treats.

- Serve non-milk sources of calcium, such as calcium-fortified soy beverages or orange juice with added calcium.

- Try a spinach salad or have fresh or cooked broccoli.

Is One Type of Milk Better than the Other?

Today, tweens, and teens have more milk choices than ever before. Most types of milk have approximately 300 mg of calcium per 8 fluid ounces (1 cup)—about 25 percent of the calcium that children and teenagers need every day. The best choices are low-fat or fat-free milk and milk products. Because these items contain little or no fat, it's easy to get enough calcium without adding extra fat to the diet. Chocolate and other flavored milks have just as much calcium as plain milk, so it is fine for young people to drink these options if they prefer the taste. Remember to choose low-fat or fat-free.

Put Calcium on the Menu at Every Meal

One way to make it easier for tweens and teens to get enough calcium is to serve low-fat or fat-free milk and other calcium-rich foods throughout the day. Putting calcium-rich foods on your family's menu at each meal is also a great way to make sure that everyone gets the calcium they need. When milk is the main beverage in the home, tweens and teens will choose it more often.

Table 21.3. Ideas for calcium-rich meals and snacks

Breakfast	Lunch	Snack	Dinner
• Pour low-fat or fat-free milk over your breakfast cereal.	• Add low-fat or fat-free cheese to a sandwich.	• Make a smoothie with fruit, ice, and low-fat or fat-free milk.	• Make a salad with dark green, leafy vegetables.
• Have a cup of low-fat or fat-free yogurt.	• Have a glass of low-fat or fat-free milk instead of soda.	• Try flavored low-fat or fat-free milk like chocolate or strawberry.	• Serve broccoli or cooked, dry beans as a side dish.
• Drink a glass of orange juice with added calcium.	• Have a pizza or macaroni and cheese.	• Have a low-fat or fat-free frozen yogurt.	• Top salads, soups, and stews with low-fat or fat-free shredded cheese.
• Add low-fat or fat-free milk instead of water to oatmeal and hot cereal.	• Add low-fat or fat-free milk instead of water to tomato soup.	• Try some pudding made with low-fat or fat-free milk.	• Toss tofu with added calcium to stir fry and other dishes.
		• Dip fruits and vegetables into low-fat or fat-free yogurt.	
		• Have some low-fat or fat-free string cheese.	

Chapter 22

Fluoride Consumption during Tooth Development

Chapter Contents

Section 22.1

Dental Fluorosis

This section includes text excerpted from "Community Water Fluoridation," Centers for Disease Control and Prevention (CDC), April 1, 2016.

The proper amount of fluoride helps prevent and control tooth decay in children and adults. Fluoride works both while the teeth are developing and every day after the teeth have emerged through the gums. Fluoride consumed during tooth development can also result in a range of visible changes to the enamel surface of the tooth. These changes have been broadly termed dental fluorosis.

What Is Dental Fluorosis?

Dental fluorosis is a condition that causes changes in the appearance of tooth enamel. It may result when children regularly consume fluoride during the teeth-forming years, age 8 and younger. Most dental fluorosis in the United States is very mild to mild, appearing as white spots on the tooth surface that may be barely noticeable and do not affect dental function. Moderate and severe forms of dental fluorosis, which are far less common, cause more extensive enamel changes. In the rare, severe form, pits may form in the teeth. The severe form hardly ever occurs in communities where the level of fluoride in water is less than 2 milligrams per liter.

What Causes Dental Fluorosis?

Dental fluorosis is caused by taking in too much fluoride over a long period when the teeth are forming under the gums. Only children aged 8 years and younger are at risk because this is when permanent teeth are developing; children older than 8 years, adolescents, and adults cannot develop dental fluorosis. The severity of the condition depends on the dose (how much), duration (how long), and timing (when consumed) of fluoride intake.

Increases in the occurrence of mostly mild dental fluorosis were recognized as more sources of fluoride became available to prevent tooth decay. These sources include drinking water with fluoride, fluoride toothpaste—especially if swallowed by young children—and dietary prescription supplements in tablets or drops (particularly if prescribed to children already drinking fluoridated water).

What Does Dental Fluorosis Look Like?

- Very mild and mild forms of dental fluorosis—teeth have scattered white flecks, occasional white spots, frosty edges, or fine, lacy chalk-like lines. These changes are barely noticeable and difficult to see except by a dental healthcare professional.

- Moderate and severe forms of dental fluorosis—teeth have larger white spots and, in the rare, severe form, rough, pitted surfaces.

What Can Parents and Caregivers Do to Reduce the Occurrence of Dental Fluorosis?

Know the Fluoride Concentration of Your Drinking Water

You should know the fluoride concentration in your primary source of drinking water, especially if you have young children. This information should help with decisions about using other fluoride products, particularly fluoride tablets or drops that your physician or dentist may prescribe for your young child. Fluoride tablets or drops should not be used at all if your drinking water has the recommended fluoride concentration of 0.7 mg/L or higher.

If you live in a state that participates in Centers for Disease Control and Prevention (CDC)'s My Water's Fluoride, you can find out your water system's fluoridation status online. If you are on a public water system, you can call the water utility company and request a copy of the utility's most recent Consumer Confidence Report.

For very young children, less than 2 years old:

Do not use fluoride toothpaste unless advised to do so by your doctor or dentist. You should clean your child's teeth as soon as the first tooth appears by brushing without toothpaste with a small, soft-bristled toothbrush and plain water.

For children aged 2 to 6 years:

Apply no more than a pea-sized amount of fluoride toothpaste to the brush and supervise their tooth brushing, encouraging the child to spit out the toothpaste rather than swallow it. Until about age 6, children have poor control of their swallowing reflex and frequently swallow most of the toothpaste placed on their brush.

Use an alternative source of water for children aged 8 years and younger if your primary drinking water contains greater than 2 mg/L of fluoride.

In some regions of the United States, public water systems and private wells contain a natural fluoride concentration of more than 2 mg/L; at this concentration, children 8 years and younger have a greater chance for developing dental fluorosis, including the moderate and severe forms. These children should have an alternative source of drinking water that contains fluoride at the recommended level.

What Can Healthcare and Public Health Professionals Do to Reduce the Occurrence of Dental Fluorosis?

Counsel Parents and Caregivers regarding Use of Fluoride Toothpaste by Young Children

Parents or caregivers should be counseled on the use of fluoride toothpaste by young children, especially those younger than 2 years. There is an increased chance for dental fluorosis for children younger than 6 years, and especially for those younger than 2 years, because they are more likely to swallow the toothpaste than older children.

For children younger than 2 years, you should consider the fluoride level in the community drinking water, other sources of fluoride, and factors likely to affect susceptibility to tooth decay when weighing the risk and benefits of using fluoride toothpaste. When assessing the risks and benefits, determine if the child may be at high risk for tooth decay because of factors such as poor hygiene, poor diet, or history of decay in the child, and in their siblings or parents.

Target Mouth Rinses to Children at High Risk for Developing Tooth Decay

Because fluoride mouth rinses have resulted in only limited reductions in tooth decay among children, especially as their exposure to other sources of fluoride has increased, their use should be targeted to individuals and groups at high risk for decay.

Children younger than 6 years should not use a fluoride mouth rinse without parents first consulting a dentist or physician because there is a possibility for dental fluorosis if these rinses are repeatedly swallowed.

Prescribe Fluoride Supplements Judiciously

Fluoride supplements can be prescribed for children at high risk for tooth decay and whose primary source of drinking water has a low fluoride level. If the children are younger than 6 years, however, then the dentist or physician should weigh the risks for developing decay without supplements with the possibility of developing dental fluorosis. Access to other sources of fluoride, especially drinking water, should be considered when determining this balance. Parents and caregivers should be informed of both the benefits and risks of fluoride supplements.

Fluoride supplements can be prescribed for persons as appropriate or used in school-based programs. When practical, supplements should be prescribed as chewable tablets or lozenges to maximize the topical effects of fluoride.

The prescription dosage of fluoride supplements should be consistent with the schedule established by the American Dental Association (ADA) Council on Scientific Affairs.

Is My Child at Increased Risk of Fluorosis If They Are on Infant Formula?

Three types of infant formula are available in the United States:

1. powdered formula, which comes in bulk or single-serve packets,

2. concentrated liquid, and

3. ready-to-feed formula.

Ready-to-feed formula contains little fluoride and does not cause dental fluorosis. The kinds of formula that must be mixed with water—powdered or liquid concentrates—may increase the chance of dental fluorosis if they are the child's main source food and if the water is fluoridated.

Section 22.2

Infant Formula and Fluorosis

This section includes text excerpted from "Overview: Infant
Formula and Fluorosis," Centers for Disease Control
and Prevention (CDC), April 20, 2015.

The proper amount of fluoride from infancy through old age helps
prevent and control tooth decay. Community water fluoridation is a
widely accepted practice for preventing and controlling tooth decay by
adding fluoride to the public water supply.

Fluoride intake from water and other fluoride sources, such as
toothpaste and mouth rinse, during the ages when teeth are forming
(from birth through age 8) can lead to changes in the appearance of
the tooth's surface called dental fluorosis. In the United States, most
dental fluorosis is mild and appears as white spots that are barely
noticeable and hard for anyone but a dentist or hygienist to see.

Because most infant formulas contain low levels of fluoride, regularly mixing powdered or liquid infant formula concentrate with
fluoridated water may increase the chance of a child developing the
faint white markings of mild fluorosis.

You can use fluoridated water to prepare infant formula. However,
if your baby is does not eat or drink anything but infant formula that
is mixed with fluoridated water, there may be an increased chance for
mild dental fluorosis. To lessen this chance, you can use low-fluoride
bottled water some of the time to mix with infant formula; these bottled
waters are labeled as de-ionized, purified, demineralized, or distilled.
If they have added fluoride, the label will say so.

What Is the Best Source of Nutrition for Infants?

Breastfeeding is ideal for infants. Breast milk is easy to digest and
contains antibodies that can protect infants from bacterial and viral
infections.

If breastfeeding is not possible, formula can be used. Parents should
speak with their pediatrician about what type of infant formula is best
for their child.

What Types of Infant Formula May Increase the Chance of Dental Fluorosis?

Three types of infant formula are available in the United States:

1. powdered formula, which comes in bulk or single-serve packets,

2. concentrated liquid, and

3. ready-to-feed formula.

Ready-to-feed formula contains little fluoride and does not cause dental fluorosis. The kinds of formula that must be mixed with water—powdered or liquid concentrates—may increase the chance of dental fluorosis if they are the child's main source food and if the water is fluoridated.

Can I Use Fluoridated Tap Water to Mix Infant Formula?

Yes, you can use fluoridated water for preparing infant formula. However, if your child is only consuming infant formula mixed with fluoridated water, there may be an increased chance for mild dental fluorosis. To lessen this chance, parents can use low-fluoride bottled water some of the time to mix infant formula; these bottled waters are labeled as de-ionized, purified, demineralized, or distilled, and without any fluoride added after purification treatment. The U.S. Food and Drug Administration (FDA) requires the label to indicate when fluoride is added.

How Can I Find out the Level (Concentration) of Fluoride in My Tap Water?

The best source of information on fluoride levels in your water system is your local water utility. Other knowledgeable sources may be a local public health department, dentist, dental hygienist, or physician. CDC's website, My Water's Fluoride, allows residents of participating states to find the amount of fluoride in their local water system.

Will Using Only Low-Fluoride Water to Mix Formula Eliminate My Child's Risk for Dental Fluorosis?

Using only water with low fluoride levels to mix formula will lower the risk for dental fluorosis but not eliminate it. Children can take in fluoride from other sources during the time that teeth are developing (birth through age 8). These sources include drinking water, foods and beverages processed with fluoridated water, and dental products, such as fluoride toothpaste, that can be swallowed by young children while brushing their teeth.

Chapter 23

Dental Caries (Cavities) Prevalence in the United States

Although dental caries has been declining in permanent teeth for many children since the 1960s, previous findings showed caries in primary teeth for preschool children increasing from 24% to 28% between 1988 and 2004. Disparities in caries continue to persist for some race and ethnic groups in the United States. Prevalence of dental sealants—applied to the tooth chewing surfaces to help prevent caries—has also varied among sociodemographic groups.

Key Findings

Data from the National Health and Nutrition Examination Survey, 2011–2012

- Approximately 23% of children aged 2–5 years had dental caries in primary teeth.

- Untreated tooth decay in primary teeth among children aged 2–8 was twice as high for Hispanic and non-Hispanic black children compared with non-Hispanic white children.

This chapter includes text excerpted from "Dental Caries and Sealant Prevalence in Children and Adolescents in the United States, 2011–2012," Centers for Disease Control and Prevention (CDC), March 5, 2015.

- Among those aged 6–11, 27% of Hispanic children had any dental caries in permanent teeth compared with nearly 18% of non-Hispanic white and Asian children.

- About three in five adolescents aged 12–19 had experienced dental caries in permanent teeth, and 15% had untreated tooth decay.

- Dental sealants were more prevalent for non-Hispanic white children (44%) compared with non-Hispanic black and Asian children (31% each) aged 6–11.

Although dental caries has been declining in permanent teeth for many children since the 1960s, previous findings showed caries in primary teeth for preschool children increasing from 24% to 28% between 1988 and 2004. Disparities in caries continue to persist for some race and ethnic groups in the United States. Prevalence of dental sealants—applied to the tooth chewing surfaces to help prevent caries—has also varied among sociodemographic groups. This report describes U.S. youth dental caries and sealant prevalence by race and Hispanic origin for 2011–2012.

How Prevalent Was Any Caries in Children's Primary Teeth?

Approximately 37% of children aged 2–8 years had experienced dental caries in primary teeth in 2011–2012. Dental caries among children aged 2–5 was nearly 23% compared with 56% among those aged 6–8. Caries prevalence was higher for Hispanic (46%) and non-Hispanic black (44%) children compared with non-Hispanic white children (31%) aged 2–8. Non-Hispanic Asian children were less likely to have experienced dental caries (36%) compared with Hispanic children (46%) aged 2–8, but were not different from non-Hispanic white or non-Hispanic black children.

In 2011–2012, 14% of children aged 2–8 had untreated tooth decay in primary teeth. Untreated caries in primary teeth was twice as high for children aged 6–8 (20%) compared with children aged 2–5 (10%). Tooth decay was significantly higher for both non-Hispanic black (21%) and Hispanic (19%) children compared with non-Hispanic white children aged 2–8 (10%). The prevalence of untreated dental caries in primary teeth in non-Hispanic Asian children did not significantly differ from that in any of the other race and Hispanic origin groups.

What Percentage of Children Had Any Dental Caries in Permanent Teeth?

In 2011–2012, 21% of children aged 6–11 had experienced dental caries in permanent teeth. Dental caries among children aged 6–8 was nearly 14% and was twice as high for children aged 9–11 (29%). Caries prevalence was higher among Hispanic children aged 6–11 (27%) compared with non-Hispanic white children (19%) or non-Hispanic Asian children (18%).

Approximately 6% of children aged 6–11 had untreated tooth decay in permanent teeth. Untreated caries in permanent teeth was twice as high for children aged 9–11 (8%) compared with children aged 6–8 years (3%). Prevalence of untreated caries was higher for Hispanic children (9%) compared with non-Hispanic white children (4%) aged 6–11 years.

Chapter 24

Preventing Tooth Decay in Children

Chapter Contents

Section 24.1

Tooth Decay and Children

This section includes text excerpted from "Brush Up on Oral Health," Early Childhood Learning and Knowledge Center (ECLKC), U.S. Department of Health and Human Services (HHS), May 2016.

Did You Know?

- Tooth decay is the number one chronic disease among children in the United States.

- As soon as a child's first tooth comes into his or her mouth, tooth decay can occur.

- Tooth decay is a disease that can spread from one person to another and from one tooth to another.

Tooth Decay in Children

Tooth decay is caused by bacteria in the mouth that use sugar in food to make acid. Acid removes minerals from the outer tooth surface (enamel). Over time, acid breaks the tooth surface down and creates a cavity (hole) in the tooth. Many factors can increase a child's risk for developing tooth decay. Likewise, many factors can lower a child's risk for developing tooth decay. This section explains why it is important to lower the factors that cause tooth decay and increase the factors that protect teeth from tooth decay. **Head Start** staff can share this information with parents.

Factors That Increase a Child's Risk for Tooth Decay

- **Parent has untreated tooth decay.** Parents with untreated tooth decay have high levels of the bacteria that cause tooth decay in their mouths. Parents can pass these bacteria to their child through saliva-sharing activities. Examples of these activities are cleaning a pacifier by mouth and giving it to a child and sharing forks or spoons.

- **Child enrolled in a public insurance plan.** Children who are enrolled in their state Medicaid or Child's Health Insurance Program may have a difficult time accessing oral healthcare because some oral health providers refuse to take public insurance.

- **Child has frequent between-meal snacks or drinks that contain sugar.** When children snack and/or drink foods or beverages containing natural or added sugar frequently, their teeth are bathed in acid for long periods of time. The acid has time to break tooth surfaces down and cause tooth decay.

- **Child is put to bed with a bottle with liquids that contain natural or added sugar.** When children are put to bed with a bottle or sippy cup containing breast milk, infant formula, or any liquid with natural or added sugar, their teeth are bathed in acid for long periods of time. The acid has time to break tooth surfaces down and cause tooth decay.

- **Child has dental plaque on teeth.** Dental plaque is a film on the surface of a tooth that is a mix of saliva, bacteria, and food. If dental plaque is not removed by brushing with fluoride toothpaste twice a day, it increases the child's risk for developing tooth decay.

- **Child has a medical condition or a disability.** Children with medical conditions, such as asthma, may take medicines that contain sugar or make their mouths dry. Children with disabilities may have oral habits that can wear or break teeth, or they may have soft diets that can lead to more dental plaque on teeth. Having one or more of these issues increases the child's risk for developing tooth decay.

- **Child has had tooth decay in the past.** Once children have had tooth decay, their risk for developing more tooth decay increases. This is true even for children who have fillings to treat earlier tooth decay.

- **Child has early signs of tooth decay.** Chalky white spots along the gum line of the upper front teeth are the beginning of tooth decay.

Factors That Lower a Child's Risk for Tooth Decay

- **Child receives fluoride.** Fluoride puts minerals back into teeth that acid has removed. It also destroys bacteria that cause tooth decay and keeps the bacteria from growing. The three main ways children can receive fluoride are:

- **Fluoridated water.** Fluoride is added to many community water supplies to protect teeth from tooth decay.

- **Fluoride toothpaste.** As soon as the first tooth comes in, brushing with the right amount of fluoride toothpaste twice a day helps to protect teeth from tooth decay.

- **Fluoride treatments.** Health staff in medical and dental offices or clinics can put fluoride varnish on a child's teeth as soon as the first tooth comes into the mouth and then every few months afterward.

- **Child has a dental home, a regular source of oral health-care.** The teeth of children with a dental home are checked regularly for early signs of tooth decay. These children also receive services to protect teeth from tooth decay and repair early stages of tooth decay.

Section 24.2

The Process of Tooth Decay

This section includes text excerpted from "The Tooth Decay Process: How to Reverse It and Avoid a Cavity," National Institute of Dental and Craniofacial Research (NIDCR), May 2013.

You probably know that a dental cavity is a hole in a tooth. But did you know that a cavity is the result of the tooth decay process that happens over time? Did you know that you can interrupt and even reverse this process to avoid a cavity? This section explains how the tooth decay process starts and how it can be stopped or even reversed to keep your child from getting cavities.

What's inside Our Mouths?

Our mouths are full of bacteria. Hundreds of different types live on our teeth, gums, tongue and other places in our mouths. Some bacteria are helpful. But some can be harmful such as those that play a role in the tooth decay process. Tooth decay is the result of an infection with certain types of bacteria that use sugars in food to make acids. Over time, these acids can make a cavity in the tooth.

What Goes on inside Our Mouths All Day?

Throughout the day, a tug of war takes place inside our mouths.

On one team are dental plaque—a sticky, colorless film of bacteria—plus foods and drinks that contain sugar or starch (such as milk, bread, cookies, candy, soda, juice, and many others). Whenever we eat or drink something that contains sugar or starch, the bacteria use them to produce acids. These acids begin to eat away at the tooth's hard outer surface, or enamel.

On the other team are the minerals in our saliva (such as calcium and phosphate) plus fluoride from toothpaste, water, and other sources. This team helps enamel repair itself by replacing minerals lost during an "acid attack."

Our teeth go through this natural process of losing minerals and regaining minerals all day long.

How Does a Cavity Develop?

When a tooth is exposed to acid frequently—for example, if you eat or drink often, especially foods or drinks containing sugar and starches—the repeated cycles of acid attacks cause the enamel to continue to lose minerals. A white spot may appear where minerals have been lost. This is a sign of early decay.

Tooth decay can be stopped or reversed at this point. Enamel can repair itself by using minerals from saliva, and fluoride from toothpaste or other sources. But if the tooth decay process continues, more minerals are lost. Over time, the enamel is weakened and destroyed, forming a cavity. A cavity is permanent damage that a dentist has to repair with a filling.

How Can We Help Teeth Win the Tug of War and Avoid a Cavity?

Use Fluoride

Fluoride is a mineral that can prevent tooth decay from progressing. It can even reverse, or stop, early tooth decay.

Fluoride works to protect teeth. It . . .

- prevents mineral loss in tooth enamel and replaces lost minerals
- reduces the ability of bacteria to make acid

You can get fluoride by:

- Drinking fluoridated water from a community water supply; about 74 percent of Americans served by a community water supply system receive fluoridated water.
- Brushing with a fluoride toothpaste

If the dentist thinks your child needs more fluoride, he or she may—

- Apply a fluoride gel or varnish to tooth surfaces
- Prescribe fluoride tablets
- Recommend using a fluoride mouth rinse

Keep an eye on how often your child eats, as well as what she eats

Your child's diet is important in preventing a cavity. Remember . . . every time we eat or drink something that contains sugar or starches, bacteria in our mouth use the sugar and starch to produce acids. These acids begin to eat away at the tooth's enamel.

Our saliva can help fight off this acid attack. But if we eat frequently throughout the day—especially foods and drinks containing sugar and starches—the repeated acid attacks will win the tug of war, causing the tooth to lose minerals and eventually develop a cavity.

That's why it's important to keep an eye on *how often* your children eat as well as *what* they eat.

Tooth-Friendly Tips

- Limit between-meal snacks. This reduces the number of acid attacks on teeth and gives teeth a chance to repair themselves.
- Save candy, cookies, soda, and other sugary drinks for special occasions.
- Limit fruit juice.
- Make sure your child doesn't eat or drink anything with sugar in it after bedtime tooth brushing. Saliva flow decreases during

sleep. Without enough saliva, teeth are less able to repair themselves after an acid attack.

Make Sure Your Child Brushes

Brushing with fluoride toothpaste is important for preventing cavities.

Here's what you should know about brushing:

1. Have your child brush two times per day.

2. Supervise young children when they brush:

- For children aged 2 to 6, you put the toothpaste on the brush. Use only a pea-sized amount of fluoride toothpaste.

  - Encourage your child to spit out the toothpaste rather than swallow it. Children under 6 tend to swallow much of the toothpaste on their brush. If children regularly consume higher-than-recommended amounts of fluoride during the teeth-forming years (age 8 and younger), their permanent teeth may develop white lines or flecks called dental fluorosis. Fluorosis is usually mild; in many cases, only a dental professional would notice it. (In children under age 2, dental experts recommend that you do not use fluoride toothpaste unless directed by a doctor or dentist.)

  - Until they are 7 or 8 years old, you will need to help your child brush. Young children cannot get their teeth clean by themselves. Try brushing your child's teeth first, then let her finish.

Talk to a Dentist about Sealants

Dental sealants are another good way to help avoid a cavity. Sealants are thin, plastic coatings painted onto the chewing surfaces of the back teeth, or molars. Here's why sealants are helpful: The chewing surfaces of back teeth are rough and uneven because they have small pits and grooves. Food and bacteria can get stuck in the pits and grooves and stay there a long time because toothbrush bristles can't easily brush them away. Sealants cover these surfaces and form a barrier that protects teeth and prevents food and bacteria from getting trapped there.

Since most cavities in children and adolescents develop in the molars (the back teeth), it's best to get these teeth sealed as soon as they come in:

- The first permanent molars—called "6 year molars"—come in between the ages of 5 and 7.

- The second permanent molars—"12 year molars"—come in when a child is between 11 and 14 years old.

Take Your Child to the Dentist for Regular Check-Ups

Visit a dentist regularly for cleanings and an examination. During the visit the dentist or hygienist will:

- Remove dental plaque

- Check for any areas of early tooth decay

- Show you and your child how to thoroughly clean the teeth

- Apply a fluoride gel or varnish, if necessary

- Schedule your next regular check-up

Section 24.3
Sugar and Tooth Decay

This section includes text excerpted from "Brush Up on Oral Health," Early Childhood Learning and Knowledge Center (ECLKC), U.S. Department of Health and Human Services (HHS), May 2013.

Did You Know?

- Sugar added to food makes up more than 13 percent of a young child's diet.

- Family income doesn't make a difference in the amount of food with added sugar that parents give a child.

- Almost two-thirds of foods with added sugar that children eat are eaten at home.

Sugar and Children's Health

Children who eat foods that are high in sugar often (for example, every hour) during the day are more likely to develop tooth decay. Parents may not know that many of the foods they give children have sugar. They may also not know that eating sugar often during the day can make it more likely that a child will develop tooth decay.

Sugar and Tooth Decay—Eating Often during the Day Matters

Sugar plays a key role in tooth decay. Most foods, like dairy products, fruit, vegetables, grains, and processed and prepared foods, contain sugar.

Bacteria that cause tooth decay breaks down food with sugar to form acid. Each time a person eats food with sugar, acid is in the mouth for 20 to 40 minutes. If a child eats food with sugar often during the day, acid will be in his or her mouth for long periods of time. The first graph (Eating Often) shows a morning where a child is fed often. The blue line below the dotted green line shows that acid is in the child's mouth almost all morning. If a child eats like this often, the child is more likely to develop tooth decay.

Children who are fed scheduled meals and snacks are at lower risk for developing tooth decay than children who are fed often during the day. The second graph (Eating on a Schedule) shows that acid is in the child's mouth for short periods of time.

Finding Hidden Sugar

Many foods contain added sugar. Sugar in foods can be listed by many different names. The best place to check for sugar is in the ingredients list on the food label. Look for words like:

- Beet sugar
- Brown sugar
- Cane sugar
- Corn sweeteners
- Corn syrup
- Cane juice
- High fructose corn syrup

- Honey
- Malt syrup
- Maple syrup
- Molasses
- Raw sugar
- White sugar

179

Section 24.4

Sealants Seal out Tooth Decay

This section contains text excerpted from the following sources: Text
beginning with the heading "What Are Dental Sealants?" is excerpted
from "Dental Sealants," Centers for Disease Control and Prevention
(CDC), July 10, 2013; Text under the heading "What Are School-
Based Sealant Programs?" is excerpted from "School-Based
Dental Sealant Programs," Centers for Disease
Control and Prevention (CDC), July 10, 2013.

What Are Dental Sealants?

Dental sealants are thin plastic coatings that are applied to the
grooves on the chewing surfaces of the back teeth to protect them from
tooth decay. Most tooth decay in children and teens occurs on these
surfaces. Sealants protect the chewing surfaces from tooth decay by
keeping germs and food particles out of these grooves.

Which Teeth Are Suitable for Sealants?

Permanent molars are the most likely to benefit from sealants. The
first molars usually come into the mouth when a child is about 6 years old.
Second molars appear at about age 12. It is best if the sealant is applied
soon after the teeth have erupted, before they have a chance to decay.

How Are Sealants Applied?

Applying sealants does not require drilling or removing tooth structure.
The process is short and easy. After the tooth is cleaned, a special gel is
placed on the chewing surface for a few seconds. The tooth is then washed
off and dried. Then, the sealant is painted on the tooth. The dentist or
dental hygienist also may shine a light on the tooth to help harden the
sealant. It takes about a minute for the sealant to form a protective shield.

Are Sealants Visible?

Sealants can only be seen up close. Sealants can be clear, white or
slightly tinted, and usually are not seen when a child talks or smiles.

Will Sealants Make Teeth Feel Different?

As with anything new that is placed in the mouth, a child may feel the sealant with the tongue. Sealants, however, are very thin and only fill the pits and grooves of molar teeth.

How Long Will Sealants Last?

A sealant can last for as long as 5 to 10 years. Sealants should be checked at your regular dental appointment and can be reapplied if they are no longer in place.

Will Sealants Replace Fluoride for Cavity Protection?

No. Fluorides, such as those used in toothpaste, mouth rinse, and community water supplies also help to prevent decay, but in a different way. Sealants keep germs and food particles out of the grooves by covering them with a safe plastic coating. Sealants and fluorides work together to prevent tooth decay.

How Do Sealants Fit into a Preventive Dentistry Program?

Sealants are one part of a child's total preventive dental care. A complete preventive dental program also includes fluoride, twice-daily brushing, wise food choices, and regular dental care.

Why Is Sealing a Tooth Better than Waiting for Decay and Filling the Cavity?

Decay damages teeth permanently. Sealants protect them. Sealants can save time, money, and the discomfort sometimes associated with dental fillings. Fillings are not permanent. Each time a tooth is filled, more drilling is done and the tooth becomes a little weaker.

What Are School-Based Sealant Programs?

School-based dental sealant delivery programs provide sealants to children unlikely to receive them otherwise. Such programs—

• Define a target population within a school district

• Verify unmet need for sealants

• Get financial, material, and policy support

- Apply rules for selecting schools and students

- Apply sealants at school or offsite in clinics

School-based sealant programs are especially important for reaching children from low-income families who are less likely to receive private dental care. Programs generally target schools by using the percentage of children eligible for federal free or reduced-cost lunch programs Tooth decay may result in pain and other problems that affect learning in school-age children.

Chapter 25

Mouth Injuries in Children

Chapter Contents

Section 25.1

Children and Oral Injuries

This section includes text excerpted from "Brush Up on Oral Health," Early Childhood Learning and Knowledge Center (ECLKC), U.S. Department of Health and Human Services (HHS), January 2014.

Did You Know?

- 18 percent of all injuries in young children involve dental trauma.

- One quarter of all oral injuries in children under age 18 occur among 1- to 2-year-olds.

- 33 percent of all 5-year-olds have injured their primary teeth.

Oral Injuries

Injuries to the head, face, and mouth happen often among young children. Because oral injuries can affect children for the rest of their lives, it is important for Head Start staff and parents to try to prevent these injuries.

Causes and Types of Oral Injuries

Most oral injuries happen when children fall. Children may stumble as they are learning to walk and being physically active. Injuries tend to happen when children trip on things, are pushed by another child, climb on stairs and furniture, or run with items in their mouths. Some children receive burns from chewing on electrical cords that are plugged into a socket. Abuse and neglect can also cause oral injuries. Children's top front teeth are injured most often. They can be chipped, pushed into the gum, pushed forward or back in the mouth, or knocked out. Bruises or cuts in or near the mouth are also common oral injuries.

Impact of Oral Injuries

Preventing oral injuries is important for many reasons. Injured primary teeth can turn brown or black, be painful, become infected, or have to be removed. Primary teeth also keep space for permanent teeth and help guide them into position. When primary teeth are lost too early, there may not be enough space for permanent teeth. Injuries to a child's primary teeth can also damage the permanent teeth that are forming under the primary teeth. If a primary tooth is pushed into the gum, it can disturb the cells that are building the permanent tooth. This can cause discolored or deformed permanent teeth or permanent teeth that decay quickly. Injuries to primary and permanent teeth can affect a child's speech, nutrition, self-esteem, and overall health.

What Parents Can Do

Parents can protect children from oral injuries by making home, play, and work areas safe and by practicing safe habits. Here are some steps to take to help prevent oral injuries in homes.

- **Do health and safety sweeps.** Tour homes and areas where children play and work. Use safety gates, and cover sharp corners on furniture. Make sure that toys and other things are regularly picked up off the floor to help prevent children from tripping. Check that there is enough uncluttered space for children to move and play, to minimize bumping and pushing. Look over playground equipment to make sure it's age-appropriate. Remove hazards or obstacles that might make a child fall.

- **Set and enforce policies and procedures.** Work with health advisory committee members, parent committees, home visitors, child-safety experts, and others to identify behaviors that could cause oral injuries, and develop policies and procedures to help prevent oral injuries. Some examples include using child safety straps on high chairs; having children wear helmets when riding wheeled toys; and keeping toys picked up from the floor, playground, and yard. The policies and procedures should also address how to handle oral injuries.

- **Record, track, and analyze oral injuries.** Head Start staff should document all injuries and inform parents if their child is injured. Keep a log of all injuries, and review the log quarterly to identify patterns where and when injuries happen. This information can be used to determine what changes are needed to help prevent injuries.

- **Educate staff, parents, and children.** Use staff training and coaching opportunities, parent meetings, newsletters, and social media to teach Head Start staff, parents, and children how to avoid oral injuries. Invite oral health providers, safety experts, and others to talk about how to prevent injuries.

Section 25.2

Preventing Oral Injuries

This section includes text excerpted from "Preventing Injuries to Your Child's Mouth," Early Childhood Learning and Knowledge Center (ECLKC), U.S. Department of Health and Human Services (HHS), 2016.

As a parent, you want to keep your child safe, but you learn that injuries can happen in a moment. Children can injure their mouths when they fall or trip. They can also injure their mouths when they climb on furniture or run with something in their mouth.

Tips for preventing injuries to your child's mouth:

- Use safety gates at the top and bottom of stairs.

- Put safety locks or latches on cabinets and drawers.

- Cover sharp corners.

- Keep one hand on your child while he is on a changing table.

- When feeding your child, put her in a high chair or booster seat. Remember to buckle the seatbelt.

- Always buckle your child into the car seat in the back seat of a car or truck.

- Pick up toys and keep floors clear so children don't trip and fall.

- Make sure rugs have nonskid pads or backing.

- Watch your child when he is on high places, like playground equipment.

- Put your baby in a front pack while shopping. Or put your child in the shopping cart and use a safety belt. Don't leave your child alone or out of reach in a shopping cart.

- Don't let your child walk or run with anything in her mouth, like sippy cups, popsicles, or toys.

In case of emergency, call your child's dental or medical clinic right away. If you can't reach them, take your child to the emergency room. Give your child's dental and medical clinic phone numbers to others who take care of your child.

First Aid for Oral Injuries

Injuries to the head, face, and mouth are common in young children. Even when parents do their best to keep children safe, oral injuries can happen. Most oral injuries happen when young children are learning to walk. The top front teeth are injured most often.

Tips to help you know what to do for common oral injuries:

- **Tongue or lip injured.** Clean the injured area. Press a clean washcloth on it to stop bleeding. Keep your child's head up and facing forward to prevent choking. Put ice, wrapped in a clean washcloth, on the area to reduce swelling. If bleeding doesn't stop after 30 minutes, take your child to your child's dentist or doctor right away. If the dentist or doctor is not available, take your child to the nearest urgent care center right away.

- **Tooth chipped or cracked.** Clean the injured area. Contact your child's dentist or an urgent care center right away. Have your child rinse with water, if possible. If there is bleeding, press a clean washcloth on the gum around the tooth to stop it.

- **Tooth knocked out.** Contact your child's dentist right away. Do not try to put a baby tooth back into the mouth. Clean the injured area. If there is bleeding, have your child bite on the area with a clean washcloth for 15 to 30 minutes to stop it.

- **Tooth knocked loose, moved, or pushed into gum.** If your child's tooth has been knocked loose, moved forward or backward, or pushed into the gum, contact your child's dentist or an urgent care center right away. Have your child rinse with water, if possible. Press a clean washcloth on the gum around the tooth to stop bleeding.

- **Toothache.** If your child has a toothache, it is likely that the tooth has a cavity. Make a dental appointment as soon as possible to find out what the problem is and get treatment.

Chapter 26

Bruxism and Non-Nutritive Sucking

Chapter Contents

Section 26.1

Oral Habits

This section includes text excerpted from "Brush Up on Oral Health,"
Early Childhood Learning and Knowledge Center (ECLKC), U.S.
Department of Health and Human Services (HHS), May 2014.

Non-nutritive sucking (for example, sucking on a thumb or a pacifier) or teeth grinding are common oral habits in young children. These habits are also common in children with special healthcare needs. Some Head Start staff and parents worry that oral habits may hurt a child's teeth or mouth or change the shape of a child's face or jaw.

Non-Nutritive Sucking and Tooth Grinding

Non-nutritive sucking: Sucking on a thumb, fingers, a hand, a pacifier, blankets, toys or other non-food items is called non-nutritive sucking. Sucking helps comfort a child when he or she is tired, nervous, upset or restless.

Tooth grinding: Tooth grinding happens most often when a child is in a deep sleep or is under stress. It is not always clear why children grind their teeth. In some cases, the child's top and bottom teeth might not be lined up correctly, so the child grinds the top and bottom teeth together to get a better fit. In other cases, the child might grind his or her teeth because of an earache or teething pain.

Strategies for Parents to Deal with Oral Habits

Using pacifiers: Pacifiers help satisfy a child's need to suck. Using pacifiers will not harm young children, as long as they are used safely. Pacifiers should never be used to replace or delay meals. Head Start staff can give parents these tips on safe pacifier use:

- Use a one-piece pacifier made of sturdy material that is firm and flexible.

- Do not place a pacifier on a ribbon or string, and never tie it to a crib or around the child's neck or hand, which can cause choking.

- Do not dip a pacifier in sugar, honey, syrup or other sweet food, which can make it more likely that the child will develop tooth decay.

- Clean pacifiers with water often, and replace them regularly. Parents should not clean a pacifier by putting it in their mouth and then giving it to the child. This practice can pass bacteria that cause tooth decay from the parent to the child.

Ending non-nutritive sucking: Most children stop non-nutritive sucking between ages 2 and 4. Children who use pacifiers usually stop sucking earlier than children who suck on a thumb, fingers or other objects. Sucking past age 4 can change the shape of the child's mouth and teeth (for example, causing buck teeth). Changes in the shape of a child's mouth and teeth can cause the child to breathe through the mouth instead of the nose and can also cause speech problems and bite problems. Here are some strategies Head Start staff can share with parents to help a child stop sucking:

- Tell the child why they want the child to stop sucking. Tell the child that they believe the child can stop.

- Use reminders when the child wants to stop sucking but needs help. Put a bandage on the child's thumb or fingers as a reminder not to suck. Putting a mitten or sock on the child's hand at night can also help.

- Give the child something to track small successes. For example, put a star on a calendar for each day the child does not suck. At the end of a certain time period, give the child a reward for not sucking. Choose a reward that is not food.

- Talk to the dental office staff, a pediatrician or a speech therapist about other strategies to help a child stop sucking.

Ending tooth grinding: Grinding rarely harms a child's teeth. The child usually stops grinding when the cause of grinding goes away. For example, when the child no longer feels stressed or has an earache or teething pain, grinding will probably stop. If grinding does not stop over time, parent should talk to the dental office staff about other strategies to help stop it.

Section 26.2

Childhood Bruxism (Teeth Grinding or Clenching)

Text in this section is excerpted from "Bruxism (Teeth Grinding or Clenching)," © 1995–2016. The Nemours Foundation/ KidsHealth®. Reprinted with permission.

What Is Bruxism?

Bruxism is the medical term for the grinding of teeth or the clenching of jaws. Many kids have it—2 to 3 out of every 10 will grind or clench, experts say, but most outgrow it. Bruxism often happens during deep sleep phases or when kids are under stress.

Causes of Bruxism

Experts aren't always sure why bruxism happens. In some cases, kids may grind because the top and bottom teeth aren't aligned properly. Others do it as a response to pain, such as from an earache or teething. Kids might grind their teeth as a way to ease the pain, just as they might rub a sore muscle. Many kids outgrow these fairly common causes for grinding.

Stress—usually nervous tension or anger—is another cause. For instance, a child might worry about a test at school or a change in routine (a new sibling or a new teacher). Even arguing with parents and siblings can cause enough stress to prompt teeth grinding or jaw clenching.

Some kids who are hyperactive also have bruxism. And sometimes kids with other medical conditions (such as cerebral palsy) or who take certain medicines can develop bruxism.

Effects of Bruxism

Many cases of bruxism go undetected with no ill effects, while others cause headaches or earaches. Usually, though, it's more bothersome to other family members because of the grinding sound. In some circumstances, nighttime grinding and clenching can wear down tooth enamel, chip teeth, increase temperature sensitivity, and cause severe facial pain and jaw problems, such as temporomandibular joint disease (TMJ). Most kids who grind, however, do not have TMJ problems unless their grinding and clenching happen a lot.

Diagnosing Bruxism

Lots of kids who grind their teeth aren't even aware of it, so it's often siblings or parents who identify the problem.

Some signs to watch for:

- grinding noises when your child is sleeping

- complaints of a sore jaw or face after waking up in the morning

- pain with chewing

If you think your child is grinding his or her teeth, visit the dentist, who will examine the teeth for chipped enamel and unusual wear and tear, and spray air and water on the teeth to check for unusual sensitivity.

If damage is found, the dentist may ask your child a few questions, such as:

- How do you feel before bed?

- Are you worried about anything at home or school?

- Are you angry with someone?

- What do you do before bed?

The exam will help the dentist determine whether the cause is anatomical (misaligned teeth) or psychological (stress), and come up with an effective treatment plan.

Treating Bruxism

Most kids outgrow bruxism, but a combination of parental observation and dental visits can help keep the problem in check until they do.

In cases where the grinding and clenching make a child's face and jaw sore or damage the teeth, dentists may prescribe a special night guard. Molded to a child's teeth, the night guard is similar to the protective mouthpieces worn by athletes. Though a mouthpiece can take some getting used to, positive results happen quickly.

Helping Kids with Bruxism

Whether the cause is physical or psychological, kids might be able to control bruxism by relaxing before bedtime—for example, by taking a warm bath or shower, listening to a few minutes of soothing music, or reading a book.

For bruxism that's caused by stress, ask about what's upsetting your child and find a way to help. For example, a kid who is worried about being away from home for a first camping trip might need reassurance that mom or dad will be nearby if needed.

If the issue is more complicated, such as moving to a new town, discuss your child's concerns and try to ease any fears. If you're concerned, talk to your doctor.

In rare cases, basic stress relievers aren't enough to stop bruxism. If your child has trouble sleeping or is acting differently than usual, your dentist or doctor may suggest further evaluation. This can help determine the cause of the stress and an appropriate course of treatment.

How Long Does Bruxism Last?

Most kids stop grinding when they lose their baby teeth. However, a few kids do continue to grind into adolescence. And if the bruxism is caused by stress, it will continue until the stress eases.

Preventing Bruxism

Because some bruxism is a child's natural reaction to growth and development, most cases can't be prevented. Stress-induced bruxism can be avoided, though. So talk with kids regularly about their feelings and help them deal with stress. Taking kids for routine dental visits can help find and treat bruxism.

Chapter 27

Oral Conditions in Children with Other Special Needs

Oral Development

Tooth eruption may be delayed, accelerated, or inconsistent in children with growth disturbances. Gums may appear red or bluish-purple before erupting teeth break through into the mouth. Eruption depends on genetics, growth of the jaw, muscular action, and other factors. Children with Down syndrome may show delays of up to 2 years. Offer information about the variability in tooth eruption patterns and refer to an oral healthcare provider for additional questions.

Malocclusion, a poor fit between the upper and lower teeth, and crowding of teeth occur frequently in people with developmental disabilities. Muscle dysfunction contributes to malocclusion, particularly in people with cerebral palsy. Teeth that are crowded or out of alignment are more difficult to keep clean, contributing to periodontal disease and dental caries. Refer to an orthodontist or pediatric dentist for evaluation and specialized instruction in daily oral hygiene.

Developmental defects appear as pits, lines, or discoloration in the teeth. Very high fever or certain medications can disturb tooth

This chapter includes text excerpted from "Oral Conditions in Children with Special Needs: A Guide for Health Care Providers," National Institute of Dental and Craniofacial Research (NIDCR), April 2015.

formation and defects may result. Many teeth with defects are prone to dental caries, are difficult to keep clean, and may compromise appearance. Refer to an oral healthcare provider for evaluation of treatment options and advice on keeping teeth clean.

Tooth anomalies are variations in the number, size, and shape of teeth. People with Down syndrome, oral clefts, ectodermal dysplasias, or other conditions may experience congenitally missing, extra, or malformed teeth. Consult an oral healthcare provider for dental treatment planning during a child's growing years.

Oral Trauma

Trauma to the face and mouth occur more frequently in people who have intellectual disability, seizures, abnormal protective reflexes, or muscle incoordination. People receiving restorative dental care should be observed closely to prevent chewing on anesthetized areas. If a tooth is avulsed or broken, take the patient and the tooth to a dentist immediately. Counsel the parent/caregiver on ways to prevent trauma and what to do when it occurs.

Oral Infections

Dental caries or tooth decay, may be linked to frequent vomiting or gastroesophageal reflux, less than normal amounts of saliva, medications containing sugar, or special diets that require prolonged bottle feeding or snacking. When oral hygiene is poor, the teeth are at increased risk for caries. Counsel the parent/caregiver on daily oral hygiene to include frequent rinsing with plain water and use of a fluoride-containing toothpaste or mouth rinse. Explain the need for supervising children to avoid swallowing fluoride. Refer to an oral healthcare provider and/or gastroenterologist for prevention and treatment. Prescribe sugarless medications when available.

Viral infections are usually due to the herpes simplex virus. Children rarely get herpetic gingivostomatitis or herpes labialis before 6 months of age. Herpetic gingivostomatitis is most common in young children, but may occur in adolescents and young adults. Viral infections can be painful and are usually accompanied by a fever. Counsel the parent/caregiver about the infectious nature of the lesions, the need for frequent fluids to prevent dehydration, and methods of symptomatic treatment.

Early, severe periodontal (gum) disease can occur in children with impaired immune systems or connective tissue disorders and inadequate oral hygiene. Simple gingivitis results from an accumulation of bacterial plaque and presents as red, swollen gums that bleed easily. Periodontitis is more severe and leads to tooth loss if not treated. Professional cleaning by an oral healthcare provider, systemic antibiotics, and instructions on home care may be needed to stop the infection. Explain that the parent/caregiver may need to help with daily toothbrushing and flossing and that frequent appointments with an oral healthcare provider may be necessary.

Gingival Overgrowth

Gingival overgrowth may be a side effect from medications such as calcium channel blockers, phenytoin sodium, and cyclosporine. Poor oral hygiene aggravates the condition and can lead to superimposed infections. Severe overgrowth can impair tooth eruption, chewing, and appearance.

Chapter 28

Finding and Visiting a Dental Clinic with Your Child

Finding a Dental Clinic for Your Child

Children need to visit the dental clinic to keep their teeth and mouth healthy. If children have regular dental visits, the dentist and dental hygienist can take care of their teeth and find oral health problems early. Here are tips for finding a dental clinic that is best for you and your child.

Tips for Finding a Dental Clinic

- Ask your child's Head Start teacher or other parents for suggestions.

- Ask your child's doctor for a referral.

This chapter contains text excerpted from the following sources: Text under the heading "Finding a Dental Clinic for Your Child" is excerpted from "Finding a Dental Clinic for Your Child," Early Childhood Learning and Knowledge Center (ECLKC), U.S. Department of Health and Human Services (HHS), September 2015; Text under the heading "Visiting the Dental Clinic with Your Child" is excerpted from "Visiting the Dental Clinic with Your Child," Early Childhood Learning and Knowledge Center (ECLKC), U.S. Department of Health and Human Services (HHS), September 2015.

Questions to Ask When Choosing a Dental Clinic

- Is your clinic taking new patients?

- Does your clinic take my child's insurance (for example, Medicaid or CHIP)?

- Do any of your staff speak my language? Can they translate so I can understand?

- Does clinic staff have training or experience treating young children?

- When is the next appointment for a new patient?

- What happens during a new patient visit?

- Is your clinic close to public transportation?

- When is your clinic open? Is it open evenings or on weekends?

- What information or forms do I need to bring to fill out your paperwork (for example, my child's insurance card or a Head Start oral health form)?

- Are there books, toys or other things for children in your waiting room?

Visiting the Dental Clinic with Your Child

At the Dental Clinic, the Dental Team Will

- Check your child's teeth and mouth.

- Talk to you about the best way to take care of your child's teeth. For example, brushing your child's teeth with fluoride toothpaste after breakfast and before bed.

- Share other ways to help prevent tooth decay (cavities). For example, putting fluoride varnish on children's teeth.

Tips for Visiting the Dental Clinic

- If your child asks what will happen at the dental clinic, give a simple answer. For example, say:

  - "They may count how many teeth you have."

  - "They may clean your teeth to make them shiny and bright!"

- If you don't like going to the dental clinic, don't tell your child. That might make your child worry about going, too.

- Set up a pretend dental chair. Pretend to be the dentist or dental hygienist. Look in your child's mouth and count her teeth; then talk to her about brushing her teeth.

- Read books or watch videos with your child about visiting the dental clinic. Don't use books or videos that have words like hurt, pain, shot, drill, afraid, or any other words that might scare your child.

- Let your child bring his favorite toy or blanket to the clinic.

- If you find out that your child will receive a small toy or new toothbrush at the end of the visit, remind your child of this reward.

- Plan a fun activity for after the clinic visit.

Part Four

Orthodontic, Endodontic, Periodontic, and Orofacial Procedures

Chapter 29

Orthodontia

Chapter Contents

Section 29.1

Orthodontia Overview

Why Do People Need Braces?

Braces are a common and almost expected part of growing up (and many adults get braces, too). To better understand why braces and other orthodontic devices are needed, it helps to talk a bit about the teeth first.

As you made your way through childhood, your "baby" teeth fell out one by one, to be replaced by permanent, adult teeth. Although some people's adult teeth grow in at the right angle and with the right spacing, many people's teeth don't. Some teeth may grow in crooked or overlapping. In other people, some teeth may grow in rotated or twisted. Some people's mouths are too small, and this crowds the teeth and causes them to shift into crooked positions. And in some cases, a person's upper jaw and lower jaw aren't the same size. When the lower half of the jaw is too small, it makes the upper jaw hang over when the jaw is shut, resulting in a condition called an **overbite.** When the opposite happens (the lower half of the jaw is larger than the upper half), it's called an **underbite.**

All of these different types of disorders go by one medical name: **Malocclusion.** This word comes from Latin and means "bad bite." In most cases, a "bad bite" isn't anyone's fault; crooked teeth, overbites, and underbites are often inherited traits, just like brown eyes or big feet are inherited traits.

In some cases, things like dental disease, early loss of baby or adult teeth, some types of medical problems, an accident, or a habit like prolonged thumb sucking can cause the disorders.

Malocclusion can be a problem because it interferes with proper chewing—crooked teeth that aren't aligned properly don't work as well as straight ones. Because chewing is the first part of eating and digestion, it's important that teeth can do the job. Teeth that aren't aligned correctly can also be harder to brush and keep clean, which can lead to tooth decay, cavities, and gum disease. And finally, many people who have crooked teeth may feel self-conscious about how they look; braces can help them feel better about their smile and entire appearance.

If a dentist suspects that someone needs braces or other corrective devices, he or she will refer the patient to an **orthodontist.** Orthodontists are dentists who have special training in the diagnosis and treatment of misaligned teeth and jaws.

Most regular dentists can tell if teeth will be misaligned once a patient's adult teeth begin to come in—sometimes as early as age 6 or 7—and the orthodontist may recommend **interceptive treatment therapy.** (Interceptive treatment therapy involves the wearing of appliances to influence facial growth and help teeth grow in better, and helps prevent more serious problems from developing.) In many cases, the patient won't be referred to an orthodontist until closer to the teen years.

Diagnosis

Before giving someone braces, the orthodontist needs to diagnose what the problem is. This means making use of several different methods, including X-rays, photographs, impressions, models, and computers.

The X-rays give the orthodontist a good idea of where the teeth are positioned and if any more teeth have yet to come through the gums. Special X-rays that are taken from 360 degrees around the head may also be ordered; this type of X-ray shows the relationships of the teeth to the jaws and the jaws to the head. The orthodontist may also take regular photographs of the patient's face to better understand these relationships.

And finally, the orthodontist may need an impression made of the patient's teeth. This is done by having the patient bite down on a soft material that is used later to form an exact model of the teeth.

Treatment

Once a diagnosis is made, the orthodontist can then decide on the right kind of treatment. In some cases, a removable retainer will be all that's necessary. In other rare cases (especially when there is an extreme overbite or underbite), an operation will be necessary. But in most cases, the answer is braces.

Braces straighten teeth because they do two very important things: stay in place for an extended amount of time, and exert steady pressure. It's this combination that allows braces to successfully change the position of teeth in a patient's mouth, through periodic adjustments by the orthodontist.

Section 29.2

Braces

Text in this section is excerpted from "Braces," © 1995–2016. The Nemours Foundation/KidsHealth®. Reprinted with permission.

Some kids can't wait to get braces. Others are a little worried about what it will be like or how they will look. It can help to learn more about braces, which straighten your teeth and make your smile even better looking.

Tooth Talk

Lots of kids don't have perfect teeth, so don't worry if yours aren't straight. Take a look at most of your classmates. Many of them probably don't have straight teeth either. Sometimes teeth just don't grow in evenly. Your teeth might be crooked or your upper and lower jaws might not be the same size. If your upper jaw is bigger than your lower jaw, that's called an overbite. If your lower jaw is bigger than your upper jaw, you have an underbite.

Either way it's called malocclusion, a word that comes from Latin and means "bad bite." Malocclusion is just a word that dentists use to describe the shape of your mouth. Your dentist might notice one of these problems during a regular visit and recommend that you see an orthodontist. This person, who also might be called a braces specialist, can determine whether you need braces.

Types of Braces

If your parents had braces, you may have seen pictures of them with their mouths full of metal. Today, braces are much less noticeable.

Metal braces are still used, but you might be able to get clear braces or braces that are the same color as your teeth. There are even braces that go behind your teeth where no one can see them.

The wires that are used in braces today are also smaller and better than they used to be, and they're made of a space-age material that straightens your teeth faster and easier. The rubber bands that go along with braces come in funky colors now, too. So you could have black and orange ones for Halloween!

How Braces Work

Braces straighten teeth by putting steady pressure on your teeth and by staying in place for a certain amount of time. Most kids just need regular braces with wires and rubber bands doing their jobs to keep pressure on the teeth. The wires on your braces help to move your teeth, and the rubber bands help to correct the **alignment,** which is the way your teeth line up.

If your teeth need a little extra help, you may have to wear head or neckgear with wires attached to your teeth. If you do have to wear headgear, don't panic! You probably will only have to wear it while you sleep or when you're at home in the evening.

Everyone has to wear braces for different lengths of time, but most people usually wear braces for about 2 years. You'll want to take special care of your teeth after the braces come off. You may need to wear a retainer, which is a small, hard piece of plastic with metal wires or a thin piece of plastic shaped like a mouthguard. Retainers make sure your teeth don't go wandering back to their original places. Your retainer will be specially molded to fit your newly straightened teeth.

After you get your retainer, your orthodontist will tell you when you have to wear it and how long—you might have to wear your retainer all day and all night for 2 years; you might have to wear it at night for 6 months; or you might have to wear it every other night for many years. It just depends on your teeth.

Life with Braces

Braces act like magnets for food, so you need to keep your teeth especially clean while you have them on. You'll want to brush after meals and be extra careful to get out any food that gets stuck in your braces.

Your orthodontist also may give you a special flosser you can use to floss in and around your braces. When your orthodontist changes your wires, ask if you can do a quick floss (it'll be easier without the wires).

You won't have to go on any special diet when you have braces, but you'll want to avoid some foods that are problems for braces. Stay away from popcorn, hard and sticky candy, and especially gum. Sugary sodas and juices can cause a problem, too, because the sugar stays on your teeth and may cause tooth decay. You can have these drinks, but be sure to brush afterward.

Because braces put pressure on your teeth, you might feel uncomfortable once in a while, especially right after the orthodontist makes adjustments. If you have pain, ask your mom or dad to give you a pain reliever.

If you ever have a loose wire or bracket, or a wire that is poking you, you should see the orthodontist right away to get it taken care of. If your orthodontist can't find a problem, he or she may give you some soft wax that you can stick on the bracket that's bothering you. Then it won't rub against your mouth.

So braces can be inconvenient, but lots of kids have them and they are definitely worth the trouble. When will you know for sure? On the day your braces are removed and you can see your new and improved smile!

Section 29.3

The Reality of Retainers

Text in this section is excerpted from "The Reality of Retainers,"
© 1995–2016. The Nemours Foundation/KidsHealth®.
Reprinted with permission.

What Is a Retainer?

A retainer is a piece of plastic and metal that is custom-made for each individual kid who needs one. It fits the top of the teeth and mouth. No two retainers are alike, even though many look similar. Retainers are really common. In fact, most people (kids and adults) who have braces have to wear a retainer for at least a little while after getting their braces taken off. Other people wear them to close gaps in their teeth, to help with speech problems, or to solve certain medical problems.

Why Do I Need to Wear a Retainer?

You might need a retainer for a few reasons. The most common reason is to help your teeth stay set in their new positions after wearing braces. It's important to wear your retainer because as your body grows, your teeth do some shifting. The retainer helps to control this shifting, which occurs naturally.

After your braces are removed, your orthodontist (a special dentist who helps straighten teeth and correct jaw problems) will fit you for a retainer and tell you how long to wear it and when. For example, you might have to wear it all day for 3 months but then only at night after that. Some kids may wear their retainer only at night right from the start, but they may have to wear it for more than a year. The retainer keeps the teeth in line and you won't even notice it while you're sleeping!

Other kids may wear retainers to close a space between their teeth or just to move one tooth. In these cases, braces aren't needed because retainers can do the job. Often, retainers will be worn for several years to close a space, for example, and then keep the gap closed by holding the teeth in place.

When you wear a retainer for any reason, certain teeth may feel pressure and might even feel sore for the first few days. If you experience this, don't worry—it's completely normal.

Retainers can help many mouth problems besides shifting teeth. Sometimes they're used to help a medical problem. For example, you may have a **tongue thrust** (a condition where your tongue sneaks through your teeth when you talk). Some retainers, known as a crib or tongue cage retainers, are designed with small metal bars that hang down from the roof of your mouth. These retainers keep your tongue from going forward in between your teeth when you speak. Your tongue is trained to go to the roof of your mouth instead of through your teeth. The length of time kids wear a tongue cage varies depending on the kid.

Another use for retainers is to help people with **temporomandibular disorder(TMD).** This disorder is usually a result of a bite problem (the teeth don't meet together properly when the jaws are closed) called **malocclusion** or **bruxism,** which is grinding your teeth while you sleep. Grinding stretches the muscles and joints in your mouth and jaws and sometimes can cause jaw pain or headaches. Retainers can help you by preventing your mouth from closing completely at night, which keeps you from grinding your teeth.

Getting Fitted for and Wearing a Retainer

This is the easy part. Your orthodontist will fit you for the retainer using a material known as **alginate.** It's a chewy, chalky kind of thick liquid that makes a mold of your teeth when you sink them into it. The fitting process is fast, painless, and doesn't even taste bad—and you can choose from different flavors.

Your finished retainer can be designed to express your style and likes. Sometimes you can have a picture such as Batman, Christmas trees, or Halloween bats on the plastic part of the retainer. Once you've been fitted for the retainer, you usually have to wait less than a week to get the real thing.

You may think your retainer feels weird at first. That's normal. But see your orthodontist for an adjustment if the retainer causes pain or cuts or rubs against your gums.

At first, you'll need to get used to talking with it in your mouth. Talking slowly at first is a good way to practice and eventually, you won't even notice it's there. Dentists advise reading aloud for several minutes each day. You may also notice an increased saliva flow (more spit in your mouth) in the first few days of wearing your new retainer, which is normal.

Caring for Your Retainer

Retainers live in your mouth along with bacteria, plaque, and left-over food particles. You should clean your retainer every day, but make sure to check with your orthodontist about how your type of retainer should be cleaned (some kinds shouldn't be cleaned with toothpaste). You can also soak it in mouthwash or a denture-cleaning agent to freshen it up and kill germs.

Because the plastic of your retainer can crack if it gets too dry, you should always soak it when it isn't in your mouth. Plastic can warp easily, so don't put it in hot water or leave it near a heat source—like on your radiator, for example. Finally, do not bend the wires. Flipping the retainer around in your mouth will cause the wires to bend.

One important way to take care of your retainer is not to lose it. They are expensive and your mom or dad might have to pay for lost or damaged retainers. Worse yet, they might ask you to help pay for a new one! So look before you dump your lunch tray and try to keep it in the same spot at home when you're not wearing it. In other words, retain your retainer!

Chapter 30

Endodontic Conditions and Treatment

Endodontics

Endodontics is a dental specialty that studies and treats the pulp of teeth. The word endodontic is derived from the Greek words endo, which means "inside," and odont, which translates as "tooth."

To understand endodontic treatment, it helps know a bit about dental anatomy. The tooth is covered by a hard layer of enamel. Another hard layer, called dentin, lies under the enamel and covers soft tissue known as the pulp, a collection of blood vessels, nerves, and connective tissue that is responsible for nourishing the tooth. The pulp is located in the center of the tooth and extends from under the crown down to the tissue under the root. Pulp is especially important during tooth growth and development, but once the tooth is fully grown, it can survive without the pulp because the surrounding tissues are able to provide nourishment.

Almost all teeth can be treated endodontically. However, in some cases treatment may not be possible. For example, this might be the case if the chambers that contain the root (called root canals) are not accessible, if the tooth is badly fractured, or if there is inadequate bone support. Endodontics has advanced so much that teeth that would have been considered lost a few years ago, can be saved today.

"Endodontic Conditions and Treatment," © 2017 Omnigraphics. Reviewed September 2016.

Root Canal Treatment

The most common type of endodontic procedure is a root canal treatment, often called simply a root canal. It is a routine procedure that relieves pain, saves millions of teeth every year, and can help improve appearance.

This procedure becomes necessary when a tooth's pulp becomes inflamed or infected. The infection may arise as a result conditions such as tooth decay, repeated dental work, or a crack in the tooth. If left untreated, the infection may lead to an abscess, a more serious infection that can be life-threating.

In root canal treatment, the pulp is fully removed from the tooth. The pulp chamber is cleaned and shaped, and the empty space is filled and sealed with an inert material. In subsequent visits, the dentist generally fixes a crown on the tooth or performs some other type of restorative work to return the tooth to its full function and appearance.

Symptoms Indicating That Root Canal May Be Necessary

Signs that root canal treatment may be needed include tooth pain, sensitivity to heat and cold, and tenderness to touch and chewing. You should also look for tooth discoloration and tenderness of lymph nodes, gum tissue, and bone. But sometimes infection requiring a root canal can be present with virtually no symptoms at all.

Root Canal Procedure

Root canal treatment generally consists of the following steps:

- The endodontist examines the tooth and X-rays it. A local anesthetic is then administered, and a sheet known as a dental dam may be placed in the mouth to isolate the tooth and keep it free of saliva.

- The endodontist drills through the crown of the tooth and uses various tools to remove the pulp.

- The space is then shaped and cleaned before it is filled with a biocompatible material, such as a rubber-like substance called gutta-percha. It is placed with adhesive cement, completely sealing the chamber. The tooth is then covered with a temporary filling, which remains in place until the next office visit.

- In the next step, the dentist or endodontist will prepare the tooth for a crown or will perform other restorative workto provide normal tooth function.

- If the tooth is incapable of holding the restoration on its own, the endodontist will fix a post inside the tooth, which will serve as an anchor.

Root Canal Treatment and Pain

Modern anesthetics and techniques are generally able to ensure that little pain is felt during a root canal procedure. But after a root canal, the tooth and surrounding area may be sensitive. This can be treated by prescription medication or by over-the-counter pain relievers. However, if pain persists for more than a few days after the treatment, consult your endodontist immediately.

Cost of Root Canal Treatment

As with any medical treatment, the cost of a root canal can depend on the complexity of the procedure. For example, molars tend to be more difficult to treat than other teeth and thus might cost more. But most dental insurance policies cover endodontic procedures, and in any case, endodontic treatment and tooth restoration is likely to be less expensive than tooth extraction, because the latter involves the additional cost of fixing an implant or bridge at the site of the extraction to restore chewing function and prevent teeth from shifting.

After Root Canal Treatment

To avoid fracture or other damage, you must not bite or chew on food with the tooth that has undergone endodontic treatment until the restoration work has been done. After the procedure is complete, it is important to practice good, basic dental hygiene, like brushing, flossing, dental checkups, and cleaning.

The restored tooth should last for a long time. But in some cases, the treated tooth might not heal and could become infected again in the future. In some cases, new trauma, decay, or a crack may result in an infection in the treated tooth. Or the endodontist may discover that complicating factors caused the tooth to be treated improperly to begin with. In such cases, a second endodontic procedure may be able to save the tooth.

Endodontic Surgery

In cases where root canal treatment will not suffice, an endodontist may recommend surgery, which can often save a tooth by providing better access for treatment. Surgery can also help the endodontist make a diagnosis that might otherwise not be possible, since some conditions do not show up in diagnostics, such as X-rays. And in some cases, a tiny fracture or canal may remain undetected in nonsurgical treatment. With surgery, the endodontist will be able to make a more thorough inspection of the area and provide the required treatment.

In addition, it can become difficult to reach the end of the root with instruments in a root canal procedure if there is calcification in the canal. With endodontic surgery, a dentist will be able to reach the end of the root to clean and seal it properly. Or, after a root canal, the tooth might not heal fully and become infected. This could occur quite some time after successful treatment. Endodontic surgery is often required to save the tooth in such cases.

Finally, endodontic surgery isoften performed to treat damage to the root surface or the surrounding bone when no other type of treatment would be effective.

Apicoectomy

An apicoectomy, also called a root-end resection or root-end filling, is the most common type of oral surgery. It generally involves the following steps:

- The gum tissue around the tooth is opened and the underlying bone is exposed.

- Any inflamed or infected tissue is then removed, along with the end of the root.

- The end of the root canal is often sealed with a filling, and the gum tissue is sutured.

- The gum tissue generally heals in a few weeks, while it may take a few months for the bone to heal fully.

Other Types of Endodontic Surgery

Other endodontic surgical procedures include dividing a tooth in half, repairing injured roots, and removing the root. Another type of endodontic surgery, intentional replantation, involves extracting the tooth, then replacing it in the socket after an endodontic procedure has been completed.

Endodontic Surgery and Pain

Endodontic surgeries are usually done under local anesthesia and aregenerally not painful during the procedure. However, pain is typically felt during healing process. The endodontist will likely prescribe medication to alleviate the pain. You will also be given postoperative instructions to follow. Talk to your endodontist if you have any queries after surgery or if the pain does not respond to medication.

After Endodontic Surgery

In many cases, patients are able to drive themselves home after endodontic surgery. But if your surgeon suggests otherwise, be sure that you make suitable arrangements for transportation.

Most patients find that they are able return to work the next day, however recovery time and postoperative effects vary from individual to individual. The endodontist will discuss recovery time with you during your consultation.

Although successful healing and full recovery are typical, there are, of course, no guarantees with any type of medical or dental treatment, including surgery. A particular procedure is recommended by an endodontist because he or she believes it offers the best possible treatment option for saving your natural tooth. An endodontist will discuss the chances of success so that you are able to make an informed decision.

Cost of Endodontic Surgery

As with root canal treatment, the cost of endodontic surgery varies with the complexity of the procedure and a number of other factors. Some insurance plans cover certain types of treatment, while others do not. Talk to your employer or insurance company to learn if your particular surgery is covered under your plan.

Endodontic Retreatment

A tooth that has undergone endodontic treatment can last a lifetime with proper care. But when a treated tooth doesnot heal properly, becomes infected, and causes pain, a second procedure may be needed to save the tooth. If you experience pain or discomfort in a tooth that was previously treated, talk to your endodontist about retreatment.

Retreatment Procedure

The endodontist will first discuss the procedure with you. If retreatment is required, the endodontist will generally follow these steps:

- Reopen the tooth to get access to the filling in the root canals by disassembling the crown, post, and filling material.

- Once the filling has been removed, the endodontist examines the canals with magnification and illumination to assess their condition.

- The canals are then cleaned and sealed with a temporary filling. If the canals are very narrow or blocked, the endodontist may suggest endodontic surgery.

- Once the retreatment is complete, you will need to make additional visits for restoration procedures in order to regain full tooth function and appearance.

Why Endodontic Retreatment May Be Required

The best possible option always is to save your natural teeth. So even if initial treatment fails, retreatment may be able to allow teeth to function properly for many years. Technological improvements are always being made in endodontics, and it is possible that retreatment may be able to employ tools and techniques that didn't even exist just a few years ago.

If nonsurgical retreatment will be ineffective, then surgical retreatment may be necessary. This will entail a process similar to that of an initial endodontic surgery, including incision, assessment, cleaning, and stitches. Your endodontist will discuss the options and necessary treatment with you.

Cost of Endodontic Retreatment

Understandably, the cost of retreatment depends on the complexity of the condition. The endodontist will need to remove the filling, assess the previous work and the underlying structures, and then redo the procedure, or use an entirely different procedure. Therefore, retreatment will likely cost more than the initial procedure, especially if surgical retreatment is necessary.

Dental insurance may cover the expenses for all or part of retreatment, but some plans cover just the initial endodontic procedure. Your employer or insurance company can help clarify this.

Alternatives to Endodontic Treatment

Tooth extraction is generally the only alternative to endodontic treatment. Once a tooth has been extracted, it must be replaced with a bridge, implant, or a partially removable denture to restore chewing function and to prevent adjacent teeth from shifting. Since extraction involves additional procedures to maintain tooth function, endodontic treatment is usually the best option, from a cost perspective, as well as for utility and appearance. Although, artificial teeth can be very effective, nothing is better than having natural teeth, and an endodontic procedure can help you retain those teeth for a long time.

References

1. "Endodontic Surgery Explained," American Association of Endodontists, n.d.

2. "Root Canals Explained," American Association of Endodontists, n.d.

3. "Endodontic Retreatment Explained," American Association of Endodontists, n.d.

4. "An Overview of Root Canals," WebMD, June 10, 2016.

5. Horne, Steven B., DDS. "Root Canal," MedicineNet, n.d.

6. "Oral Surgery," WebMD, July 28, 2016.

Chapter 31

Periodontal (Gum) Disease

Chapter Contents

Section 31.1

Facts about Periodontal Disease

This section includes text excerpted from "Gum
(Periodontal) Disease," NIHSeniorHealth, National
Institutes of Health (NIH), March 2013.

Gum (Periodontal) Disease: An Overview

An Infection of the Gums and Surrounding Tissues

Gum (periodontal) disease is an infection of the gums and surrounding tissues that hold teeth in place. The two forms of gum disease are gingivitis, a mild form that is reversible with good oral hygiene, and periodontitis, a more severe form that can damage the soft tissues and bone that support teeth. If left untreated, periodontitis can lead to tooth loss.

In its early stages, gum disease is usually painless, and many people are not aware that they have it. In more advanced cases, gum disease can cause sore gums and pain when chewing.

Not a Normal Part of Aging

The good news is that gum disease can be prevented. It does not have to be a part of growing older. With thorough brushing and flossing and regular professional cleanings by your dentist, you can reduce your risk of developing gum disease as you age. If you have been treated for gum disease, sticking to a proper oral hygiene routine and visiting your dentist for regular cleanings can minimize the chances that it will come back.

Plaque Buildup Can Form Tartar

Gum disease is typically caused by poor brushing and flossing habits that allow dental plaque—a sticky film of bacteria—to build up on the teeth. Plaque that is not removed can harden and form tartar that brushing doesn't clean. Only a professional cleaning by a dentist or dental hygienist can remove tartar.

Gum disease can range from simple gum inflammation to serious disease. The two forms of gum disease are gingivitis and periodontitis.

Gingivitis and Periodontitis

In gingivitis, the gums become red, swollen and can bleed easily. Gingivitis can usually be reversed with daily brushing and flossing, and regular cleaning by a dentist or dental hygienist. This form of gum disease does not include any loss of bone and tissue that hold teeth in place.

When gingivitis is not treated, it can advance to periodontitis. In periodontitis, gums pull away from the teeth and form spaces (called "pockets") that become infected. The body's immune system fights the bacteria as the plaque spreads and grows below the gum line. Bacterial toxins and the body's natural response to infection start to break down the bone and connective tissue that hold teeth in place. If not treated, the bones, gums, and tissue that support the teeth are destroyed. The teeth may eventually become loose and may have to be removed.

Section 31.2

Older Adults and Gum Disease

This section includes text excerpted from "Gum (Periodontal) Disease," NIHSeniorHealth, National Institutes of Health (NIH), March 2013.

What Is Gum (Periodontal) Disease?

Gum disease is an infection of the tissues that hold your teeth in place. In its early stages, it is usually painless, and many people are not aware that they have it. But in more advanced stages, gum disease can lead to sore or bleeding gums, painful chewing problems, and even tooth loss.

Is Gum Disease a Normal Part of Aging?

No, gum disease does not have to be a part of growing older. With proper dental hygiene and regular dental visits, people can reduce their chance of developing periodontal disease as they age.

What Happens If Gum Disease Is Not Treated?

If left untreated, gum disease can lead to tooth loss. Gum disease is the leading cause of tooth loss in older adults.

Can Gum Disease Cause Problems beyond the Mouth?

In some studies, researchers have observed that people with periodontal disease (when compared to people without periodontal disease) were more likely to develop heart disease or have difficulty controlling their blood sugar. But so far, it has not been determined whether periodontal disease is the cause of these conditions.

There may be other reasons people with periodontal disease sometimes develop additional health problems. For example, something else may be causing both the gum disease and the other condition, or it could be a coincidence that gum disease and other health problems are present together.

More research is needed to clarify whether gum disease actually causes health problems beyond the mouth, and whether treating gum disease can keep other health conditions from developing.

In the meantime, it's a fact that controlling periodontal disease can save your teeth—a very good reason to take care of your teeth and gums.

Are There Ways to Prevent Gum Disease?

Yes, you can prevent gum disease with proper dental hygiene and regular cleanings by your dentist or dental hygienist. Specifically, you should:

- brush your teeth twice a day (with a fluoride toothpaste).

- floss regularly to remove plaque from between teeth. Or use a device such as a special pick recommended by a dental professional.

- visit the dentist routinely for a check-up and professional cleaning.

- not smoke.

- eat a well-balanced diet.

If I Have Trouble Cleaning My Teeth and Gums Because of Arthritis or a Physical Disability, What Can I Do?

If your hands have become stiff because of arthritis or if you have a physical disability, you may find it difficult to use your toothbrush or dental floss. The following tips might make it easier for you to clean your teeth and gums:

- Make the toothbrush easier to hold. The same kind of Velcro® strap used to hold food utensils is helpful for some people.

- Make the toothbrush handle bigger. You can cut a small slit in the side of a tennis ball and slide it onto the handle of the toothbrush.

- You can also buy a toothbrush with a large handle, or you can slide a bicycle grip onto the handle. Attaching foam tubing, available from home healthcare catalogs, is also helpful.

- Try other toothbrush options. A power toothbrush might make brushing easier. Some people may find that it takes time to get used to a power toothbrush.

- A floss holder can make it easier to hold the dental floss.

Also, talk with your dentist about whether an oral irrigation system, special small brushes, or other instruments that clean between teeth are right for you. Be sure to check with your dentist, though, before using any of these methods since they may injure the gums if used improperly.

Are Medications Used to Treat Gum Disease?

Medications may be used with treatment that includes scaling and root planing. Depending on how far the disease has progressed, the dentist or periodontist may also suggest surgical treatment. Long-term studies are needed to find out if using medications reduces the need for surgery and whether they are effective over a long period of time.

When Is Surgery Used to Treat Gum Disease?

Surgery might be necessary if inflammation and deep pockets remain following treatment with deep cleaning and medications.

A periodontist may perform flap surgery to remove tartar deposits in deep pockets or to reduce the periodontal pocket and make it easier for the patient, dentist, and hygienist to keep the area clean. This common surgery involves lifting back the gums and removing the tartar. The gums are then sutured back in place so that the tissue fits snugly around the tooth again.

Section 31.3

Causes and Risk Factors of Gum Disease

This section includes text excerpted from "Periodontal (Gum) Disease: Causes, Symptoms, and Treatments," National Institute of Dental and Craniofacial Research (NIDCR), September 2013.

If you have been told you have periodontal (gum) disease, you're not alone. Many adults in the United States have some form of the disease. Periodontal diseases range from simple gum inflammation to serious disease that results in major damage to the soft tissue and bone that support the teeth. In the worst cases, teeth are lost. Whether your gum disease is stopped, slowed or gets worse depends a great deal on how well you care for your teeth and gums every day, from this point forward.

What Causes Gum Disease?

Our mouths are full of bacteria. These bacteria, along with mucus and other particles, constantly form a sticky, colorless "plaque" on teeth. Brushing and flossing help get rid of plaque. Plaque that is not removed can harden and form "tartar" that brushing doesn't clean. Only a professional cleaning by a dentist or dental hygienist can remove tartar.

Gingivitis

The longer plaque and tartar are on teeth, the more harmful they become. The bacteria cause inflammation of the gums that is called "gingivitis." In gingivitis, the gums become red, swollen and can bleed easily. Gingivitis is a mild form of gum disease that can usually be reversed with daily brushing and flossing, and regular cleaning by a dentist or dental hygienist. This form of gum disease does not include any loss of bone and tissue that hold teeth in place.

Periodontitis

When gingivitis is not treated, it can advance to "periodontitis" (which means "inflammation around the tooth"). In periodontitis, gums pull away from the teeth and form spaces (called "pockets") that become infected. The body's immune system fights the bacteria as the plaque spreads and grows below the gum line. Bacterial toxins and the body's natural response to infection start to break down the bone and connective tissue that hold teeth in place. If not treated, the bones, gums, and tissue that support the teeth are destroyed. The teeth may eventually become loose and have to be removed.

Risk Factors

- **Smoking.** Need another reason to quit smoking? Smoking is one of the most significant risk factors associated with the development of gum disease. Additionally, smoking can lower the chances for successful treatment.

- **Hormonal changes in girls/women.** These changes can make gums more sensitive and make it easier for gingivitis to develop.

- **Diabetes.** People with diabetes are at higher risk for developing infections, including gum disease.

- **Other illnesses and their treatments.** Diseases such as AIDS and its treatments can also negatively affect the health of gums, as can treatments for cancer.

- **Medications.** There are hundreds of prescription and over the counter medications that can reduce the flow of saliva, which has a protective effect on the mouth. Without enough saliva, the mouth is vulnerable to infections such as gum disease. And some medicines can cause abnormal overgrowth of the gum tissue; this can make it difficult to keep teeth and gums clean.

- **Genetic susceptibility.** Some people are more prone to severe gum disease than others.

Who Gets Gum Disease?

People usually don't show signs of gum disease until they are in their 30s or 40s. Men are more likely to have gum disease than women. Although teenagers rarely develop periodontitis, they can develop gingivitis, the milder form of gum disease. Most commonly, gum disease develops when plaque is allowed to build up along and under the gum line.

How Do I Know If I Have Gum Disease?

Symptoms of gum disease include:

• Bad breath that won't go away

• Red or swollen gums

• Tender or bleeding gums

• Painful chewing

• Loose teeth

• Sensitive teeth

• Receding gums or longer appearing teeth

Any of these symptoms may be a sign of a serious problem, which should be checked by a dentist. At your dental visit the dentist or hygienist should:

• Ask about your medical history to identify underlying conditions or risk factors (such as smoking) that may contribute to gum disease.

• Examine your gums and note any signs of inflammation.

• Use a tiny ruler called a "probe" to check for and measure any pockets. In a healthy mouth, the depth of these pockets is usually between 1 and 3 millimeters. This test for pocket depth is usually painless.

The dentist or hygienist may also:

• Take an X-ray to see whether there is any bone loss.

• Refer you to a periodontist. Periodontists are experts in the diagnosis and treatment of gum disease and may provide you with treatment options that are not offered by your dentist.

How Can I Keep My Teeth and Gums Healthy?

- Brush your teeth twice a day (with a fluoride toothpaste).

- Floss regularly to remove plaque from between teeth. Or use a device such as a special brush or wooden or plastic pick recommended by a dental professional.

- Visit the dentist routinely for a check-up and professional cleaning.

- Don't smoke.

Section 31.4

Treatment of Gum Disease

This section includes text excerpted from "Gum (Periodontal) Disease," NIHSeniorHealth, National Institutes of Health (NIH), March 2013.

Controlling the Infection

The main goal of treatment is to control the infection. The number and types of treatment will vary, depending on how far the disease has advanced. Any type of treatment requires the patient to keep up good daily care at home. The doctor may also suggest changing certain behaviors, such as quitting smoking, as a way to improve treatment outcome.

Treatments may include deep cleaning, medications, surgery, and bone and tissue grafts.

Deep Cleaning (Scaling and Planing)

In deep cleaning, the dentist, periodontist or dental hygienist removes the plaque through a method called scaling and root planing. Scaling means scraping off the tartar from above and below the gum line. Root planing gets rid of rough spots on the tooth root where the germs gather, and helps remove bacteria that contribute to the disease.

In some cases a laser may be used to remove plaque and tartar. This procedure can result in less bleeding, swelling, and discomfort compared to traditional deep cleaning methods.

Medications

Medications may be used with treatment that includes scaling and root planing, but they cannot always take the place of surgery. Depending on how far the disease has progressed, the dentist or periodontist may still suggest surgical treatment. Long-term studies are needed to find out if using medications reduces the need for surgery and whether they are effective over a long period of time.

Table: 31.1. Medications for Gum Disease

Medications	What is it?	Why is it used?	How is it used?
Prescription antimicrobial mouthrinse	A prescription mouthrinse containing an antimicrobial called chlorhexidine	To control bacteria when treating gingivitis and after gum surgery	It's used like a regular mouthwash.
Antiseptic chip	A tiny piece of gelatin filled with the medicine chlorhexidine	To control bacteria and reduce the size of periodontal pockets	After root planing, it's placed in the pockets where the medicine is slowly released over time.
Antibiotic gel	A gel that contains the antibiotic doxycycline	To control bacteria and reduce the size of periodontal pockets	The periodontist puts it in the pockets after scaling and root planing. The antibiotic is released slowly over a period of about seven days.
Antibiotic microspheres	Tiny, round particles that contain the antibiotic minocycline	To control bacteria and reduce the size of periodontal pockets	The periodontist puts the microspheres into the pockets after scaling and root planing. The particles release minocycline slowly over time.

Table: 31.1. Continued

Medications	What is it?	Why is it used?	How is it used?
Enzyme suppressant	A low dose of the medication doxycycline that keeps destructive enzymes in check	To hold back the body's enzyme response — If not controlled, certain enzymes can break down gum tissue	This medication is in tablet form. It is used in combination with scaling and root planing.
Oral antibiotics	Antibiotic tablets or capsules	For the short term treatment of an acute or locally persistent periodontal infection	These come as tablets or capsules and are taken by mouth.

Flap Surgery

Surgery might be necessary if inflammation and deep pockets remain following treatment with deep cleaning and medications. A dentist or periodontist may perform flap surgery to remove tartar deposits in deep pockets or to reduce the periodontal pocket and make it easier for the patient, dentist, and hygienist to keep the area clean. This common surgery involves lifting back the gums and removing the tartar. The gums are then sutured back in place so that the tissue fits snugly around the tooth again. After surgery, the gums will shrink to fit more tightly around the tooth. This sometimes results in the teeth appearing longer.

Bone and Tissue Grafts

In addition to flap surgery, your periodontist or dentist may suggest procedures to help regenerate any bone or gum tissue lost to periodontitis.

- **Bone grafting**, in which natural or synthetic bone is placed in the area of bone loss, can help promote bone growth. A technique that can be used with bone grafting is called guided tissue regeneration. In this procedure, a small piece of mesh-like material is inserted between the bone and gum tissue. This keeps the gum tissue from growing into the area where the bone should be, allowing the bone and connective tissue to regrow.

- **Growth factors**—proteins that can help your body naturally regrow bone—may also be used. In cases where gum tissue has been lost, your dentist or periodontist may suggest a soft tissue graft, in which synthetic material or tissue taken from another area of your mouth is used to cover exposed tooth roots.

Since each case is different, it is not possible to predict with certainty which grafts will be successful over the long-term. Treatment results depend on many things, including how far the disease has progressed, how well the patient keeps up with oral care at home, and certain risk factors, such as smoking, which may lower the chances of success. Ask your periodontist what the level of success might be in your particular case.

Treatment Results

Treatment results depend on many things, including how far the disease has progressed, how well the patient keeps up with home care, and certain risk factors, such as smoking, which may lower the chances of success. Ask your periodontist what the likelihood of success might be in your particular case.

Consider Getting a Second Opinion

When considering any extensive dental or medical treatment options, you should think about getting a second opinion. To find a dentist or periodontist for a second opinion, call your local dental society. They can provide you with names of practitioners in your area. Also, dental schools may sometimes be able to offer a second opinion. Call the dental school in your area to find out whether it offers this service.

Section 31.5

Public Health Implications of Chronic Periodontal Infections in Adults

This section includes text excerpted from "Public Health Implications of Chronic Periodontal Infections in Adults," Centers for Disease Control and Prevention (CDC), July 10, 2013.

Periodontitis is a chronic infectious disease that affects approximately 34% of the U.S. population over age 30 (about 36 million persons), and it a major cause of tooth loss in about 13% of adults. The disease begins as an acute inflammation of the gingival tissue known as gingivitis, manifested by bleeding, especially during tooth brushing. In susceptible individuals, gingivitis progresses to periodontitis, in which the destructive inflammatory process extends into the deeper periodontal tissues. Clinical signs of periodontitis are gingival bleeding, loss of periodontal attachment as detected by increasing probing depth around the necks of the teeth, and radiographic loss of alveolar bone. As the disease advances, the teeth may become loose, periodontal abscesses may form, and the affected teeth may be lost.

Periodontitis is caused by a small group of predominantly gram-negative anaerobic bacteria among which Porphyromonas gingivalis is especially important. Biofilms containing these pathogenic bacteria form on the tooth surfaces and extend apically between the surface of the tooth root and gingiva to cause a destructive inflammation that destroys the attachment of gingival tissue to the tooth. Consequently, periodontal pockets form and collagenous fibers of the periodontal ligament and the bony housing of the tooth roots are destroyed.

Lipopolysaccharide, antigenic bacterial components, and intact bacteria have ready access through the ulcerated pocket wall into the inflamed tissue, where they may enter the circulation and become systemically disseminated. Bacteria and their components stimulate a dense infiltrate of inflammatory cells including neutrophilic granulocytes, macrophages, and lymphoid cells. Bacterial substances activate macrophages and neutrophilic granulocytes to produce and release large quantities of proinflammatory cytokines and prostanoids especially interleukin-1 (IL-1), tumor necrosis factor-alpha (TNF-alpha), prostaglandin E2 (PGE2) and matrix metalloproteinases. Resident connective tissue fibroblasts also are involved in this process. Binding of the C1 component of complement and cytokines such as IL-1 and TNF-alpha causes the fibroblasts to contribute to the growing concentrations of proinflammatory cytokines, prostaglandins, and matrix metalloproteinases. PGE2 mediates alveolar bone destruction, and the matrix metalloproteinases destroy the collagens and other connective tissue components of the gingiva and periodontal ligament.

A growing body of evidence suggests that periodontitis, in addition to being a major cause of tooth loss in adults, also enhances risk for several potentially deadly systemic diseases and conditions. This enhanced risk may be related to the systemic dissemination of gram-negative anaerobic bacteria and their components present in subgingival biofilms as well as inflammatory mediators that reach very high levels in the diseased periodontal tissues.

Chapter 32

Dental Implants

Dental implants are metal posts or frames that are surgically implanted in the gums. They fuse to the jawbone and serve as permanent anchors or roots for dental prosthetics—including crowns, bridges, and dentures—that replace missing natural teeth.

Dental implants offer many advantages over conventional tooth-replacement techniques. Most patients find that bridges and dentures placed on implants fit securely, feel comfortable and natural, and do not shift while eating or speaking. Ordinary dentures that rest on top of the gums, in contrast, often affect speech, create problems while eating, or cause sore gums by moving around. An advantage over ordinary bridges is that dental implants do not require adjacent teeth to be ground down in order to provide an attachment point to hold the replacement teeth in place.

Dental implants also play an important role in stabilizing and preserving the alveolar bone in the jaw. When teeth are missing, the underlying bone that once connected and supported them breaks down as part of a natural process called resorption. Studies have shown that the bone width can decrease by 25% in the first year after a tooth is lost. As the bone loss progresses, it can lead to aesthetic and functional problems in the mouth. Dental implants fuse to the bone and provide stimulation that helps to keep the bone healthy and strong.

The main disadvantage of dental implants is their cost, which is generally higher than other methods of tooth replacement and not as likely to be covered by insurance. In addition, to be eligible to receive dental

"Dental Implants," © 2017 Omnigraphics. Reviewed September 2016.

implants, a patient must be in good health and have adequate bone to support the implants. Medical conditions such as uncontrolled gum disease, diabetes, or cancer—as well as lifestyle factors such as smoking or alcoholism—can prevent dental implants from fusing to the bone. Finally, patients who receive dental implants must commit to practicing good oral hygiene and making regular dental visits to keep the structures healthy.

Getting Dental Implants

Getting dental implants is a multi-step process that involves a team of specialists. The implant dentistry team is likely to include a periodontist, oral surgeon, or general dentist with training in implant surgery; a dental laboratory technician with training in fabrication of crowns, bridgework, and dentures that attach to implants; and a restorative dentist with training in planning and placing tooth restorations. The team works together to assess and plan the placement of the dental implants and the design of the tooth restorations.

To begin the process, the team will typically conduct a detailed assessment of the patient's teeth, jaws, and bite to determine the exact positioning of the dental implants. This assessment will likely involve specialized X-rays and computerized tomography (CT) scans to create a three-dimensional model of the patient's mouth. Once the assessment is complete, the periodontist uses the information to guide the precise surgical placement of the implants. Channels are created in the jawbone, and metal posts are fitted into the sites. In cases where resorption of the bone has occurred, additional surgery may be needed to graft bone into tooth sockets or regenerate bone that has been lost in order to provide a sufficient base for anchoring the implants.

The bone will generally fuse with the implants within two to six months of the surgery. Temporary healing caps may be placed on the implants until they are fully fused. At that point, tooth restorations are fabricated in a dental laboratory to match the patient's existing teeth. Finally, the artificial teeth are screwed or cemented onto the implants. Once the restorations are attached, they are virtually indistinguishable in appearance and function from the patient's original teeth.

Types of Dental Implants

There are two main types of dental implants:

1. Endosteal implants
2. Subperiosteal implants.

Endosteal implants are artificial roots or anchors that are surgically placed into the jawbone. Once they fuse with the bone and the surrounding gum tissue heals, metal posts are connected to the implants to hold tooth restorations.

Subperiosteal implants consist of a metal frame that is surgically fitted on the jawbone beneath the gum tissue. Once the frame fuses with the jawbone, metal posts are attached to it to hold tooth restorations.

Dental implants can be used to replace a single tooth, multiple teeth, or an entire upper or lower set of teeth. In single-tooth replacement, a single implant serves as the anchor for a custom-made, artificial tooth form called a crown. In multiple-tooth replacement, multiple implants serve as the anchors for a permanent, custom-made bridge that contains several artificial teeth. For patients who are missing all of their upper or lower teeth, four to six implants may be used to support a removable denture that snaps or clips into place.

Since dental implants are made of metal, they are not subject to dental decay in the same way as the roots of natural teeth. In addition, crowns, bridges, and other prosthetic tooth restorations can be replaced by a dentist if they suffer excessive wear or damage without affecting the implants supporting them. However, people with dental implants must commit to practicing good oral hygiene to control bacterial biofilm on the tissues surrounding the implants. Otherwise, the patient may develop an inflammatory response called peri-implantitis, which can cause disintegration of the bone surrounding the implant. Finally, people with dental implants must visit a dentist regularly to ensure the continued stability and function of the implants.

References

1. "Understanding Dental Implants." ICOI, 2016.

2. "What Are Dental Implants?" Colgate Oral Care Center, 2016.

3. "What Types of Dental Implants Are Available?" Gordon West, DDS, 2013.

Chapter 33

Facial Trauma

Facial trauma describes any type of injury to the face, ranging from cuts and bruises to fractures of facial bones, such as the jaw, nose, eye socket, cheek, or forehead. Some of the most common causes of facial trauma include sports injuries, automobile and motorcycle accidents, falls, and violence. Children sustain facial injuries more frequently than adults, but they are less likely to break facial bones.

Symptoms of Facial Trauma

Although many facial injuries are minor, they should always be taken seriously. After all, the face plays a critical role in breathing, eating, speaking, and seeing, as well as personal identity and self-esteem. Prompt treatment of a facial laceration by a cosmetic surgeon, for instance, may prevent the formation of an embarrassing or disfiguring scar. In addition, facial trauma often coincides with injuries to the head, spine, eye, mouth, or teeth, so people who show symptoms of facial trauma should also be evaluated for signs of concussion or other potentially serious injuries.

Some of the common symptoms of facial trauma include bleeding, swelling, bruising, numbness, and facial bones that appear uneven or out of place. If these symptoms are severe, or are accompanied by any of the following symptoms, the patient should seek immediate medical attention:

- loss of consciousness
- seizure

"Facial Trauma," © 2017 Omnigraphics. Reviewed September 2016.

- weakness, numbness, or tingling on one side of the body
- severe headache
- dizziness, light headedness, or trouble standing or walking
- confusion, irritability, or abnormal behavior
- eye pain or vision problems, such as blurring or double vision
- ear pain or hearing problems
- missing teeth, tooth pain, or trouble chewing
- pain or other symptoms that get worse rather than steadily improving

Treatment of Facial Injuries

Minor facial injuries can often be treated at home using basic first aid techniques. To stop bleeding, put firm but gentle pressure on the wound with a sterile gauze pad or clean cloth. Avoid taking aspirin, which may prolong bleeding. Apply an ice or cold pack to relieve pain and minimize swelling. Avoid things that might increase swelling—such as heating pads, hot showers, or drinking hot fluids—for the first 48 hours. Keep the head of the bed elevated while sleeping. Avoid smoking, which can prolong the healing process.

More serious facial injuries should be examined by a physician or treated in an emergency room. An X-ray or computerized tomography (CT) scan of the head and neck may be used to check for fractures in the facial bones. Treatment of facial trauma depends on the location, type, and severity of the injury, as well as the overall health condition of the patient. Surgery may be needed if the injury affects the normal functioning of the eyes, nose, or mouth or if the injury poses a risk of scarring or deformity.

Fractures of the jaw, palate, or cheekbones may require treatment by an oral and maxillofacial surgeon to restore the patient's ability to speak, chew, and swallow. Wiring or plating techniques may be used to hold the facial bones in the correct position until they heal. The jaws may be wired shut for up to six weeks, during which time the patient will need to eat a nutritional liquid or pureed diet.

Prevention of Facial Trauma

Many facial injuries are preventable with proper attention to safety. Some tips for reducing the risk of facial trauma include the following:

- wear seatbelts and place children in age-appropriate car safety seats

- wear a helmet while participating in such activities as bicycling, skateboarding, skiing, snowboarding, horseback riding, or rock climbing

- wear a mouth guard while participating in contact sports

- wear appropriate protective clothing, such as safety goggles, face shields, or hard hats, while working with power tools

- remove loose rugs, fix loose boards, and remove other hazards that could cause a fall in the home

- never keep loaded guns in the home

- never dive into shallow water

- use child safety gates to prevent children from falling down stairs

- never allow children to walk around while using a bottle or sippy cup

- never leave babies or toddlers unattended on a couch, bed, table, porch, or deck

References

1. "Facial Injuries," WebMD, November 14, 2014.

2. Jothi, Sumana. "Facial Trauma," MedlinePlus, August 5, 2015.

3. "Treatment of Facial Injuries," American Association of Oral and Maxillofacial Surgeons, 2016.

Chapter 34

Corrective Jaw Surgery

Corrective jaw surgery—formally known as orthognathic surgery—is performed to address skeletal and dental irregularities that cannot be remedied through orthodontic treatment alone. In most cases, corrective jaw surgery is used to adjust the supporting bones of the jaw so that fixed orthodontic braces can effectively align the teeth and bite. Orthognathic surgery can correct a varietyof functional problems affecting the teeth and jaws, leading to improvements in chewing, speaking, and breathing as well as appearance. It is performed by an oral and maxillofacial surgeon, a specialist whose training includes four years of surgical residency in addition to four years of dental school.

Some of the problems that are commonly treated with corrective jaw surgery include the following:

- severe under bites or overbites

- congenital abnormalities or birth defects affecting jaw development, such as cleft palate

- facial asymmetries or unbalanced facial appearance

- protruding jaw or receding chin

- chronic jaw or temporomandibular joint (TMJ) pain

- difficulty in biting, chewing, or swallowing food

- facial injury or trauma

- chronic mouth breathing or dry mouth
- obstructive sleep apnea

Undergoing Corrective Jaw Surgery

Patients are likely to be referred to an oral and maxillofacial surgeon for corrective jaw surgery by a dentist or orthodontist who has determined that an irregularity in the structure of the jaws makes it impossible for orthodontic treatment alone to provide effective results. The process of orthognathic surgery begins with consultation and planning among members of the dental team, including the oral and maxillofacial surgeon, the orthodontist, and the general or restorative dentist. These professionals will use diagnostic imaging to create three-dimensional models of the patient's mouth and jaws to develop a step-by-step treatment plan.

In preparation for orthognathic surgery, most patients will have fixed orthodontic braces installed to align their teeth and move them into the best possible position for the necessary surgical adjustment to the jaws. The braces are typically applied around 18 months prior to the surgery and remain in place both during and after the procedure. In some cases, patients may also need to have their wisdom teeth extracted prior to surgery if they obstruct the area of the jaw on which the surgeon will be operating. Two weeks before the surgery date, the orthodontist will attach hooks to the braces to facilitate the procedure.

Corrective jaw surgery generally involves making a planned fracture of the jaw in order to reset the bone in a new position. Small plates and screws are inserted into the bone to hold it in the desired position. Wires or strong elastic bands may also be used to help maintain the new jaw position and guide the teeth into alignment. Since the work is completed inside the mouth, there are usually no visible scars on the patient's face. The procedure generally takes 3 to 6 hours. It is usually performed in a hospital with the patient under general anesthesia, although in some cases it may be performed in the oral and maxillofacial surgeon's office. Depending on the complexity of the procedure, the patient may remain in the hospital for 2 to 3 days.

Recovering from Corrective Jaw Surgery

Immediately after undergoing corrective jaw surgery, patients are likely to experience jaw soreness and stiffness and facial swelling. Pain medications are usually prescribed for the first few weeks to reduce the discomfort. Since it takes 4 to 6 weeks for bones in the jaw to heal, patients who undergo orthognathic surgery cannot chew solid food and must follow a nutritional liquid or pureed diet. They should also practice good oral hygiene to reduce the risk of infection and avoid smoking or drinking alcohol, which can prolong the healing process.

Many patients who have surgery on their lower jaw experience numbness in the lower lip or chin, while patients who have surgery on their upper jaw may experience numbness in the upper lip or cheek. The numbness is usually temporary, but it is important to avoid biting or burning the lips during this time. Patients may experience a tingling sensation as the feeling gradually returns to the area over the course of several weeks.

Many patients need at least four weeks of recovery time before they can return to work or school.

In addition, people who have orthognathic surgery may need to avoid air travel for at least six weeks due to potential complications from changes in air pressure. Finally, patients should avoid playing contact sports or doing other activities that put strain on the jaw for at least 10 to 12 weeks following surgery.

Beginning about one week after undergoing corrective jaw surgery, patients must make regular visits to the orthodontist to check and adjust the fixed braces. The braces will remain in place for 6 to 9 months after the surgery to further align the teeth and prevent the jaw from moving back to its original position. Even after the braces are removed, the patient will likely need to wear retainers to maintain the alignment of the teeth and jaw. In most cases the plates and screws that were inserted by the oral surgeon will remain in place for life.

References

1. "Corrective Jaw Surgery." Christopher M. Brieden, DDS, 2016.

2. "What Is Corrective Jaw Surgery?" NHS Foundation Trust, 2016.

Part Five

Oral Diseases and Disorders

Chapter 35

Bad Breath (Halitosis)

You lean over to whisper something to your friend and you can tell by the look on your friend's face that something is up. Could it be your breath? Maybe you shouldn't have put extra onions on your hamburger at lunch. What's one with smelly breath to do?

The good news is that bad breath happens to everyone once in a while. Let's find out how to detect it, prevent it, and even treat it.

What's That Smell?

Bad breath is the common name for the medical condition known as halitosis. Many different things can cause halitosis—from not brushing your teeth to certain medical conditions.

Sometimes, a person's bad breath can blow you away—and he or she may not realize there's a problem. There are tactful (nice) ways of letting someone know about bad breath. You could offer mints or sugarless gum without having to say anything.

If you need to tell a friend he or she has bad breath, you could say that you understand foods can cause bad breath because you've had it before yourself. By letting someone know that bad breath isn't something unusual, you'll make your friend feel more comfortable and less embarrassed about accepting your piece of chewing gum.

This chapter contains text excerpted from the following sources: Text in this chapter begins with excerpts from "Bad Breath," © 1995–2016. The Nemours Foundation/KidsHealth®; Text beginning with the heading "Tips for Preventing Bad Breath" is excerpted from "Bad Breath," Office on Women's Health (OWH), U.S. Department of Health and Human Services (HHS), April 15, 2014.

If you suspect your own breath is foul, ask someone who will give you an honest answer without making fun of you. (Just don't ask your brother or sister—they just might tell you your breath stinks even when it doesn't!)

Although everyone gets bad breath sometimes, if you have bad breath a lot, you may need to visit your dentist or doctor.

What Causes Bad Breath?

Here are three common causes of bad breath:

1. foods and drinks, such as garlic, onions, cheese, orange juice, and soda

2. poor dental hygiene, meaning not brushing and flossing regularly

3. smoking and other tobacco use

Poor oral hygiene leads to bad breath because when food particles are left in your mouth, they can rot and start to smell. The food bits may begin to collect bacteria, which can be smelly, too.

Not brushing your teeth regularly will let plaque (a sticky, colorless film) build up on your teeth. Plaque is a great place for bacteria to live and yet another reason why breath can turn foul.

Tips for Preventing Bad Breath

- **Brush your teeth** (and tongue!) for at least two minutes twice a day with fluoride toothpaste, especially after meals and at bedtime.

- **Ask your dentist how to floss correctly.** Flossing can remove tiny bits of food that can rot and smell bad.

- **Replace your toothbrush** every three to four months.

- **Visit your dentist twice a year.** He or she will help keep your teeth and your mouth healthy.

- **Eat smart.** Avoid foods and drinks that can leave behind strong smells, like cabbage, garlic, raw onions, and coffee. If you're trying to lose weight, remember that not eating enough or cutting out certain foods (such as carbohydrates) can cause bad breath.

- **Don't smoke!** You'll smell sweeter—and be lots healthier.

- **Drink enough fluids.** Drinking helps wash away tiny bits of food and bacteria, which can smell bad.

If your bad breath doesn't go away, be sure to talk to your dentist, doctor, or nurse. It could be a sign of a medical problem, such as a sinus infection or gum disease. You may feel a little funny talking about bad breath, but it's very common and you can get help.

Tips for Keeping Your Mouth Healthy

A lot of the tips for keeping your mouth healthy are the same as the tips for stopping bad breath, such as brushing and flossing. Below are some more tips for good oral hygiene, which is just a fancy way to say taking care of your teeth and mouth. Do you feel like they are a pain? Well, they are a lot less of a pain than the dentist's drill!

- **Eat smart.** Avoid sugary foods and drinks. This helps prevent damage to your teeth and is great for your overall health.

- **Brush after sweets.** If you eat or drink sugary stuff, try to brush right after. If you can't brush, at least rinse your mouth with water.

- **Definitely don't smoke.** Smoking doesn't just smell bad and stain your teeth. It also can increase your risk of gum disease and tooth decay.

Chapter 36

Burning Mouth Syndrome (BMS)

What Is Burning Mouth Syndrome (BMS)?[1]

Burning mouth syndrome (BMS) is characterized by long-lasting burning sensations of the mouth. The pain may affect the tongue, gums, lips, palate, throat, or the entire mouth. Burning mouth syndrome may be primary or secondary. Experts believe that the primary form may be caused by damage to the nerves that control pain and taste. The secondary form is caused by an underlying medical condition. In many cases, the underlying cause in unknown. Treatment depends on the symptoms present and aims to control them.

What Are the Symptoms of Burning Mouth Syndrome?[1]

Symptoms of burning mouth syndrome may include severe burning or tingling in the mouth which may persist or come and go over the course of months to years. The tongue is usually affected, but the pain may also be in the lips, gums, palate, throat or whole mouth. The

This chapter contains text excerpted from documents published by two public domain sources. Text under headings marked 1 are excerpted from "Burning Mouth Syndrome," Genetic and Rare Diseases (GARD) Information Center, National Institutes of Health (NIH), March 28, 2016; Text under headings marked 2 are excerpted from "Burning Mouth Syndrome," National Institute of Dental and Craniofacial Research (NIDCR), April 2015.

burning sensation may be absent in the morning and increase over the course of the day, start first thing in the morning and last all day, or come and go all day long. For many, the pain is reduced when eating or drinking. Other symptoms may include a sensation of dry mouth with increased thirst, a bitter or metallic taste, or loss of taste.

What Causes Burning Mouth Syndrome?[1]

Burning mouth syndrome can be primary or secondary. Some research suggests that primary burning mouth syndrome is caused by damage to the nerves that control pain and taste. Secondary burning mouth syndrome is usually caused by an underlying medical condition. Some of the problems that have been linked to secondary burning mouth syndrome include:

- Dry mouth, which can be caused by various medications or underlying health problems

- Other oral conditions, such as fungal infections, oral lichen planus, or geographic tongue

- Nutritional deficiencies, such as lack of iron, zinc, folic acid, thiamin, riboflavin, pyridoxine, and cobalamin

- Dentures, especially if they don't fit well and irritate the mouth

- Allergies or reactions to foods, additives, dyes or dental work

- Certain medications, in particular those for high blood pressure

- Oral habits such as tooth grinding, tongue thrusting, or biting of the tongue

- Endocrine disorders, such as diabetes or hypothyroidism

- Excessive mouth irritation which may result from over-brushing, use of abrasive toothpastes, overuse of mouthwashes, or drinking too many acidic drinks

- Psychological factors, such as anxiety, depression, or stress

For many people, the underlying cause of burning mouth syndrome can not be identified.

Diagnosis[2]

BMS is hard to diagnose. One reason is that people with BMS often don't have a mouth problem that the doctor or dentist can see during an exam. Your dentist or doctor may refer you to a specialist. Specialists who diagnose BMS include dentists who specialize in oral medicine or oral surgery. Other specialists include doctors who are ear, nose, and throat specialists; gastroenterologists; or dermatologists. The dentist or doctor will review your medical history and examine your mouth. A lot of tests may be needed. Tests may include:

- Blood tests to check for certain medical problems
- Oral swab tests
- Allergy tests
- Salivary flow test
- Biopsy of tissue
- Imaging tests

Primary and Secondary BMS[2]

Primary BMS

If tests do not reveal an underlying medical problem, the diagnosis is primary BMS. Experts believe that primary BMS is caused by damage to the nerves that control pain and taste.

Secondary BMS

Certain medical conditions can cause BMS. Treating the medical problem will cure the secondary BMS. Common causes of secondary BMS include:

- Hormonal changes (such as from diabetes or thyroid problem)
- Allergies to dental products, dental materials (usually metals), or foods
- Dry mouth, which can be caused by certain disorders (such as Sjögren's syndrome) and treatments (such as certain drugs and radiation therapy)
- Certain medicines, such as those that reduce blood pressure
- Nutritional deficiencies (such as a low level of vitamin B or iron)
- Infection in the mouth, such as a yeast infection
- Acid reflux

How Might Burning Mouth Syndrome Be Treated?[1]

If the underlying cause of burning mouth syndrome is determined, treatment is aimed at the triggering factor(s). If no cause can be found, treatment can be challenging. The following are potential therapies for burning mouth syndrome; we strongly recommend that you work with your healthcare provider in determining which therapy is right for you.

- A lozenge-type form of the anticonvulsant medication clonazepam (Klonopin)
- Oral thrush medications
- Medications that block nerve pan
- Certain antidepressants
- B vitamins
- Cognitive behavioral therapy
- Special oral rinses or mouth washes
- Saliva replacement products
- Capsaicin

In addition to these medications, the following measures may be helpful in reducing symptoms of burning mouth syndrome:

- Sip water frequently
- Suck on ice chips
- Chew sugarless gum
- Avoid irritating substances like tobacco, hot or spicy foods, alcoholic beverages, mouthwashes that contain alcohol, and products high in acid, like citrus fruits and juices, as well as cinnamon or mint.

Helpful Tips[2]

To help ease the pain of BMS, sip a cold beverage, suck on ice chips, or chew sugarless gum. Avoid irritating substances, such as:

- Tobacco
- Hot, spicy foods

- Alcoholic beverages
- Mouthwashes that contain alcohol
- Products high in acid, such as citrus fruits and juices

Ask your dentist and doctor for other helpful tips.

Chapter 37

Cleft Lip and Cleft Palate

Chapter Contents

Section 37.1

Understanding Craniofacial Defects

This section includes text excerpted from "Birth Defects," Centers for Disease Control and Prevention (CDC), November 21, 2014.

Craniofacial defects—such as orofacial clefts, craniosynostosis, and microtia and anotia—have a significant public health impact. You can learn more below about what the Centers for Disease Control and Prevention (CDC) is doing to identify the causes of craniofacial defects and help improve the lives of infants and children with these conditions.

Craniofacial defects are conditions present at birth that affect the structure and function of a baby's head and face. Two of the most common craniofacial defects are orofacial clefts, which occur when the lip and mouth do not form properly, and craniosynostosis, which happens when the bones in the baby's skull fuse too early. Microtia is when the external portion of the ear does not form properly, and anotia occurs when the external portion of the ear is missing. Treatments and services for children with craniofacial defects can vary depending on the severity of the defect; the presence of associated syndromes or other birth defects, or both; as well as the child's age and other medical or developmental needs. Children with certain craniofacial defects can have a greater risk for physical, learning, developmental, or social challenges, or a mix of these. Craniofacial defects have significant effects on families and the healthcare system:

- Each year, about 4,400 infants in the United States are born with a cleft lip with or without a cleft palate and about 2,700 infants are born with a cleft palate alone.

- About 4 infants per 10,000 live-births in the metropolitan Atlanta, Georgia, area are born with craniosynostosis.

- Recent studies have found that direct medical and healthcare use and average costs per child were a lot higher for children with orofacial clefts than for children of the same age without these conditions.

CDC is working to learn more about craniofacial defects by monitoring and doing research to guide prevention efforts. CDC and its partners also work to better understand healthcare use and improve access to services and the quality of life of infants and children with these conditions.

Surveillance of Craniofacial Defects

CDC helps support state-based birth defects programs surveillance systems to track and monitor birth defects, including craniofacial defects. Many states in the United States have birth defects surveillance programs that include some craniofacial defects in their monitoring efforts. Information from these programs and CDC partners is used to:

- Understand the risk factors for craniofacial defects.

- Identify disparities in the occurrence of craniofacial defects.

- Help ensure children with craniofacial defects get medical care and services when they need them, including referral to cleft and craniofacial teams, early intervention services (e.g., services, support and education to young children with an established condition or special need or who are "at risk" for developing a delay or special need), and special education.

- Examine associated health service use and costs.

- Better understand and help improve the quality of life and outcomes of infants and children with craniofacial defects.

Healthcare programs, state and local health departments, and policy makers can use this information to plan for services for children and families. Information from birth defects surveillance systems also can provide a basis for research studies designed to identify possible causes of and opportunities for preventing craniofacial defects.

Identifying Preventable Causes

CDC funds the National Birth Defects Prevention Study (NBDPS), the largest population-based study in the United States to identify the risk factors for and potential causes of birth defects, including orofacial clefts, craniosynostosis, and microtia and anotia. Population-based means that the researchers look at all babies with selected birth defects that live in the study region to get a complete picture of what is happening within the population. Population-based studies like the NBDPS determine the frequency of disease across a wide group of people, which is important to make sure that study results relate to the entire population of the United States.

Recently, CDC researchers and NBDPS partners have reported important findings about some risk factors for craniofacial defects:

- Diabetes? Women who have diabetes before they get pregnant have been shown to be more at risk of having a baby with anotia or microtia or a cleft lip with or without cleft palate.

- Smoking? Women who smoke anytime during the month before they get pregnant through the end of the third month of pregnancy have been shown to be more likely to have a baby with a cleft lip with or without cleft palate.

- Maternal thyroid disease? Women with thyroid disease or who are treated for thyroid disease while they are pregnant have been shown to be at higher risk of having an infant with craniosynostosis.

- Certain medications? Women who report using clomiphene citrate (a fertility medication) just before or early in pregnancy have been shown to be more likely to have a baby with craniosynostosis.

Section 37.2

Facts about Cleft Lip and Cleft Palate

This section includes text excerpted from "Facts about
Cleft Lip and Cleft Palate," Centers for Disease Control and
Prevention (CDC), November 12, 2015.

Cleft lip and cleft palate are birth defects that occur when a baby's
lip or mouth do not form properly during pregnancy. Together, these
birth defects commonly are called "orofacial clefts."

What Is Cleft Lip?

The lip forms between the fourth and seventh weeks of pregnancy.
As a baby develops during pregnancy, body tissue and special cells
from each side of the head grow toward the center of the face and
join together to make the face. This joining of tissue forms the facial
features, like the lips and mouth. A cleft lip happens if the tissue that
makes up the lip does not join completely before birth. This results in
an opening in the upper lip. The opening in the lip can be a small slit or
it can be a large opening that goes through the lip into the nose. A cleft
lip can be on one or both sides of the lip or in the middle of the lip, which
occurs very rarely. Children with a cleft lip also can have a cleft palate.

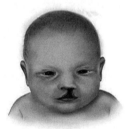

Figure 37.1. *Baby with Cleft Lip*

What Is Cleft Palate?

The roof of the mouth (palate) is formed between the sixth and
ninth weeks of pregnancy. A cleft palate happens if the tissue that

makes up the roof of the mouth does not join together completely during pregnancy. For some babies, both the front and back parts of the palate are open. For other babies, only part of the palate is open.

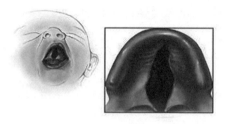

Figure 37.2. *Baby with the Left Cleft Palate*

Other Problems

Children with a cleft lip with or without a cleft palate or a cleft palate alone often have problems with feeding and speaking clearly and can have ear infections. They also might have hearing problems and problems with their teeth.

Causes and Risk Factors

The causes of orofacial clefts among most infants are unknown. Some children have a cleft lip or cleft palate because of changes in their genes. Cleft lip and cleft palate are thought to be caused by a combination of genes and other factors, such as things the mother comes in contact with in her environment, or what the mother eats or drinks, or certain medications she uses during pregnancy.

Like the many families of children with birth defects, CDC wants to find out what causes them. Understanding the factors that are more common among babies with a birth defect will help us learn more about the causes. CDC funds the Centers for Birth Defects Research and Prevention, which collaborate on large studies such as the National Birth Defects Prevention Study (NBDPS; births 1997–2011) and the Birth Defects Study To Evaluate Pregnancy exposures (BD-STEPS; began with births in 2014), to understand the causes of and risks for birth defects, including orofacial clefts.

Recently, CDC reported on important findings from research studies about some factors that increase the chance of having a baby with an orofacial cleft:

- Smoking? Women who smoke during pregnancy are more likely to have a baby with an orofacial cleft than women who do not smoke.

- Diabetes? Women with diabetes diagnosed before pregnancy have an increased risk of having a child with a cleft lip with or without cleft palate, compared to women who did not have diabetes.

- Use of certain medicines? Women who used certain medicines to treat epilepsy, such as topiramate or valproic acid, during the first trimester (the first 3 months) of pregnancy have an increased risk of having a baby with cleft lip with or without cleft palate, compared to women who didn't take these medicines.

CDC continues to study birth defects, such as cleft lip and cleft palate, and how to prevent them. If you are pregnant or thinking about becoming pregnant, talk with your doctor about ways to increase your chances of having a healthy baby.

Diagnosis

Orofacial clefts, especially cleft lip with or without cleft palate, can be diagnosed during pregnancy by a routine ultrasound. They can also be diagnosed after the baby is born, especially cleft palate. However, sometimes certain types of cleft palate (for example, submucous cleft palate and bifid uvula) might not be diagnosed until later in life.

Management and Treatment

Services and treatment for children with orofacial clefts can vary depending on the severity of the cleft; the child's age and needs; and the presence of associated syndromes or other birth defects, or both.

Surgery to repair a cleft lip usually occurs in the first few months of life and is recommended within the first 12 months of life. Surgery to repair a cleft palate is recommended within the first 18 months of life or earlier if possible. Many children will need additional surgical procedures as they get older. Surgical repair can improve the look and appearance of a child's face and might also improve breathing, hearing, and speech and language development. Children born with orofacial clefts might need other types of treatments and services, such as special dental or orthodontic care or speech therapy.

Because children with orofacial clefts often require a variety of services that need to be provided in a coordinated manner throughout childhood and into adolescence and sometimes adulthood, the American Cleft Palate—Craniofacial Association recommends services and treatment by cleft and craniofacial teams. Cleft and craniofacial teams provide a coordinated approach to care for children with orofacial clefts. These teams usually consist of experienced and qualified physicians and healthcare providers from different specialties. Cleft and craniofacial teams and centers are located throughout the United States and other countries.

With treatment, most children with orofacial clefts do well and lead a healthy life. Some children with orofacial clefts may have issues with self-esteem if they are concerned with visible differences between themselves and other children. Parent-to-parent support groups can prove to be useful for families of babies with birth defects of the head and face, such as orofacial clefts.

Occurrence

CDC recently estimated that, each year in the United States, about 2,650 babies are born with a cleft palate and 4,440 babies are born with a cleft lip with or without a cleft palate. Isolated orofacial clefts, or clefts that occur with no other major birth defects, are one of the most common types of birth defects in the United States. Depending on the cleft type, the rate of isolated orofacial clefts can vary from 50% to 80%.

Section 37.3

Smoking during Pregnancy Can Cause Clefts

This section includes text excerpted from "Smoking Can Cause Clefts," Centers for Disease Control and Prevention (CDC), July 7, 2014.

Smoking and Clefts

Although we don't know the causes of most orofacial clefts (clefts of the lip or palate) in babies, the 2014 Surgeon General's Report confirmed that smoking in early pregnancy can cause orofacial clefts in babies. This highlights an important prevention opportunity to improve the health of babies. Research has shown that about 6% of orofacial clefts in the United States are caused by smoking during early pregnancy. This means that over 400 babies could be born without orofacial clefts each year in the United States if women did not smoke early in pregnancy. Because these conditions often require numerous surgeries for repair, preventing orofacial clefts caused by smoking could save an estimated $40 million in healthcare costs each year for children up to age 10 years. Orofacial cleft defects happen very early in pregnancy, so quitting smoking before becoming pregnant is best.

Other Health Concerns

Most people know that smoking leads to cancer, heart disease, and other major health problems. However, women who smoke during pregnancy place themselves—and their unborn babies—at risk for even more health problems. Some of the dangers of smoking during pregnancy include premature birth, certain birth defects (like cleft lip and/or cleft palate and possibly some heart defects), and Sudden Infant Death Syndrome (SIDS). Even being around cigarette smoke puts a woman and her baby at risk for health problems.

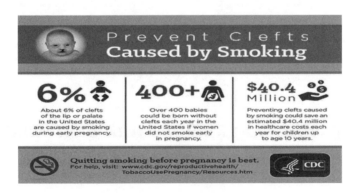

Figure 37.3. *Prevent Clefts Caused by Smoking*

Quit Now

Quitting smoking before becoming pregnant is best. But for women who are already pregnant, it is never "too late" to quit smoking. Quitting after becoming pregnant can still help protect against some health problems, such as the baby being born at a low birth weight (less than 5 ½ pounds).

Quit for Good

It is important to quit smoking for good. Some women might think it is safe to start smoking again after their baby is born, but their babies are not out of harm's way. Babies who are around cigarette smoke have weaker lungs than babies who aren't around cigarette smoke. They are also more likely to have other health problems, such as infections and frequent asthma attacks. Being around cigarette smoke can also increase the risk of SIDS.

Quitting Smoking Can Be Hard, but It Is One of the Best Ways a Woman Can Protect Herself and Her Baby's Health

If you or someone you know wants to quit smoking, talk to your healthcare provider about strategies. For support in quitting, including free quit coaching, a free quit plan, free educational materials, and referrals to local resources, please call 1-800-QUIT-NOW (1-800-784-8669); TTY 1-800-332-8615. More free help and support resources are available for pregnant women and others who want to quit for good.

Section 37.4

Breastfeeding Children with Cleft Palate

"Breastfeeding Children with Cleft Palate,"
© 2017 Omnigraphics. Reviewed September 2016.

Cleft palate and cleft lip—known collectively as orofacial clefts—rank among the most common types of birth defects in the United States. According to the Centers for Disease Control and Prevention (CDC), around 2,650 babies are born with a cleft palate in the United States each year, while around 4,440 babies are born with a cleft lip. Orofacial clefts occur early in the gestation process, when the tissues that grow around the sides of the head to form the face fail to meet in the middle. Left untreated, they can have a significant impact on a child's breathing, hearing, eating, and speech. As a result, most babies born with orofacial clefts undergo surgery within the first year of life to repair the cleft and improve the function of the mouth.

Prior to the surgical repair, orofacial clefts can greatly complicate breastfeeding efforts. Experts have compared breastfeeding with a cleft palate to drinking through a straw with a hole in it. The cleft allows air to enter the mouth and prevents the baby from getting adequate suction. The feeding process becomes physically taxing, and the baby may swallow a great deal of air. As a result of these complications, the breastfeeding advocacy group La Leche League International warns that most babies with uncorrected cleft palate are not able to get the nutrition they need through breastfeeding exclusively. Since research has shown that breastfeeding offers a number of important benefits to a baby's health and well-being, this news is upsetting to many mothers of babies with a cleft palate.

Feeding Options for Babies with Cleft Palate

Babies born with a cleft lip only (not a cleft palate) are often able to breastfeed successfully before surgery. The mother usually needs to experiment with different nursing positions to help the baby's lips form a seal over the nipple. Lactation consultants often recommend holding the baby in an upright position, perhaps with the support of a nursing pillow.

Babies born with a cleft palate, on the other hand, are rarely able to breastfeed successfully before surgery. Although this situation can be deeply disappointing for mothers, there are still many options available to help them share the benefits of breastfeeding with their babies. Some of the main options include the following:

- Use a hospital-grade breast pump to express breast milk and feed it to the baby using a cleft palate feeding system, which includes specialized bottles and nipples. Feeding breast milk from a bottle ensures that the baby gets all the nutritional benefits of nursing.

- To experience the physical intimacy and emotional bonding aspects of breastfeeding, make as much eye contact and skin contact with the baby as possible while bottle feeding.

- Once bottle feeding has been established successfully, put the baby on the mother's breast for non-nutritive sucking. This action not only helps develop muscles in the baby's mouth and tongue but can also stimulate milk production in mothers who pump.

- After the baby undergoes surgery to repair the cleft palate, it may be possible to reintroduce breastfeeding.

Using a pump to express milk can be challenging and time consuming for new mothers, as can learning to feed a baby with a cleft palate. It is important that mothers have the support of friends and family members as they figure out the best feeding methods for themselves and their babies. Even though breast milk is widely viewed as the best food for newborns, formula has nourished millions of healthy children. Overwhelmed mothers of babies with orofacial clefts may simply decide that pumping is too difficult given the demands of work and family, and they should not feel guilty about lovingly feeding their babies with formula.

References

1. Condon, Susan. "How Do I Breastfeed a Baby with Cleft Lip or Palate?" Baby Center, April 2015.

2. "What about Breastfeeding?" Cleft Palate Foundation, July 15, 2009.

Section 37.5

Use of Topiramate in Pregnancy and Risk of Oral Clefts

This section includes text excerpted from "FDA Drug Safety Communication: Risk of Oral Clefts in Children Born to Mothers Taking Topamax (Topiramate)," U.S. Food and Drug Administration (FDA), August 4, 2016.

Facts about Topiramate

- An anticonvulsant medication U.S. Food and Drug Administration (FDA)-approved for use alone or with other medications to treat patients with epilepsy who have certain types of seizures.

- FDA-approved for use to prevent migraine headaches, but not to relieve the pain of migraine headaches when they occur.

- Has been used off-label (for unapproved uses) for other conditions, some of which may not be considered serious.

- From January 2007 through December 2010, approximately 32.3 million topiramate prescriptions were dispensed and approximately 4.3 million patients filled topiramate prescriptions from the outpatient retail pharmacies in the United States.

Think Twice

The benefits and the risks of topiramate should be carefully weighed when prescribing this drug to women of childbearing age, particularly for conditions not usually associated with permanent injury or death. Alternative medications that have a lower risk of oral clefts and other adverse birth outcomes should be considered for these patients. If the decision is made to use topiramate in women of childbearing age, effective birth control should be used. Oral clefts occur in the first trimester of pregnancy before many women know they are pregnant.

Topiramate was previously classified as a Pregnancy Category C drug, which means that data from animal studies suggested potential fetal risks, but no adequate data from human clinical trials or studies were available at the time of approval. However, because of new human data that show an increased risk for oral clefts, topiramate is being placed in Pregnancy Category D. Pregnancy Category D means there is positive evidence of human fetal risk based on human data but the potential benefits from use of the drug in pregnant women may be acceptable in certain situations despite its risks.

Data Summary

Data from the North American Antiepileptic Drug (NAAED) Pregnancy Registry indicate an increased risk of oral clefts in infants exposed to topiramate monotherapy during the first trimester of pregnancy. The prevalence of oral clefts was 1.4% compared to a prevalence of 0.38%–0.55% in infants exposed to other antiepileptic drugs (AEDs), and a prevalence of 0.07% in infants of mothers without epilepsy or treatment with other AEDs. The relative risk of oral clefts in topiramate-exposed pregnancies in the NAAED Pregnancy Registry was 21.3 as compared to the risk in a background population of untreated women (95% Confidence Interval: 7.9–57.1). The UK Epilepsy and

Pregnancy Register reported a similarly increased prevalence of oral clefts (3.2%) among infants exposed to topiramate monotherapy, a 16-fold increase in risk compared to the risk in their background population (0.2%).

The benefits and the risks of topiramate should be carefully weighed when prescribing this drug for women of childbearing age, particularly when topiramate is considered for a condition not usually associated with permanent injury or death. Appropriate alternative treatment should be considered. Inform women of childbearing age of the increased risk for having a baby with an oral cleft if they become pregnant while using topiramate.

Cleft lip and cleft palate range from a small notch in the lip to a groove that runs into the roof of the mouth and nose, possibly leading to problems with eating, talking and ear infections. Surgery is often used to close the lip and palate. With treatment, most children with cleft lip or palate do well.

Additional Information for Patients

- If you take topiramate during pregnancy, there is a higher risk that your baby will develop a cleft lip and/or cleft palate. Oral clefts happen early in pregnancy, before many women even know they are pregnant. For this reason, women of childbearing age should talk to their healthcare professionals about other treatment options.

- Women of childbearing age who do decide to take topiramate and are not planning a pregnancy should use effective birth control (contraception) while taking topiramate. Women should talk to their healthcare professionals about the best kind of birth control to use while taking topiramate.

- Before you start topiramate, you should tell your healthcare professional if you are pregnant or are planning to become pregnant. Healthcare professionals may discuss other treatment options with you.

- You should tell your healthcare professional right away if you become pregnant while taking topiramate. You and your healthcare provider should decide if you will continue to take topiramate while you are pregnant.

- Topiramate should not be stopped without talking to a healthcare professional, even in pregnant women. Stopping topiramate suddenly can cause serious problems. Not treating epilepsy during pregnancy can be harmful to women and their developing babies.

- If you become pregnant while taking topiramate, you should talk to your healthcare professional about registering with the North American Antiepileptic Drug Pregnancy Registry. You can enroll in this registry by calling 1-888-233-2334.

- Topiramate passes into breast milk, but its effects on developing babies remain unknown. You should talk to your healthcare professional about the best way to feed your baby if you take topiramate.

- You should read the Medication Guide when picking up a prescription for topiramate. It will help you understand the potential risks and benefits of this medication.

Chapter 38

Dentinogenesis Imperfecta

What Is Dentinogenesis Imperfecta?

Dentinogenesis imperfecta is a disorder of tooth development. This condition causes the teeth to be discolored (most often a blue-gray or yellow-brown color) and translucent. Teeth are also weaker than normal, making them prone to rapid wear, breakage, and loss. These problems can affect both primary (baby) teeth and permanent teeth.

Researchers have described three types of dentinogenesis imperfecta with similar dental abnormalities. Type I occurs in people who have osteogenesis imperfecta, a genetic condition in which bones are brittle and easily broken. Dentinogenesis imperfecta type II and type III usually occur in people without other inherited disorders. A few older individuals with type II have had progressive high-frequency hearing loss in addition to dental abnormalities, but it is not known whether this hearing loss is related to dentinogenesis imperfecta.

Some researchers believe that dentinogenesis imperfecta type II and type III, along with a condition called dentin dysplasia type II, are actually forms of a single disorder. The signs and symptoms of

This chapter contains text excerpted from the following sources: Text beginning with the heading "What Is Dentinogenesis Imperfecta?" is excerpted from "Dentinogenesis imperfecta," Genetics Home Reference (GHR), National Institutes of Health (NIH), November 2009. Reviewed September 2016; Text beginning with the heading "How Do People Inherit Dentinogenesis Imperfecta?" is excerpted from "DSPP," Genetics Home Reference (GHR), National Institutes of Health (NIH), November 2009. Reviewed September 2016.

dentin dysplasia type II are very similar to those of dentinogenesis imperfecta. However, dentin dysplasia type II affects the primary teeth much more than the permanent teeth.

How Common Is Dentinogenesis Imperfecta?

Dentinogenesis imperfecta affects an estimated 1 in 6,000 to 8,000 people.

What Genes Are Related to Dentinogenesis Imperfecta?

Mutations in the dentin sialophosphoprotein (*DSPP*) gene have been identified in people with dentinogenesis imperfecta type II and type III. Mutations in this gene are also responsible for dentin dysplasia type II. Dentinogenesis imperfecta type I occurs as part of osteogenesis imperfecta, which is caused by mutations in one of several other genes (most often the *COL1A1* or *COL1A2* genes).

The *DSPP* gene provides instructions for making two proteins that are essential for normal tooth development. These proteins are involved in the formation of dentin, which is a bone-like substance that makes up the protective middle layer of each tooth. *DSPP* gene mutations alter the proteins made from the gene, leading to the production of abnormally soft dentin. Teeth with defective dentin are discolored, weak, and more likely to decay and break. It is unclear whether *DSPP* gene mutations are related to the hearing loss found in a few older individuals with dentinogenesis imperfecta type II.

How Do People Inherit Dentinogenesis Imperfecta?

This condition is inherited in an autosomal dominant pattern, which means one copy of the altered gene in each cell is sufficient to cause the disorder. In most cases, an affected person has one parent with the condition.

What Is the Normal Function of the DSPP Gene?

The *DSPP* gene provides instructions for making a protein called dentin sialophosphoprotein. Soon after it is produced, this protein is cut into two smaller proteins: dentin sialoprotein and dentin phosphoprotein. These proteins are components of dentin, which is a bone-like substance that makes up the protective middle layer of each tooth. A third smaller protein produced from dentin sialophosphoprotein, called dentin glycoprotein, was identified in pigs but has not been found in humans.

Although the exact functions of the *DSPP*-derived proteins are unknown, these proteins appear to be essential for normal tooth development. Dentin phosphoprotein is thought to be involved in the normal hardening of collagen, the most abundant protein in dentin. Specifically, dentin phosphoprotein may play a role in the deposition of mineral crystals among collagen fibers (mineralization).

The *DSPP* gene is also active in the inner ear, although it is unclear whether it plays a role in normal hearing.

How Are Changes in the DSPP Gene Related to Health Conditions?

More than 20 mutations in the *DSPP* gene have been identified in people with dentinogenesis imperfecta. These genetic changes are responsible for two forms of this disorder, type II and type III. Mutations in this gene also cause dentin dysplasia type II, a disorder with signs and symptoms very similar to those of dentinogenesis imperfecta. However, dentin dysplasia type II affects the primary (baby) teeth much more than the permanent teeth. Some researchers believe that this type of dentin dysplasia and dentinogenesis imperfecta types II and III are actually forms of a single disorder.

About half of *DSPP* gene mutations affect dentin sialoprotein, altering its transport in cells. The remaining mutations affect dentin phosphoprotein, interfering with its normal production and/or secretion. As a result of these abnormalities of *DSPP*-related proteins, teeth have abnormally soft dentin. Teeth with defective dentin are discolored, weak, and prone to breakage and decay.

Although the *DSPP* gene is active in the inner ear, it is unclear whether *DSPP* gene mutations are related to the hearing loss found in a few older individuals with dentinogenesis imperfecta type II.

Chapter 39

Dry Mouth Disorders

Chapter Contents

Section 39.1

Dry Mouth: Overview

This section contains text excerpted from the following sources: Text
beginning with the heading "What Is Dry Mouth?" is excerpted from
"Dry Mouth," NIHSeniorHealth, National Institutes of Health (NIH),
October 2015; Text beginning with the heading "Treatment for Dry
Mouth" is excerpted from "Dry Mouth? Don't Delay Treatment," U.S.
Food and Drug Administration (FDA), August 31, 2015.

What Is Dry Mouth?

Dry mouth is the feeling that there is not enough saliva in the
mouth. Everyone has dry mouth once in a while—if they are nervous,
upset, under stress, or taking certain medications. But if you have dry
mouth all or most of the time, see a dentist or physician. Many older
adults have dry mouth, but it is not a normal part of aging.

Why Saliva Is Important

Saliva does more than keep your mouth wet. It protects teeth from
decay, helps heal sores in your mouth, and prevents infection by controlling bacteria, viruses, and fungi in the mouth.

Saliva helps digest food and helps us chew and swallow. Saliva is
involved in taste perception as well. Each of these functions of saliva
is hampered when a person has dry mouth.

How Dry Mouth Feels

Dry mouth can be uncomfortable. Some people notice a sticky, dry
feeling in the mouth. Others notice a burning feeling or difficulty while
eating. The throat may feel dry, too, making swallowing difficult and
choking common. Also, people with dry mouth may get mouth sores,
cracked lips, and a dry, rough tongue.

What Causes Dry Mouth?

People get dry mouth when the glands in the mouth that make
saliva are not working properly. Because of this, there might not be

enough saliva to keep your mouth healthy. There are several reasons why these glands, called salivary glands, might not work right.

Medicines and Dry Mouth

More than 400 medicines, including some over-the-counter medications, can cause the salivary glands to make less saliva, or to change the composition of the saliva so that it can't perform the functions it should. As an example, medicines for urinary incontinence, allergies, high blood pressure, and depression often cause dry mouth.

Diseases That Can Cause Dry Mouth

Some diseases can affect the salivary glands. Dry mouth can occur in patients with diabetes. Dry mouth is also the hallmark symptom of the fairly common autoimmune disease Sjögren's syndrome.

Sjögren's syndrome can occur either by itself or with another autoimmune disease like rheumatoid arthritis or lupus. Salivary and tear glands are the major targets of the syndrome and the result is a decrease in production of saliva and tears. The disorder can occur at any age, but the average person with the disorder at the Sjögren's Syndrome Clinic of the National Institute of Dental and Craniofacial Research (NIDCR) is in his or her late 50s. Women with the disorder outnumber men 9 to

Cancer Treatments and Dry Mouth

Certain cancer treatments can affect the salivary glands. Head and neck radiation therapy can cause the glands to produce little or no saliva. Chemotherapy may cause the salivary glands to produce thicker saliva, which makes the mouth feel dry and sticky.

Injury to the head or neck can damage the nerves that tell salivary glands to make saliva.

Treatment for Dry Mouth

Your doctor or dentist may recommend oral rinses and moisturizers, or prescribe an artificial saliva.

Also called saliva substitutes, artificial salivas are regulated by U.S. Food and Drug Administration (FDA) as medical devices. "Unlike drugs, artificial salivas have no chemical action," says Susan Runner, D.D.S., chief of FDA's dental devices branch. "Their action is mechanical. They moisten and lubricate the mouth but do not stimulate the salivary glands to make saliva."

While not a cure, artificial salivas can provide short-term relief of the symptoms of dry mouth. "They can also help minimize discomfort after an oral procedure," says Runner.

Artificial salivas come in a variety of forms, including rinses, sprays, swabs, gels, and tablets that dissolve in the mouth. Some are available by prescription only; others can be bought over-the-counter.

FDA has also approved several prescription drugs to relieve dry mouth caused by certain medical treatments or conditions, such as Sjögren's syndrome and radiation for head or neck cancer.

Advice for Consumers

If you have persistent dry mouth:

- Talk to your doctor, who may change your medications or adjust the doses.

- Talk to your dentist and provide a list of the medicines you take as well as any medical conditions or treatments you've had. The American Dental Association recommends seeing your dentist at least twice a year.

Tips for Relieving Dry Mouth

- Sip water or sugarless drinks, or suck on ice chips.

- Avoid irritants, such as alcohol, tobacco, and caffeine. Remember that caffeine is found in many sodas as well as in coffee and tea.

- Chew sugar-free gum or suck on sugar-free candy.

- Avoid salty or spicy foods, which may irritate the mouth.

- Use a humidifier in your bedroom at night.

- Consider using saliva substitutes.

Section 39.2

Sialadenitis

This section includes text excerpted from "Sialadenitis," Genetic
and Rare Diseases (GARD) Information Center, National
Institutes of Health (NIH), September 17, 2014.

What Is Sialadenitis?

Sialadenitis is an infection of the salivary glands. It is usually
caused by a virus or bacteria. The parotid (in front of the ear) and
submandibular (under the chin) glands are most commonly affected.
Sialadenitis may be associated with pain, tenderness, redness, and
gradual, localized swelling of the affected area. There are both acute
and chronic forms. Although it is quite common among elderly adults
with salivary gland stones, sialadenitis can also occur in other age
groups, including infants during the first few weeks of life. Without
proper treatment, sialadenitis can develop into a severe infection,
especially in people who are debilitated or elderly.

What Causes Sialadenitis?

Sialadenitis usually occurs after hyposecretion (reduced flow from
the salivary glands) or duct obstruction, but may develop without
an obvious cause. Saliva flow can be reduced in people who are sick
or recovering from surgery, or people who are dehydrated, malnourished, or immunosuppressed. A stone or a kink in the salivary duct
can also diminish saliva flow, as can certain medications (such as
antihistamines, diuretics, psychiatric medications, beta-blockers, or
barbiturates). It often occurs in chronically ill people with xerostomia
(dry mouth), people with Sjogren syndrome, and in those who have
had radiation therapy to the oral cavity.

The most common causative organism in the infection is *Staphylococcus aureus*; others include streptococci, coliforms, and various
anaerobic bacteria. Although less common than bacteria, several
viruses have also been implicated in sialadenitis. These include the
mumps virus, HIV, coxsackievirus, parainfluenza types I and II, influenza A, and herpes.

What Are the Signs and Symptoms of Sialadenitis?

Signs and symptoms of sialadenitis may include fever, chills, and unilateral pain and swelling in the affected area. The affected gland may be firm and tender, with redness of the overlying skin. Pus may drain through the gland into the mouth.

How Might Sialadenitis Be Treated?

The initial treatment for sialadenitis is antibiotics active against *Staphylococcus aureus*. Hydration, ingesting things that trigger saliva flow (such as lemon juice or hard candy), warm compresses, gland massage, and good oral hygiene are also important. Abscesses need to be drained. Occasionally, in cases of chronic or relapsing sialadenitis, a superficial parotidectomy or submandibular gland excision is needed.

What Is the Long-Term Outlook for People with Sialadenitis?

With prompt diagnosis and appropriate treatment, the long-term outlook (prognosis) for people with sialadenitis is very good. Those with chronic sialadenitis often have a relapsing and remitting course. Complications are not common, but may occur and can include abscess of the salivary gland or localized spreading of bacterial infection (such as cellulitis or Ludwig's angina).

Section 39.3

Sjögren's Syndrome

This section includes text excerpted from "Sjögren's Syndrome," National Institute of Arthritis and Musculoskeletal and Skin Diseases (NIAMS), April 2016.

What Is Sjögren's Syndrome?

Sjögren's syndrome is an autoimmune disease; that is, a disease in which the immune system turns against the body's own cells.

Normally, the immune system works to protect us from disease by destroying harmful invading organisms like viruses and bacteria. In the case of Sjögren's syndrome, disease-fighting cells attack various organs, most notably the glands that produce tears and saliva. Damage to these glands causes a reduction in both the quantity and quality of their secretions. This results in symptoms that include dry eyes and dry mouth.

Sjögren's syndrome is also a rheumatic disease. These are diseases characterized by inflammation (signs include redness or heat, swelling, and symptoms such as pain) and loss of function of one or more connecting or supporting structures of the body. They especially affect joints, tendons, ligaments, bones, and muscles.

Primary versus Secondary Sjögren's Syndrome

Sjögren's syndrome is classified as either primary or secondary. The primary form occurs in people who do not have other rheumatic diseases. The secondary form occurs in people who already have another rheumatic disease, most commonly rheumatoid arthritis (RA) or systemic lupus erythematosus (SLE). These people then develop dry eyes or dry mouth.

What Are the Symptoms of Sjögren's Syndrome?

Sjögren's syndrome can cause many symptoms. The main ones are:

- **Dry eyes.** Eyes affected by Sjögren's syndrome may burn or itch. Some people say it feels like they have sand in their eyes. Others have trouble with blurry vision, or are bothered by bright light, especially fluorescent lighting.

- **Dry mouth.** Dry mouth may feel chalky or like your mouth is full of cotton. It may be difficult to swallow, speak, or taste. Because you lack the protective effects of saliva, you may develop more dental decay (cavities) and mouth infections.

Sjögren's syndrome can also affect other parts of the body, causing symptoms such as:

- multiple sites of joint and muscle pain

- prolonged dry skin

- skin rashes on the extremities

- chronic dry cough

- vaginal dryness
- numbness or tingling in the extremities
- prolonged fatigue that interferes with daily life

Who Gets Sjögren's Syndrome?

Sjögren's syndrome can affect people of either sex and of any age, but most cases occur in women. The average age for onset is late forties, but in rare cases, Sjögren's syndrome is diagnosed in children.

What Causes Sjögren's Syndrome?

Researchers think Sjögren's syndrome is caused by a combination of genetic and environmental factors. Several different genes appear to be involved, but scientists are not certain exactly which ones are linked to the disease, because different genes seem to play a role in different people.

Scientists think that the trigger may be a viral or bacterial infection. The possibility that the endocrine and nervous systems play a role in the disease is also under investigation.

How Is Sjögren's Syndrome Diagnosed?

Your doctor will diagnose Sjögren's syndrome based on your medical history, a physical exam, and results from clinical or laboratory tests. During the exam, your doctor will check for clinical signs of Sjögren's syndrome, such as indications of mouth dryness or signs of other connective tissue diseases.

Depending on what your doctor finds during the history and exam, he or she may want to perform some tests or refer you to a specialist to establish the diagnosis of Sjögren's syndrome and/or to see how severe the problem is and whether the disease is affecting other parts of the body as well.

Because there are many causes of dry eyes and dry mouth (including many common medications, other diseases, or previous treatment such as radiation of the head or neck), the doctor needs a thorough history from the patient, and additional tests to see whether other parts of the body are affected.

Blood tests can determine the presence of antibodies common in Sjogren's syndrome, including anti-SSA and anti-SSB antibodies or rheumatoid factor. Other tests can identify decreases in tear and saliva production. Biopsy of the saliva glands and other specialized tests can also help to confirm the diagnosis.

What Type of Doctor Diagnoses and Treats Sjögren's Syndrome?

Because the symptoms of Sjögren's syndrome develop gradually and are similar to those of many other diseases, getting a diagnosis can take time. A person could see a number of doctors, any of whom could diagnose the disease and be involved in its treatment. These might include a rheumatologist (a doctor who specializes in diseases of the joints, muscles, and bones), a primary care physician, internist, ophthalmologist (eye specialist), otolaryngologist (ear, nose, and throat specialist), or another specialist. Usually a rheumatologist will coordinate treatment among a number of specialists.

How Is Sjögren's Syndrome Treated?

Treatment can vary from person to person, depending on what parts of the body are affected.

Treatments for Dry Eyes

There are many treatments you can try or your doctor can prescribe for dry eyes. Here are some that might help:

- **Artificial tears.** Available by prescription or over the counter under many brand names, these products keep eyes moist by replacing natural tears. Artificial tears come in different thicknesses, so you may have to experiment to find the right one. Some drops contain preservatives that might irritate your eyes. Drops without preservatives usually don't bother the eyes.

- **Ointments.** Ointments are thicker than artificial tears. Because they moisturize and protect the eye for several hours, and may blur your vision, they are most effective during sleep.

- **Other therapies.** Other therapies such as plugging or blocking the tear ducts, anti-inflammatory medication, or surgery may be needed in more severe cases.

Treatments for Dry Mouth

There are many remedies for dry mouth. You can try some of them on your own. Your doctor may prescribe others. Here are some many people find useful:

- **Chewing gum and hard candy.** If your salivary glands still produce some saliva, you can stimulate them to make more by chewing gum or sucking on hard candy. However, gum and candy must be sugar-free, because dry mouth makes you extremely prone to progressive dental decay (cavities).

- **Water.** Take sips of water or another sugar-free, noncarbonated drink throughout the day to wet your mouth, especially when you are eating or talking. Note that drinking large amounts of liquid throughout the day will not make your mouth any less dry and will make you urinate more often. You should only take small sips of liquid, but not too often. If you sip liquids every few minutes, it may reduce or remove the mucus coating inside your mouth, increasing the feeling of dryness.

- **Lip balm.** You can soothe dry, cracked lips by using oil- or petroleum-based lip balm or lipstick. If your mouth hurts, your doctor may give you medicine in a mouth rinse, ointment, or gel to apply to the sore areas to control pain and inflammation.

- **Other therapies.** Other therapies such as saliva substitutes or medications that stimulate the salivary glands to produce saliva are sometimes indicated.

Treatments for Symptoms in Other Parts of the Body

If you have extraglandular involvement, that is, a problem that extends beyond the moisture-producing glands of your eyes and mouth, your doctor—or the appropriate specialist—may also treat those problems using nonsteroidal anti-inflammatory drugs (NSAIDs)*, or immune-modifying drugs.

*__Warning__: Side effects of NSAIDs include stomach problems; skin rashes; high blood pressure; fluid retention; and liver, kidney, and heart problems. The longer a person uses NSAIDs, the more likely he or she is to have side effects, ranging from mild to serious. Many other drugs cannot be taken when a patient is being treated with NSAIDs, because NSAIDs alter the way the body uses or eliminates these other drugs. Check with your healthcare provider or pharmacist before you take NSAIDs. NSAIDs should only be used at the lowest dose possible for the shortest time needed.

The Importance of Oral Hygiene

Natural saliva contains substances that rid the mouth of the bacteria that cause dental decay (cavities) and mouth infections, so good oral hygiene is extremely important when you have dry mouth. Here's what you can do to prevent cavities and infections:

- Visit a dentist regularly, at least twice a year, to have your teeth examined and cleaned.
- Rinse your mouth with water several times a day. Don't use mouthwash that contains alcohol, because alcohol is drying.
- Use toothpaste that contains fluoride to gently brush your teeth, gums, and tongue after each meal and before bedtime. Nonfoaming toothpaste is less drying.
- Floss your teeth every day.
- Avoid sugar between meals. That means choosing sugar-free gum, candy, and soda. If you do eat or drink sugary foods, brush your teeth immediately afterward.
- See a dentist right away if you notice anything unusual or have continuous burning or other oral symptoms.
- Ask your dentist whether you need to take fluoride supplements, use a fluoride gel at night, or have a varnish put on your teeth to protect the enamel.

Protect Your Voice

People with Sjögren's syndrome can develop hoarseness if their vocal cords become inflamed as part of the disease or become irritated from throat dryness or coughing. To prevent further strain on your vocal cords, try not to clear your throat before speaking. Instead, take a sip of water, chew sugar-free gum, or suck on sugar-free candy. Or else make an "h" sound, hum, or laugh to gently bring the vocal cords together so you can get sound out. Clearing your throat does the same thing, but it's hard on the vocal cords, and you want to avoid irritating them further.

Other Diseases Linked to Sjögren's Syndrome

Patients who have an autoimmune connective tissue disease other than Sjögren's syndrome (see list below) may subsequently develop the dry eyes and or dry mouth of Sjögren's syndrome. They would then be diagnosed as having secondary Sjögren's syndrome, along with their primary connective tissue disease. These other autoimmune connective tissue diseases include:

- **Polymyositis.** An inflammation of the muscles that causes weakness and pain, difficulty moving, and, in some cases, problems breathing and swallowing. If the skin is inflamed too, it's called dermatomyositis.

- **Rheumatoid arthritis (RA).** A form of arthritis that is characterized by severe inflammation of the joints. This inflammation can eventually damage the surrounding bones (fingers, hands, knees, etc.). Rheumatoid arthritis can also damage muscles, blood vessels, and major organs.

- **Scleroderma.** A disease in which the body accumulates too much collagen, a protein commonly found in the skin. The result is thick, tight skin and possibly damage to muscles, joints, and internal organs such as the esophagus, intestines, lungs, heart, kidneys, and blood vessels.

- **Systemic lupus erythematosus (SLE).** A disease that causes joint and muscle pain, weakness, skin rashes, and, in more severe cases, heart, lung, kidney, and nervous system problems.

Does Sjögren's Syndrome Cause Lymphoma?

A small percentage of people with Sjögren's syndrome develop lymphoma, which involves salivary glands, lymph nodes, the gastrointestinal tract, or the lungs. Persistent enlargement of a major salivary gland should be carefully and regularly observed by your doctor and investigated further if it changes in size in a short period of time. Other symptoms may include the following: (Note that many of these can be symptoms of other problems, including Sjögren's syndrome itself. Nevertheless, it is important to see your doctor if you have any of these symptoms so that any problem can be diagnosed and treated as early as possible.)

- unexplained fever

- night sweats

- constant fatigue

- unexplained weight loss

- itchy skin

- reddened patches on the skin.

If you're worried that you might develop lymphoma, talk to your doctor to learn more about the disease, the symptoms to watch for, any special medical care you might need, and what you can do to relieve your worry.

Chapter 40

Jaw Problems

Chapter Contents

Section 40.1

Temporomandibular Joint and Muscle (TMJ) Disorders

This section includes text excerpted from "TMJ Disorders," National Institute of Dental and Craniofacial Research (NIDCR), August 2013.

Temporomandibular joint and muscle disorders, commonly called "TMJ," are a group of conditions that cause pain and dysfunction in the jaw joint and the muscles that control jaw movement. We don't know for certain how many people have TMJ disorders, but some estimates suggest that over 10 million Americans are affected. The condition appears to be more common in women than men.

For most people, pain in the area of the jaw joint or muscles does not signal a serious problem. Generally, discomfort from these conditions is occasional and temporary, often occurring in cycles. The pain eventually goes away with little or no treatment. Some people, however, develop significant, long-term symptoms.

If you have questions about TMJ disorders, you are not alone. Researchers, too, are looking for answers to what causes these conditions and what the best treatments are. Until we have scientific evidence for safe and effective treatments, it's important to avoid, when possible, procedures that can cause permanent changes in your bite or jaw. This booklet provides information you should know if you have been told by a dentist or physician that you have a TMJ disorder.

What Is the Temporomandibular Joint?

The temporomandibular joint connects the lower jaw, called the mandible, to the bone at the side of the head—the temporal bone. If you place your fingers just in front of your ears and open your mouth, you can feel the joints. Because these joints are flexible, the jaw can move smoothly up and down and side to side, enabling us to talk, chew and yawn. Muscles attached to and surrounding the jaw joint control its position and movement.

When we open our mouths, the rounded ends of the lower jaw, called condyles, glide along the joint socket of the temporal bone. The condyles slide back to their original position when we close our mouths. To keep this motion smooth, a soft disc lies between the condyle and the temporal bone. This disc absorbs shocks to the jaw joint from chewing and other movements.

The temporomandibular joint is different from the body's other joints. The combination of hinge and sliding motions makes this joint among the most complicated in the body. Also, the tissues that make up the temporomandibular joint differ from other load-bearing joints, like the knee or hip. Because of its complex movement and unique makeup, the jaw joint and its controlling muscles can pose a tremendous challenge to both patients and healthcare providers when problems arise.

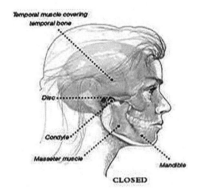

Figure 40.1. *Temporomandibular Joint*

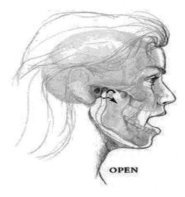

Figure 40.2. *Temporomandibular Joint*

What Are TMJ Disorders?

Disorders of the jaw joint and chewing muscles—and how people respond to them—vary widely. Researchers generally agree that the conditions fall into three main categories:

1. Myofascial pain involves discomfort or pain in the muscles that control jaw function.

2. Internal derangement of the joint involves a displaced disc, dislocated jaw, or injury to the condyle.

3. Arthritis refers to a group of degenerative/inflammatory joint disorders that can affect the temporomandibular joint.

A person may have one or more of these conditions at the same time. Some people have other health problems that co-exist with TMJ disorders, such as chronic fatigue syndrome, sleep disturbances or fibromyalgia, a painful condition that affects muscles and other soft tissues throughout the body. These disorders share some common symptoms, which suggests that they may share similar underlying mechanisms of disease. However, it is not known whether they have a common cause.

Rheumatic disease, such as arthritis, may also affect the temporomandibular joint as a secondary condition. Rheumatic diseases refer to a large group of disorders that cause pain, inflammation, and stiffness in the joints, muscles, and bone. Arthritis and some TMJ disorders involve inflammation of the tissues that line the joints. The exact relationship between these conditions is not known.

How jaw joint and muscle disorders progress is not clear. Symptoms worsen and ease over time, but what causes these changes is not known. Most people have relatively mild forms of the disorder. Their symptoms improve significantly, or disappear spontaneously, within weeks or months. For others, the condition causes long-term, persistent and debilitating pain.

What Causes TMJ Disorders?

Trauma to the jaw or temporomandibular joint plays a role in some TMJ disorders. But for most jaw joint and muscle problems, scientists don't know the causes. Because the condition is more common in women than in men, scientists are exploring a possible link between female hormones and TMJ disorders.

For many people, symptoms seem to start without obvious reason. Research disputes the popular belief that a bad bite or orthodontic braces can trigger TMJ disorders.

There is no scientific proof that sounds—such as clicking—in the jaw joint lead to serious problems. In fact, jaw sounds are common in the general population. Jaw noises alone, without pain or limited jaw movement, do not indicate a TMJ disorder and do not warrant treatment.

What Are the Signs and Symptoms?

A variety of symptoms may be linked to TMJ disorders. Pain, particularly in the chewing muscles and/or jaw joint, is the most common symptom. Other likely symptoms include:

- radiating pain in the face, jaw, or neck,

- jaw muscle stiffness,

- limited movement or locking of the jaw,

- painful clicking, popping or grating in the jaw joint when opening or closing the mouth,

- a change in the way the upper and lower teeth fit together.

How Are TMJ Disorders Diagnosed?

There is no widely accepted, standard test now available to correctly diagnose TMJ disorders. Because the exact causes and symptoms are not clear, identifying these disorders can be difficult and confusing. Currently, healthcare providers note the patient's description of symptoms, take a detailed medical and dental history, and examine problem areas, including the head, neck, face, and jaw. Imaging studies may also be recommended.

You may want to consult your doctor to rule out other known causes of pain. Facial pain can be a symptom of many conditions, such as sinus or ear infections, various types of headaches, and facial neuralgias (nerve-related facial pain). Ruling out these problems first helps in identifying TMJ disorders.

How Are TMJ Disorders Treated?

Because more studies are needed on the safety and effectiveness of most treatments for jaw joint and muscle disorders, experts strongly recommend using the most conservative, reversible treatments possible. Conservative treatments do not invade the tissues of the face, jaw, or joint, or involve surgery. Reversible treatments do not cause permanent changes in the structure or position of the jaw or teeth. Even when TMJ disorders have become persistent, most patients still do not need aggressive types of treatment.

Conservative Treatments

Because the most common jaw joint and muscle problems are temporary and do not get worse, simple treatment may be all that is necessary to relieve discomfort.

Self-Care Practices

There are steps you can take that may be helpful in easing symptoms, such as:

- eating soft foods,
- applying ice packs,
- avoiding extreme jaw movements (such as wide yawning, loud singing, and gum chewing),
- learning techniques for relaxing and reducing stress,
- practicing gentle jaw stretching and relaxing exercises that may help increase jaw movement. Your healthcare provider or a physical therapist can recommend exercises if appropriate for your particular condition.

Pain Medications

For many people with TMJ disorders, short-term use of over-the-counter pain medicines or nonsteroidal anti-inflammatory drugs (NSAIDs), such as ibuprofen, may provide temporary relief from jaw discomfort. When necessary, your dentist or physician can prescribe stronger pain or anti-inflammatory medications, muscle relaxants, or anti-depressants to help ease symptoms.

Stabilization Splints

Your physician or dentist may recommend an oral appliance, also called a stabilization splint or bite guard, which is a plastic guard that fits over the upper or lower teeth. Stabilization splints are the most widely used treatments for TMJ disorders. Studies of their effectiveness in providing pain relief, however, have been inconclusive. If a stabilization splint is recommended, it should be used only for a short time and should not cause permanent changes in the bite. If a splint causes or increases pain, or affects your bite, stop using it and see your healthcare provider.

The conservative, reversible treatments described are useful for temporary relief of pain—they are not cures for TMJ disorders. If symptoms continue over time, come back often, or worsen, tell your doctor.

Botox

Botox® (botulinum toxin type A) is a drug made from the same bacterium that causes food poisoning. Used in small doses, Botox injections can actually help alleviate some health problems and have been approved by the Food and Drug Administration (FDA) for certain disorders. However, Botox is currently not approved by the FDA for use in TMJ disorders.

Results from recent clinical studies are inconclusive regarding the effectiveness of Botox for treatment of chronic TMJ disorders. Additional research is under way to learn how Botox specifically affects jaw muscles and their nerves. The findings will help determine if this drug may be useful in treating TMJ disorders.

Irreversible Treatments

Irreversible treatments that have not been proven to be effective—and may make the problem worse—include orthodontics to change the bite; crown and bridge work to balance the bite; grinding down teeth to bring the bite into balance, called "occlusal adjustment"; and repositioning splints, also called orthotics, which permanently alter the bite.

Surgery

Other types of treatments, such as surgical procedures, invade the tissues. Surgical treatments are controversial, often irreversible, and should be avoided where possible. There have been no long-term clinical trials to study the safety and effectiveness of surgical treatments for TMJ disorders. Nor are there standards to identify people who would most likely benefit from surgery. Failure to respond to conservative treatments, for example, does not automatically mean that surgery is necessary. If surgery is recommended, be sure to have the doctor explain to you, in words you can understand, the reason for the treatment, the risks involved, and other types of treatment that may be available.

Implants

Surgical replacement of jaw joints with artificial implants may cause severe pain and permanent jaw damage. Some of these devices may fail to function properly or may break apart in the jaw over time. If you have already had temporomandibular joint surgery, be very cautious about considering additional operations. Persons undergoing multiple surgeries on the jaw joint generally have a poor outlook for normal, pain-free joint function. Before undergoing any surgery on the jaw joint, it is extremely important to get other independent opinions and to fully understand the risks.

The U.S. Food and Drug Administration (FDA) monitors the safety and effectiveness of medical devices implanted in the body, including artificial jaw joint implants.

If You Think You Have a TMJ Disorder...

Remember that for most people, discomfort from TMJ disorders will eventually go away on its own. Simple self-care practices are often effective in easing symptoms. If treatment is needed, it should be based on a reasonable diagnosis, be conservative and reversible, and be customized to your special needs. Avoid treatments that can cause permanent changes in the bite or jaw. If irreversible treatments are recommended, be sure to get a reliable, independent second opinion.

Because there is no certified specialty for TMJ disorders in either dentistry or medicine, finding the right care can be difficult. Look for a healthcare provider who understands musculoskeletal disorders (affecting muscle, bone and joints) and who is trained in treating pain conditions. Pain clinics in hospitals and universities are often a good source of advice, particularly when pain continues over time and interferes with daily life. Complex cases, often marked by prolonged, persistent and severe pain; jaw dysfunction; co-existing conditions; and diminished quality of life, likely require a team of experts from various fields, such as neurology, rheumatology, pain management and others, to diagnose and treat this condition.

Hope for the Future

The challenges posed by TMJ disorders span the research spectrum, from causes to diagnosis through treatment and prevention. Researchers throughout the health sciences are working together not only to gain a better understanding of the temporomandibular joint and muscle disease process, but also to improve quality of life for people affected by these disorders.

Section 40.2

Osteonecrosis of the Jaw

This section contains text excerpted from the following sources: Text in this section begins with excerpts from "Expert Panel Recommendation for the Prevention, Diagnosis, and Treatment of Osteonecrosis of the Jaw," U.S. Food and Drug Administration (FDA), March 4, 2005. Reviewed September 2016; Text beginning with the heading "A Background on Pathophysiology and Clinical Studies of Osteonecrosis of the Jaw (ONJ)" is excerpted from "Pathophysiology and Clinical Studies of Osteonecrosis of the Jaw (ONJ)," National Institute of Dental and Craniofacial Research (NIDCR), February 26, 2014.

Osteonecrosis of the jaws is a rare potential complication in cancer patients receiving radiation, chemotherapy, or other cancer treatment regimens, or in patients with tumors/infectious embolic events.

Clinical Presentation and Diagnosis of Osteonecrosis of the Jaws

- Osteonecrosis of the jaws may remain asymptomatic for many weeks or months and may only be recognized by the presence of the exposed bone in the oral cavity. These lesions are most frequently symptomatic when sites become secondarily infected or there is trauma to the soft tissues via the sharp edges of the exposed bone, which may occur spontaneously or, more commonly, at the site of previous tooth extraction. Some patients may present with atypical complaints, such as "numbness," the feeling of a "heavy jaw," and various dysesthesias.

- Typical signs and symptoms include pain, soft-tissue swelling and infection, loosening of teeth, drainage.

- Signs and symptoms that may occur before the development of clinical osteonecrosis include a sudden change in the health of periodontal or mucosal tissues, failure of the oral mucosa to heal, undiagnosed oral pain, loose teeth, or soft-tissue infection.

- If osteonecrosis is suspected, panoramic and tomographic imaging may be performed to rule out other etiologies (eg., cysts or impacted teeth). Smaller intraoral films can also be used to demonstrate subtle bone changes.

- Microbial cultures may provide a differential diagnosis for comorbid oral infections.

Tissue biopsy should be performed only if metastatic disease is suspected. If a biopsy is performed to rule out metastatic tumor, microbial cultures (aerobic and anaerobic) may provide identification of the pathogens causing secondary infections. (Note: actinomyces organisms are often seen microscopically or identified upon culture)

Potential Risk Factors for the Development of Osteonecrosis of the Jaws

- The precise risk factors for osteonecrosis of the jaws have not been identified. Risk factors may include:

  - Concomitant therapy with steroids, chemotherapy, and IV bisphosphonates (in few instances after short dosing)

  - Dental extraction, infectious disease, and/or trauma

Occasionally the concomitant risk factors may not be apparent, other risk factors that have been previously identified for osteonecrosis (not limited to the jaws) include:

- Head and neck radiotherapy, chemotherapy, immunotherapy, or other cancer treatment regimens

- Female gender, coagulopathies, infections, periodontal disease, bony exostosis, previous invasive dental procedures, dental prostheses, arthritis, blood dyscrasias, vascular disorders, alcohol abuse, smoking, and malnutrition. Controversially, anesthetics with vasoconstrictors (i.e., novocaine) have been reported as potentially contributing to some cases of osteonecrosis

Dental Treatment for Patients Currently Receiving Bisphosphonate Therapy

- Maintain excellent oral hygiene to reduce the risk of dental and periodontal infections.

- Check and adjust removable dentures for potential soft-tissue injury, especially tissue overlying bone.

- Perform routine dental cleanings, being sure to avoid soft-tissue injury

- Aggressively manage dental infections nonsurgically with root canal treatment if possible or with minimal surgical intervention.

- Endodontic (root canal) therapy is preferable to extractions when possible. It may be necessary to carry out coronal amputation with subsequent root canal therapy on retained roots to avoid the need for tooth extraction and, therefore, the potential development of osteonecrosis.

A Background on Pathophysiology and Clinical Studies of Osteonecrosis of the Jaw (ONJ)

The bisphosphonates are a class of drugs that inhibit the activities and functions of osteoclasts (bone resorbing cells) and perturb the differentiation of osteoblasts (bone forming cells). Intravenous bisphosphonates are used primarily to treat the pain, bone resorption and hypercalcemia associated with cancer metastasis and multiple myeloma. Oral bisphosphonates are used to prevent bone loss and are prescribed for patients with osteoporosis, osteopenia, and Paget's disease.

In 2003, reports appeared in the literature that suggested an association of ONJ with bisphosphonate use in a subset of patients. Patients with ONJ present with painful, exposed necrotic bone of the maxilla or mandible. These slow or non-healing lesions often develop following invasive dental procedures, but they may develop spontaneously. Secondary infection of the necrotic bone can result in a localized osteomyelitis. Various reports have estimated the incidence and prevalence of this condition, but the range is large and the estimates need to be verified. Most cases are related to intravenous bisphosphonate use in cancer patients, but many cases are reported in those using oral bisphosphonates to prevent or treat osteoporosis. Currently, there are no

303

evidence-based treatments for ONJ. Patients may be treated non-invasively with antibiotics and chlorhexidine mouth rinses to prevent secondary infection. Surgical interventions such as local debridement or resection of necrotic bone have not been evaluated for their effectiveness. Taking "drug holidays" is an option to be explored and should only be approached with caution to balance the benefits and risks of bisphosphonate use. While ONJ affects relatively few patients taking oral bisphosphonates, the oral forms are used long term by millions of patients world-wide. Very recent data suggest newer biological agents that inhibit osteoclast-mediated bone resorption may be associated with ONJ. Therefore, ONJ research has the potential to have broad health impact.

Chapter 41

Mouth Sores

Chapter Contents

Section 41.1

Canker Sores

What Is a Canker Sore?

If you've ever had those open, shallow sores in your mouth and taken a gulp of orange juice, you know what a pain canker sores can be. Canker sores are fairly common: About 1 in 5 people get them on a regular basis. The good news is, they usually go away on their own without treatment. Canker sores (also known as **aphthous ulcers**) only happen inside the mouth. You can get them on or under the tongue and on the inside of the cheeks and lips—the parts of the mouth that can move. They usually pop up alone, but sometimes they show up in small clusters.

Signs It's a Canker Sore

Your mouth might tingle or burn before a canker sore appears. Soon, a small red bump rises. Then after a day or so it bursts, leaving an open, shallow white or yellowish wound with a red border. The sores are often painful and can be up to half an inch across, although most of them are much smaller. A person who has canker sores doesn't usually have the fever or swollen lymph nodes that can show up with some other kinds of sores. Aside from the annoying pain in the mouth, you'll generally feel OK.

The good news is that canker sores are not contagious like some other mouth sores, such as cold sores. You can't get canker sores by sharing food or kissing someone.

If you have a sore and you're wondering if it's a cold sore or a canker sore, just look at where it shows up: Cold sores usually appear outside the mouth, around the lips, chin or nostrils. Canker sores are always found *inside* the mouth.

You can also get spots in your mouth when you have an infection like chickenpox or measles. In some cases of these diseases, the rash actually spreads into the mouth. If you have chickenpox or measles, you'll find spots on other parts of your body as well, so you'll know they're not canker sores.

Causes

Canker sores usually begin showing up between the ages of 10 and 20, although they can happen at any time in a person's life. No one knows exactly what causes them. One thing that doctors have noticed is that although the sores are not contagious, they can run in families. That means if your parents or siblings get canker sores, the genes you share with them make it more likely that you'll develop the sores, too.

There may be a connection between canker sores and stress. If you get canker sores around exam time or some other big event in your life, it may be a sign of how much stress you're under. In addition, about twice as many women as men get them. Doctors think that may be due to the differences in male and female hormones, especially because women often get them during certain times in their menstrual cycle.

Some research suggests that using products containing sodium lauryl sulfate (SLS) can be associated with canker sores. SLS is a foaming agent found in most toothpastes and mouthwashes. Finally, not getting the right nutrition, such as not getting enough iron or vitamin B12, may also contribute to some cases of canker sores.

What You Can Do

Most canker sores will heal on their own in a few days to a couple of weeks. While you're waiting for them to disappear, you can take over-the-counter pain relievers like ibuprofen or acetaminophen for the pain. You'll also want to watch what you eat. Spicy foods and acidic foods such as lemons or tomatoes can be extremely painful on these open wounds. Stay away from hard, scratchy, or crunchy foods like nuts, toast, pretzels, or potato chips for a while. They can poke or rub the sore.

Be careful when you brush your teeth. Brush and rinse with toothpastes and mouthwashes that don't contain sodium lauryl sulfate. And avoid brushing the sore itself with a toothbrush, which will make it worse.

There are lots of "home remedies" for canker sores out there, but no evidence to show that they help sores heal faster. If you have canker sores that do not get better after a few weeks, if the sores keep coming back, or if they make you feel so sick that you don't want to eat, call your doctor or dentist. He or she may prescribe a topical medicine or special mouthwash to help heal the sores.

For medications that are applied directly to the sore, first blot the area dry with a tissue. Use a cotton swab to apply a small amount of the medication, and do not eat or drink for at least 30 minutes to make sure that the medicine is not immediately washed away.

In some cases, doctors may want to do blood tests to find out if another condition—such as a vitamin deficiency, a problem with your immune system, or even a food allergy—could be contributing to the sores.

Although they can certainly be a pain, in most cases canker sores aren't serious and should go away on their own.

Section 41.2

Cold Sores

Text in this section is excerpted from "Coping with Cold Sores," © 1995–2016. The Nemours Foundation/KidsHealth®. Reprinted with permission.

What Is a Cold Sore?

Cold sores are small blisters that is reddish and a little painful. They are usually on the outer edge of the lip or inside the mouth. Cold sores can appear one at a time or in little bunches. They are filled with fluid but crust over and form a scab before they go away. They last a week or two and usually don't require any special treatment.

Although they're called cold sores, you don't need to have a cold to get one. Some people call them fever blisters, but you don't have to have a fever to have one, either. (Cold sores **aren't** the same as canker sores, which are small white sores that are always found inside the mouth.)

What Causes Cold Sores?

Cold sores are caused by a virus called **herpes.** Herpes is one of the most common viral infections in the world. The medical name for the specific virus that causes cold sores is herpes simplex.

There are two types of herpes simplex infection: herpes simplex virus one (called **HSV-1** for short) and herpes simplex virus two (called **HSV-2** for short). Although both can cause cold sores around a person's mouth, most are caused by HSV-1.

HSV-1 is so common that most Americans get infected with it, although many never have any symptoms. People can catch HSV-1 by kissing a person with a cold sore or sharing a drinking glass or utensils, so it's easy to see why there are so many cold sores around.

Kids who get infected with HSV-1 may get cold sores occasionally for the rest of their lives. That's because even after the sores themselves dry up and go away, the virus stays in the body, waiting around for another time to come out and cause more sores. When a cold sore reappears, it is often in the same place as the previous one.

How Can I Keep from Getting Cold Sores?

Although HSV-1 isn't a big deal, it's a good idea to try to keep cold sores as far away as possible. If someone you know has a cold sore, don't kiss him or her and don't drink out of the same glass or use the same knife, fork, or spoon. Sharing towels, washcloths, or napkins is off-limits, too, because the virus may survive on the fabric.

If you've had cold sores before, it can be hard to tell what might make them come back. For some kids, too much stress, too much time in the sun, or getting sick can cause cold sores to reappear. Eating well, getting enough rest, and learning how to deal with stress are important things for any kid to do, especially a kid who is likely to get cold sores.

Putting on sunblock lip balm and sunscreen on the face before going out in the sun may help prevent cold sores from reappearing in kids who tend to get them.

Treating Cold Sores

For most kids, the sores go away on their own without any special treatment from a doctor. If you get a cold sore, try holding some ice wrapped in cloth on the sore. It also might help to eat a popsicle.

Sometimes, if the cold sores are making a kid sick, a doctor may prescribe a special medicine that fights the herpes simplex virus. Some kids may take acetaminophen or ibuprofen if their sores are painful.

While you're waiting for the cold sore to go away, wash your hands regularly and don't pick at it. You'll only get in the way of your body's natural healing process. Picking at a cold sore is also bad news because it's easy to spread the virus to other parts or your body, like your fingers or eyes. Worse yet, you might spread the virus to other people. No one will thank you for giving them a cold sore!

Chapter 42

Oral Allergy Syndrome

What Is Food Allergy?

Food allergy is an abnormal response to a food triggered by the body's immune system. There are several types of immune responses to food. This booklet focuses on one type of adverse reaction to food—that in which the body produces a specific type of antibody called immunoglobulin E (IgE). The binding of IgE to specific molecules present in a food triggers the immune response. The response may be mild or in rare cases it can be associated with the severe and life- threatening reaction called anaphylaxis, which is described in this chapter. Therefore, if you have a food allergy, it is extremely important for you to work with your healthcare professional to learn what foods cause your allergic reaction. Sometimes, a reaction to food is not an allergy at all but another type of reaction called food intolerance. A description of food intolerance appears later in this chapter.

What Is an Allergic Reaction to Food?

A food allergy occurs when the immune system responds to a harmless food as if it were a threat. The first time a person with food allergy is exposed to the food, no symptoms occur; but the first exposure primes the body to respond the next time. When the person eats the food again, an allergic response can occur.

This chapter includes text excerpted from "Food Allergy: An Overview," National Institute of Allergy and Infectious Diseases (NIAID), July 2012. Reviewed September 2016.

What Is a First Exposure to Food?

Usually, the way you are first exposed to a food is when you eat it. But sometimes a first exposure or subsequent exposure can occur without your knowledge. This may be true in the case of peanut allergy. A person who experiences anaphylaxis on the first known exposure to peanut may have previously

- Touched peanuts
- Used a peanut-containing skin care product
- Breathed in peanut dust in the home or when close to other people eating peanuts

The Allergic Reaction Process An allergic reaction to food is a two-step process.

Step 1: The first time you are exposed to a food allergen, your immune system reacts as if the food were harmful and makes specific IgE antibodies to that allergen. The antibodies circulate through your blood and attach to mast cells and basophils. Mast cells are found in all body tissues, especially in areas of your body that are typical sites of allergic reactions. Those sites include your nose, throat, lungs, skin, and gastrointestinal (GI) tract. Basophils are found in your blood and also in tissues that have become inflamed due to an allergic reaction.

Step 2: The next time you are exposed to the same food allergen, it binds to the IgE antibodies that are attached to the mast cells and basophils. The binding signals the cells to release massive amounts of chemicals such as histamine. Depending on the tissue in which they are released, these chemicals will cause you to have various symptoms of food allergy. The symptoms can range from mild to severe. A severe allergic reaction can include a potentially life-threatening reaction called anaphylaxis. Generally, you are at greater risk for developing a food allergy if you come from a family in which allergies are common. These allergies are not necessarily food allergies but perhaps other allergic diseases, such as asthma, eczema (atopic dermatitis), or allergic rhinitis (hay fever). If you have two parents who have allergies, you are more likely to develop food allergy than someone with one parent who has allergies. An allergic reaction to food usually takes place within a few minutes to several hours after exposure to the allergen. The process of eating and digesting food and the location of mast cells both affect the timing and location of the reaction.

Symptoms of Food Allergy

If you are allergic to a particular food, you may experience all or some of the following symptoms:

- Itching in your mouth

- Swelling of lips and tongue

- GI symptoms, such as vomiting, diarrhea, or abdominal cramps and pain

- Hives

- Worsening of eczema

- Tightening of the throat or trouble breathing

- Drop in blood pressure

Oral Allergy Syndrome (OAS)

Oral allergy syndrome is an allergic reaction to certain raw fruits and vegetables, such as apples, cherries, kiwis, celery, tomatoes, melons, and bananas. Oral allergy syndrome occurs in people with hay fever, or cold-like symptoms caused by allergies. The syndrome is most likely to occur in those allergic to birch, grass and ragweed pollens because some of the protein allergens in these types of pollen are similar in structure to the proteins of certain fruits.

Those with oral allergy syndrome generally do not experience life-threatening reactions, but they can experience a rash, itching, swelling and sneezing if they eat or even just hold these raw fruits and vegetables. Similar to the experimental baked food approach to treating other food allergies, symptoms typically do not occur after consuming cooked or baked fruits and vegetables, as cooking or processing fruits and vegetables easily breaks down the proteins that cause oral allergy syndrome.

Eosinophilic Esophagitis

Eosinophilic esophagitis, or EoE, is a chronic disease that can be associated with food allergies. It is increasingly being diagnosed in children and adults. EoE is characterized by immune cells called eosinophils building up in the esophagus.

Symptoms of EoE include nausea, vomiting, and abdominal pain after eating. A person may also have symptoms that resemble acid reflux from the stomach, known as heartburn. In older children and adults, EoE can cause more severe symptoms, such as difficulty swallowing solid food, or solid food getting stuck in the esophagus and requiring removal by a physician. In infants, this disease may be associated with failure to thrive.

National Institute of Allergy and Infectious Diseases (NIAID)-funded researchers have found several genes associated with the development of EoE and have evaluated treatment with swallowed anti-inflammatory drugs called corticosteroids. A person diagnosed with EoE is usually tested for food allergies. Oftentimes, those that have both food allergy and EoE can avoid EoE symptoms by avoiding their allergen. NIAID currently funds studies investigating the effectiveness of food avoidance diets and other, experimental approaches to controlling EoE.

Conditions Often Mistaken for Food Allergy

People can feel ill after eating specific foods for reasons other than food allergy. Though these disorders may have some symptoms in common, these illnesses should not be confused with food allergy.

A problem often confused with food allergy is food intolerance, which is also an abnormal response to a food product, but differs from an allergy. A common example is an intolerance to lactose, a sugar found in many milk products that can cause an uncomfortable buildup of gas in the gastrointestinal tract. Gluten intolerance, or celiac disease, occurs when the immune system responds abnormally to gluten, a component of barley, wheat, and rye. However, unlike food allergies, these disorders do not involve IgE antibodies. The National Institute of Diabetes and Digestive and Kidney Disorders (NIDDK) currently conducts research on lactose and gluten intolerance.

Foodborne illness, or food poisoning, can also be confused with food allergy because of similar symptoms, such as abdominal cramping. Foodborne illness, however, is caused by microbes, microbial products, and other toxins that can contaminate foods that were improperly preserved or processed.

Preventing and Treating Food Allergy Prevention

There is currently no cure for food allergies. You can only prevent the symptoms of food allergy by avoiding the allergenic food. After you and your healthcare professional have identified the food(s) to which you are sensitive, you must remove them from your diet.

Read food labels You must read the list of ingredients on the label of each prepared food that you are considering eating. Many allergens, such as peanut, egg, and milk, appear in prepared foods you normally would not associate with those foods. Since 2006, U.S. food manufacturers have been required by law to list the ingredients of prepared foods. In addition, food manufacturers must use plain language to disclose whether their products contain any of the top eight allergenic foods—egg, milk, peanut, tree nuts, soy, wheat, shellfish, and fish. Be aware that some labels say "may contain."

Keep clean Simple measures of cleanliness can remove most allergens from the environment of a person with food allergy. For example, simply washing your hands with soap and water will remove peanut allergens, and most household cleaners will remove allergens from surfaces.

Treatment of a Food Allergy Reaction

Unintentional exposure When you have food allergies, you must be prepared to treat an unintentional exposure. Talk to your healthcare professional and develop a plan to protect yourself in case of an unintentional exposure to the food. For example, you should

- Wear a medical alert bracelet or necklace
- Carry an auto-injector device containing epinephrine (adrenaline)

Seek medical help immediately Mild symptoms Talk to your healthcare professional to find out what medicines may relieve mild food allergy symptoms that are not part of an anaphylactic reaction. However, be aware that it is very hard for you to know which reactions are mild and which may lead to anaphylaxis.

Chapter 43

Oral Cancer

Chapter Contents

Section 43.1

What You Need to Know about Oral Cancer

This section includes text excerpted from "Oral Cancer," National
Institute of Dental and Craniofacial Research (NIDCR), August 2014.

Oral cancer includes cancers of the mouth and the pharynx (the
back of the throat). Oral cancer accounts for roughly two percent of
all cancers diagnosed annually in the United States. Approximately
42,000 people will be diagnosed with oral cancer each year and about
8,000 will die from the disease. On average, 60 percent of those with
the disease will survive more than 5 years. Oral cancer most often
occurs in people over the age of 40 and affects more than twice as
many men as women.

What Puts Someone at Risk?

Tobacco and alcohol use. Tobacco use of any kind, including
cigarette smoking, puts you at risk. Heavy alcohol use also increases
your chances of developing the disease. And using tobacco plus alcohol
poses a much greater risk than using either substance alone.

HPV. Infection with the sexually transmitted human papillomavirus (specifically the HPV 16 type) has been linked to a subset of oral
cancers.

Age. Risk increases with age. Oral cancer most often occurs in
people over the age of 40.

Sun Exposure. Cancer of the lip can be caused by sun exposure.

Diet. A diet low in fruits and vegetables may play a role in oral
cancer development.

Possible Signs and Symptoms

See a dentist or physician if any of the following symptoms lasts
for more than 2 weeks.

- A sore, irritation, lump or thick patch in your mouth, lip, or throat
- A white or red patch in your mouth
- A feeling that something is caught in your throat
- Difficulty chewing or swallowing
- Difficulty moving your jaw or tongue
- Numbness in your tongue or other areas of your mouth
- Swelling of your jaw that causes dentures to fit poorly or become uncomfortable
- Pain in one ear without hearing loss

Early Detection

It is important to find oral cancer as early as possible when it can be treated more successfully. An oral cancer examination can detect early signs of cancer. The exam is painless and takes only a few minutes. Your regular dental check-up is an excellent opportunity to have the exam. During the exam, your dentist or dental hygienist will check your face, neck, lips, and entire mouth for possible signs of cancer. Some parts of the pharynx are not visible during an oral cancer exam. Talk to your dentist about whether a specialist should check your pharynx.

Section 43.2

Detecting Oral Cancer

This section includes text excerpted from "Detecting Oral Cancer: A Guide for Health Care Professionals," National Institute of Dental and Craniofacial Research (NIDCR), July 2013.

The Importance of Early Detection

With early detection and timely treatment, deaths from oral cancer could be dramatically reduced. The 5-year survival rate for those with localized disease at diagnosis is 83 percent compared with only 32 percent for those whose cancer has spread to other parts of the body. Early detection of oral cancer is often possible. Tissue changes in the mouth that might signal the beginnings of cancer often can be seen and felt easily.

Warning Signs

Lesions That Might Signal Oral Cancer

Two lesions that could be precursors to cancer are leukoplakia (white lesions) and erythroplakia (red lesions). Although less common than leukoplakia, erythroplakia and lesions with erythroplakic components have a much greater potential for becoming cancerous. Any white or red lesion that does not resolve itself in 2 weeks should be reevaluated and considered for biopsy to obtain a definitive diagnosis.

Other Possible Signs and Symptoms

Possible signs and symptoms of oral cancer that your patients may report include: a lump or thickening in the oral soft tissues, soreness or a feeling that something is caught in the throat, difficulty chewing or swallowing, ear pain, difficulty moving the jaw or tongue, hoarseness, numbness of the tongue or other areas of the mouth, or swelling of the jaw that causes dentures to fit poorly or become uncomfortable.

If these problems persist for more than 2 weeks, a thorough clinical examination and laboratory tests, as necessary, should be performed to obtain a definitive diagnosis. If a diagnosis cannot be obtained, referral to the appropriate specialist is indicated.

Risk Factors

Tobacco / Alcohol Use

Most cases of oral cancer are linked to cigarette smoking, heavy alcohol use, or the use of both tobacco and alcohol together. Using tobacco plus alcohol poses a much greater risk than using either substance alone.

HPV

Infection with the sexually transmitted human papillomavirus (specifically the HPV 16 type) has been linked to a subset of oral cancers.

Age

Risk increases with age. Oral cancer most often occurs in people over the age of 40.

Sun Exposure

Cancer of the lip can be caused by sun exposure.

Diet

A diet low in fruits and vegetables may play a role in oral cancer development.

What You Can Do

A thorough head and neck examination should be a routine part of each patient's dental visit and general medical examination. Clinicians should be particularly vigilant in checking those who use tobacco or excessive amounts of alcohol.

- **Examine** your patients using the head and neck exam illustrated in this program.
- **Take a history** of their alcohol and tobacco use.
- **Inform** your patients of the association between tobacco use, alcohol use, and oral cancer.
- **Follow-up** to make sure a definitive diagnosis is obtained on any possible signs or symptoms of oral cancer.

The Exam

This **exam** is abstracted from the standardized oral examination method recommended by the World Health Organization. The method is consistent with those followed by the Centers for Disease Control and Prevention and the National Institutes of Health. It requires adequate lighting, a dental mouth mirror, two 2" x 2" gauze squares, and gloves; it should take no longer than 5 minutes.

The Exam Review

The examination is conducted with the patient seated. Any intraoral prostheses are removed before starting. The extraoral and perioral tissues are examined first, followed by the intraoral tissues.

I. The Extraoral Examination

Face: The extraoral assessment includes inspection of the face, head, and neck. The face, ears, and neck are observed, noting any asymmetry or changes on the skin such as crusts, fissuring, growths, and/or color change. The regional lymph node areas are bilaterally palpated to detect any enlarged nodes. If enlargement is detected, the examiner should determine the mobility and consistency of the nodes. A recommended order of examination includes the preauricular, submandibular, anterior cervical, posterior auricular, and posterior cervical regions.

II. Perioral and Intraoral Soft Tissue Examination

The perioral and intraoral examination procedure follows a seven-step systematic assessment of the lips; labial mucosa and sulcus; commissures, buccal mucosa, and sulcus; gingiva and alveolar ridge; tongue; floor of the mouth; and hard and soft palate.

Lips: Begin examination by observing the lips with the patient's mouth both closed and open. Note the color, texture and any surface abnormalities of the upper and lower vermilion borders.

Labial mucosa: With the patient's mouth partially open, visually examine the labial mucosa and sulcus of the maxillary vestibule and frenum and the mandibular vestibule. Observe the color, texture, and any swelling or other abnormalities of the vestibular mucosa and gingiva.

Bussal mucosa: Retract the buccal mucosa. Examine first the right then the left buccal mucosa extending from the labial commissure and back to the anterior tonsillar pillar. Note any change in pigmentation, color, texture, mobility, and other abnormalities of the mucosa, making sure that the commissures are examined carefully and are not covered by the retractors during the retraction of the cheek.

Gingiva: First, examine the buccal and labial aspects of the gingiva and alveolar ridges (processes) by starting with the right maxillary posterior gingiva and alveolar ridge and then move around the arch to the left posterior area. Drop to the left mandibular posterior gingiva and alveolar ridge and move around the arch to the right posterior area.

Second, examine the palatal and lingual aspects as had been done on the facial side, from right to left on the palatal (maxilla) and left to right on the lingual (mandible).

Tongue: With the patient's tongue at rest, and mouth partially open, inspect the dorsum of the tongue for any swelling, ulceration, coating, or variation in size, color, or texture. Also note any change in the pattern of the papillae covering the surface of the tongue and examine the tip of the tongue. The patient should then protrude the tongue, and the examiner should note any abnormality of mobility or positioning.

With the aid of mouth mirrors, inspect the right and left lateral margins of the tongue.

Grasping the tip of the tongue with a piece of gauze will assist full protrusion and will aid examination of the more posterior aspects of the tongue's lateral borders.

Then examine the ventral surface. Palpate the tongue to detect growths.

Floor: With the tongue still elevated, inspect the floor of the mouth for changes in color, texture, swellings, or other surface abnormalities.

Palate: With the mouth wide open and the patient's head tilted back, gently depress the base of the tongue with a mouth mirror. First inspect the hard and then the soft palate.

Examine all soft palate and oropharyngeal tissues.

Bimanually palpate the floor of the mouth for any abnormalities. All mucosal or facial tissues that seem to be abnormal should be palpated.

Section 43.3

Smokeless Tobacco's Connection to Cancer

This section contains text excerpted from the following sources:
Text beginning with the heading "Smokeless Tobacco's Connection
to Cancer" is excerpted from "Smokeless Tobacco: Health Effects,"
Centers for Disease Control and Prevention (CDC), February 18,
2016; Text beginning with the heading "Types of Smokeless Tobacco"
is excerpted from "Types of Smokeless Tobacco," Centers for Disease
Control and Prevention (CDC), July 13, 2016.

Smokeless Tobacco and Its Effects

Smokeless tobacco is associated with many health problems. Using
smokeless tobacco:

- Can lead to nicotine addiction

- Causes cancer of the mouth, esophagus (the passage that connects the throat to the stomach), and pancreas (a gland that
  helps with digestion and maintaining proper blood sugar levels)

- Is associated with diseases of the mouth

- Can increase risks for early delivery and stillbirth when used
  during pregnancy

- Can cause nicotine poisoning in children

- May increase the risk for death from heart disease and stroke

Addiction to Smokeless Tobacco

- Smokeless tobacco contains nicotine, which is highly addictive.

- Because young people who use smokeless tobacco can become
  addicted to nicotine, they may be more likely to also become cigarette smokers.

Smokeless Tobacco and Cancer

- Many smokeless tobacco products contain cancer-causing
  chemicals.

- The most harmful chemicals are tobacco-specific nitrosa-mines, which form during the growing, curing, fermenting, and aging of tobacco. The amount of these chemicals varies by product.

- The higher the levels of these chemicals, the greater the risk for cancer.

- Other chemicals found in tobacco can also cause cancer. These include:

- A radioactive element (polonium-210) found in tobacco fertilizer

- Chemicals formed when tobacco is cured with heat (polynu-clear aromatic hydrocarbons—also known as polycyclic aro-matic hydrocarbons)

- Harmful metals (arsenic, beryllium, cadmium, chromium, cobalt, lead, nickel, mercury)

- Smokeless tobacco causes cancer of the mouth, esophagus, and pancreas.

Smokeless Tobacco and Oral Disease

- Smokeless tobacco can cause white or gray patches inside the mouth (leukoplakia) that can lead to cancer.

- Smokeless tobacco can cause gum disease, tooth decay, and tooth loss.

Reproductive and Developmental Risks

- Using smokeless tobacco during pregnancy can increase the risk for early delivery and stillbirth.

- Nicotine in smokeless tobacco products that are used during pregnancy can affect how a baby's brain develops before birth.

Other Risks

- Using smokeless tobacco increases the risk for death from heart disease and stroke.

- Smokeless tobacco can cause nicotine poisoning in children.

- Additional research is needed to examine long-term effects of newer smokeless tobacco products, such as dissolvables and U.S. snus.

Types of Smokeless Tobacco

Chewing tobacco comes in the form of loose leaf, plug, or twist.

- Most people who use smokeless tobacco put the product between their cheek and gums and suck or chew on the tobacco.

- The saliva and tobacco juice that form may be spit out or swallowed.

- Smokeless tobacco products may appeal to youth because they come in flavors such as cinnamon, berry, vanilla, and apple.

Table 43.1. Smokeless Tobacco

Form	Description	Use
Loose leaf	Cured (aged) tobacco, typically sweetened and packaged in foil pouches	Piece taken from pouch and placed between cheek and gums
Plug	Cured tobacco leaves pressed together into a cake or "plug" form and wrapped in a tobacco leaf	Piece taken from pouch and placed between cheek and gums
Twist or roll	Cured (aged) tobacco leaves twisted together like a rope	Piece cut off from twist and placed between cheek and gums

Snuff is finely ground tobacco that can be dry, moist, or packaged in pouches or packets (U.S. snus).

- Some types of snuff are sniffed or inhaled into the nose; 2 other types are placed in the mouth.

Table 43.2. Types of Snuff

Form	Description	Use
Moist	Cured (aged) and fermented tobacco processed into fine particles and often packaged in round cans	Pinch or "dip" is placed between cheek or lip and gums; requires spitting

Table 43.2. (Continued)

Form	Description	Use
Dry	Fire-cured tobacco in powder form	Pinch of powder is put in the mouth or inhaled through the nose; may require spitting
U.S snus	Moist snuff packaged in ready-to-use pouches that resemble small tea bags	Pouch is placed between cheek or teeth and gums; does not require spitting

Dissolvables are finely ground tobacco pressed into shapes such as tablets, sticks, or strips.

- Dissolvable tobacco products slowly dissolve in the mouth.

- These products may appeal to youth because they come in attractive packaging, look like candy or small mints, and can be easily hidden from view.

Table 43.3. Dissolvables Tobacco Products

Form	Description
Lozenges	Resemble pellets or tablets
Orbs	Resemble small mints
Sticks	Have a toothpick-like appearance
Strips	Thin sheets that work like dissolvable breath strips or medication strips

Chapter 44

Taste Disorders

Chapter Contents

Section 44.1

Problems with Taste

This section includes text excerpted from "Problems with Taste," NIHSeniorHealth, National Institutes of Health (NIH), January 2014.

Taste or gustation, is one of our most robust senses. Although there is a small decline in taste in people over 60, most older people will not notice it because normal aging does not greatly affect our sense of taste. Problems with taste occur less frequently than problems with smell.

How Our Sense of Taste Works

Our sense of taste, along with our sense of smell, is part of our chemical sensing system. Normal taste occurs when tiny molecules released by chewing or the digestion of food stimulate special sensory cells in the mouth and throat. These taste cells, or gustatory cells, send messages through three specialized taste nerves to the brain, where specific tastes are identified. Damage to these nerves following head injury can lead to taste loss.

The taste cells are clustered within the taste buds of the tongue and roof of the mouth, and along the lining of the throat. Many of the small bumps that can be seen on the tip of the tongue contain taste buds. At birth, we have about 10,000 taste buds scattered on the back, sides, and tip of the tongue. After age 50, we may start to lose taste buds.

Five Taste Sensations

We can experience five basic taste sensations: sweet, sour, bitter, salty, and umami, or savory. Umami is the taste we get from glutamate, a building block of protein found in chicken broth, meat stock, and some cheeses. Umami is also the taste associated wtih MSG (monosodium glutamate) that is often added to foods as a flavor enhancer.

The five taste qualities combine with other oral sensations, such as texture, spiciness, temperature, and aroma to produce what is commonly referred to as flavor. It is flavor that lets us know whether we are eating an apple or a pear.

Flavors and the Sense of Smell

Many people are surprised to learn that we recognize flavors largely through our sense of smell. Try holding your nose while eating chocolate. You will be able to distinguish between its sweetness and bitterness, but you can't identify the chocolate flavor. That's because the distinguishing characteristic of chocolate is largely identified by our sense of smell as aromas are released during chewing. Food flavor is affected by a head cold or nasal congestion because the aroma of food does not reach the sensory cells that detect odors.

Smell and Taste Closely Linked

Smell and taste are closely linked senses. Many people mistakenly believe they have a problem with taste, when they are really experiencing a problem with smell. It is common for people who lose their sense of smell to say that food has lost its taste. This is incorrect; the food has lost its aroma, but taste remains. In older people, there is a normal decline in the sense of smell and the taste of food shifts toward blandness. This is why people often believe they have a taste problem.

When Taste Is Impaired

Problems with taste can have a big impact on an older person's life. Because taste affects the amount and type of food we eat, when there are problems with taste, a person may change his or her eating habits. Some people may eat too much and gain weight, while others may eat too little and lose weight. A loss of appetite, especially in older adults, can lead to loss of weight, poor nutrition, weakened immunity, and even death.

Taste helps us detect spoiled food or liquids and it also helps some people detect ingredients they are allergic to. A problem with taste can weaken or remove an early warning system that most of us take for granted.

A distorted sense of taste can be a serious risk factor for illnesses that require sticking to a specific diet. Loss of taste can cause us to eat too much sugar or salt to make our food taste better. This can be a problem for people with such illnesses as diabetes or high blood pressure. In severe cases, loss of taste can lead to depression.

Taste Problems Are Often Temporary

When an older person has a problem with taste, it is often temporary and minor. True taste disorders are uncommon. When a problem with taste exists, it is usually caused by medications, disease, some cancer treatments, or injury.

Many older people believe that there is nothing they can do about their weakened sense of taste. If you think you have a problem with your sense of taste, see your doctor. Depending on the cause of your problem, your doctor may be able to suggest ways to regain your sense of taste or to cope with the loss of taste.

Section 44.2

Facts on Taste Disorders

This section includes text excerpted from "Taste Disorders,"
National Institute on Deafness and Other Communication
Disorders (NIDCD), January 5, 2014.

How Common Are Taste Disorders?

Many of us take our sense of taste for granted, but a taste disorder can have a negative effect on your health and quality of life. If you are having a problem with your sense of taste, you are not alone. More than 200,000 people visit a doctor each year for problems with their ability to taste or smell. Scientists believe that up to 15 percent of adults might have a taste or smell problem, but many don't seek a doctor's help.

The senses of taste and smell are very closely related. Most people who go to the doctor because they think they have lost their sense of taste are surprised to learn that they have a smell disorder instead.

How Does Your Sense of Taste Work?

Your ability to taste comes from tiny molecules released when you chew, drink, or digest food; these molecules stimulate special sensory cells in the mouth and throat. These taste cells, or gustatory cells, are clustered within the taste buds of the tongue and roof of the mouth, and along the lining of the throat. Many of the small bumps on the tip of your tongue contain taste buds. At birth, you have about 10,000 taste buds, but after age 50, you may start to lose them.

When the taste cells are stimulated, they send messages through three specialized taste nerves to the brain, where specific tastes are identified. Taste cells have receptors that respond to one of at least five basic taste qualities: sweet, sour, bitter, salty, and umami. Umami, or savory, is the taste you get from glutamate, which is found in chicken broth, meat extracts, and some cheeses. A common misconception is that taste cells that respond to different tastes are found in separate regions of the tongue. In humans, the different types of taste cells are scattered throughout the tongue.

Taste quality is just one way that you experience a certain food. Another chemosensory mechanism, called the common chemical sense, involves thousands of nerve endings, especially on the moist surfaces of the eyes, nose, mouth, and throat. These nerve endings give rise to sensations such as the coolness of mint and the burning or irritation of chili peppers. Other specialized nerves create the sensations of heat, cold, and texture. When you eat, the sensations from the five taste qualities, together with the sensations from the common chemical sense and the sensations of heat, cold, and texture, combine with a food's aroma to produce a perception of flavor. It is flavor that lets you know whether you are eating a pear or an apple.

Most people who think they have a taste disorder actually have a problem with smell. When you chew food, aromas are released that activate your sense of smell by way of a special channel that connects the roof of the throat to the nose. If this channel is blocked, such as when your nose is stuffed up by a cold or flu, odors can't reach sensory cells in the nose that are stimulated by smells. As a result, you lose much of our enjoyment of flavor. Without smell, foods tend to taste bland and have little or no flavor.

What Are the Taste Disorders?

The most common taste disorder is phantom taste perception: a lingering, often unpleasant taste even though there is nothing in your mouth. People can also experience a reduced ability to taste sweet, sour, bitter, salty, and umami—a condition called hypogeusia. Some people can't detect any tastes, which is called ageusia. True taste loss, however, is rare. Most often, people are experiencing a loss of smell instead of a loss of taste.

In other disorders of the chemical senses, an odor, a taste, or a flavor may be distorted. Dysgeusia is a condition in which a foul, salty, rancid, or metallic taste sensation persists in the mouth. Dysgeusia is sometimes accompanied by burning mouth syndrome, a condition in which a person experiences a painful burning sensation in the mouth. Although it can affect anyone, burning mouth syndrome is most common in middle-aged and older women.

How Are Taste Disorders Diagnosed?

Both taste and smell disorders are diagnosed by an otolaryngologist (sometimes called an ENT), a doctor of the ear, nose, throat, head, and neck. An otolaryngologist can determine the extent of your taste disorder by measuring the lowest concentration of a taste quality that you can detect or recognize. You may be asked to compare the tastes of different substances or to note how the intensity of a taste grows when a substance's concentration is increased.

Scientists have developed taste tests in which the patient responds to different chemical concentrations. This may involve a simple "sip, spit, and rinse" test, or chemicals may be applied directly to specific areas of the tongue.

An accurate assessment of your taste loss will include, among other things, a physical examination of your ears, nose, and throat; a dental examination and assessment of oral hygiene; a review of your health history; and a taste test supervised by a healthcare professional.

Can Taste Disorders Be Treated?

Diagnosis by an otolaryngologist is important to identify and treat the underlying cause of your disorder. If a certain medication is the cause, stopping or changing your medicine may help eliminate the problem. (Do not stop taking your medications unless directed by your doctor, however.) Often, the correction of a general medical problem can correct the loss of taste. For example, people who lose their sense of taste because of respiratory infections or allergies may regain it when these conditions resolve. Occasionally, a person may recover his or her sense of taste spontaneously. Proper oral hygiene is important to regaining and maintaining a well-functioning sense of taste. If your taste disorder can't be successfully treated, counseling may help you adjust to your problem.

If you lose some or all of your sense of taste, here are things you can try to make your food taste better:

• Prepare foods with a variety of colors and textures.

• Use aromatic herbs and hot spices to add more flavor; however, avoid adding more sugar or salt to foods.

• If your diet permits, add small amounts of cheese, bacon bits, butter, olive oil, or toasted nuts on vegetables.

• Avoid combination dishes, such as casseroles, that can hide individual flavors and dilute taste.

Are Taste Disorders Serious?

Taste disorders can weaken or remove an early warning system that most of us take for granted. Taste helps you detect spoiled food or liquids and, for some people, the presence of ingredients to which they are allergic.

Loss of taste can create serious health issues. A distorted sense of taste can be a risk factor for heart disease, diabetes, stroke, and other illnesses that require sticking to a specific diet. When taste is impaired, a person may change his or her eating habits. Some people may eat too little and lose weight, while others may eat too much and gain weight.

Loss of taste can cause you to add too much sugar or salt to make food taste better. This can be a problem for people with certain medical conditions, such as diabetes or high blood pressure. In severe cases, loss of taste can lead to depression.

If you are experiencing a taste disorder, talk with your doctor.

Section 44.3

Symptoms and Diagnosis of Taste Disorders

This section includes text excerpted from "Problems
with Taste," NIHSeniorHealth, National Institutes of
Health (NIH), January 2014.

There are several types of taste disorders depending on how the
sense of taste is affected. People who have taste disorders usually lose
their ability to taste or can no longer perceive taste in the same way.
True taste disorders are rare. Most changes in the perception of food
flavor result from the loss of smell.

Phantom Taste Perception. The most common taste complaint
is "phantom taste perception"—tasting something when nothing is in
the mouth.

Hypogeusia. Some people have hypogeusia, or the reduced ability
to taste sweet, sour, bitter, salty, and savory, or umami. This disorder
is usually temporary.

Dysgeusia. Dysgeusia is a condition in which a foul, salty, rancid,
or metallic taste sensation will persist in the mouth. Dysgeusia is
sometimes accompanied by burning mouth syndrome, a condition in
which a person experiences a painful burning sensation in the mouth.
Although it can affect anyone, burning mouth syndrome is most common in middle-aged and older women.

Ageusia. Other people can't detect taste at all, which is called
ageusia. This type of taste disorder can be caused by head trauma;
some surgical procedures, such as middle ear surgery or extraction of
the third molar; radiation therapy; and viral infections.

Why a Diagnosis Is Important

If you think you have a taste disorder, see your doctor. Loss of the
sense of taste can lead to depression and a reduced desire to eat. Loss
of appetite can lead to loss of weight, poor nutrition and weakened

immunity. In some cases, loss of taste can accompany or signal conditions such as diabetes. Sometimes, a problem with taste can be a sign of a disease of the nervous system, such multiple sclerosis, Alzheimer's disease, or Parkinson's disease.

Do You Have a Taste Disorder?

If you think you have a taste disorder, try to identify and record the circumstances surrounding it. Ask yourself the following questions:

- When did I first become aware of it?
- What changes in my taste do I notice?
- Do all foods and drinks taste the same?
- Have there been any changes in my sense of smell?
- Does the change in taste affect my ability to eat normally?
- What medications do I take? What are the names of the medications? How much do I take? What is the health condition for which I take them?
- Have I recently had a cold or the flu?

Talking with Your Doctor

Bring this information with you when you visit the doctor. He or she may refer you to an otolaryngologist, a specialist in diseases of the ear, nose, and throat. An accurate assessment of your taste loss will include, among other things

- a physical examination of your ears, nose, and throat
- a dental examination and assessment of oral hygiene
- a review of your health history
- a taste test supervised by a healthcare professional.

Tests for Taste Disorders

Some tests are designed to measure the lowest concentration of a substance that a person can detect or recognize. Your doctor may ask you to compare the tastes of different substances or to note how the intensity of a taste grows when a substance's concentration is increased.

Scientists have developed taste tests in which the patient responds to different concentrations of a substance. This may involve a simple "sip, spit, and rinse" test or the application of a substance directly to your tongue using an eyedropper. By using these tests, your doctor can determine if you have a true taste disorder and what type it is.

If your doctor suspects that nerves in your mouth or head may be affected, he or she may order an X-ray, usually a CAT scan, to look further into the head and neck area.

Once the cause of a taste disorder is found, your doctor may be able to treat it. Many types of taste disorders are reversible, but if not, counseling and self-help techniques may help you cope.

Section 44.4

What Causes Taste Disorders?

This section includes text excerpted from "Problems with Taste," NIHSeniorHealth, National Institutes of Health (NIH), January 2014.

Causes of Taste Disorders

Loss of taste may be permanent or temporary, depending on the cause. As with vision and hearing, people gradually lose their ability to taste as they get older, but it is usually not as noticeable as loss of smell. Medications and illness can make the normal loss of taste worse.

Problems with taste are caused by anything that interrupts the transfer of taste sensations to the brain, or by conditions that affect the way the brain interprets the sensation of taste. Some people are born with taste disorders, but most develop them after an injury or illness. Among the causes of taste problems are:

- medications

- upper respiratory and middle ear infections

- radiation for treatment of head and neck cancers

- exposure to certain chemicals

- head injury

- some surgeries

- poor oral hygiene and dental problems

- smoking

In many cases, people regain their sense of taste when they stop taking medications or when the illness or injury clears up.

Medications. Taking medications can affect our ability to taste. Some antibiotics and antihistamines as well as other medications can cause a bad taste in the mouth or a loss of taste. One type of taste disorder is characterized by a persistent bad taste in the mouth, such as a bitter or salty taste. This is called dysgeusia and it occurs in older people, usually because of medications or oral health problems.

Upper Respiratory and Middle Ear Infections. Respiratory infections such as the flu can lead to taste disorders.

Radiation for Head and Neck Cancers. People with head and neck cancers who receive radiation treatment to the nose and mouth regions commonly experience problems with their sense of smell and taste as an unfortunate side effect. Older people who have lost their larynx or voice box commonly complain of poor ability to smell and taste.

Exposure to Certain Chemicals. Sometimes exposure to certain chemicals, such as insecticides and solvents, can impair taste. Avoid contact with these substances, and if you do come in contact with them and experience a problem, see your doctor.

Head Injury. Previous surgery or trauma to the head can impair your sense of taste because the taste nerves may be cut, blocked or physically damaged.

Some Surgeries. Some surgeries to the ear nose and throat can impair taste. These include third molar—wisdom tooth—extraction and middle ear surgery.

Poor Oral Hygiene and Dental Problems. Gum disease can cause problems with taste and so can can dentures and inflammation or infections in the mouth. If you take several medications, your mouth may produce less saliva. This causes dry mouth, which can make swallowing and digestion difficult and increase dental problems. Practice good oral hygiene, keep up to date with your dental appointments, and tell your dentist if you notice any problems with your sense of taste.

Smoking. Tobacco smoking is the most concentrated form of pollution that most people are exposed to. Smokers often report an improved sense of taste after quitting.

When to See the Doctor

Be sure to see your doctor if you have had a taste problem for a while or if you notice that your problem with taste is associated with other symptoms. Let your doctor know if you are taking any medications that might affect your sense of taste. You may be able to change or adjust your medicine to one that will not cause a problem with taste. Your doctor will work with you to get the medicine you need while trying to reduce unwanted side effects.

Section 44.5

Preventing Taste Disorders

This section includes text excerpted from "Problems with Taste," NIHSeniorHealth, National Institutes of Health (NIH), January 2014.

Protecting Your Sense of Taste

Taste, or gustation, is one of our most robust senses. Taste helps us recognize when food is good or bad for us. But, even more important, loss of taste can cause a loss of appetite, especially in older adults, which can lead to loss of weight, poor nutrition, weakened immunity, and even death.

These steps may help you protect your sense of taste.

Avoid Upper Respiratory and Middle Ear Infections

You can help prevent problems with taste caused by respiratory infections such as the flu by washing your hands frequently, especially during the winter months. Also, get a flu shot every year to prevent influenza and other serious respiratory conditions that can result from the flu.

Review Your Medications

If you are taking medications such as certain antibiotics or antihistamines or other medications and notice a persistent bad taste in your mouth, talk to your doctor. You may be able to adjust or change your medicine to one that will not cause a problem with taste. In many cases, people regain their sense of taste when they stop taking medications or when the illness or injury clears up.

Avoid Head Injuries

Previous surgery or trauma to the head can impair your sense of taste because the taste nerves may be cut, blocked or physically damaged.

To reduce the risk of injuries to the head, everyone should wear a seatbelt when riding in a car. People who participate in sports, such as bicycling, should wear protective helmets.

Avoid Exposure to Toxic Substances

Sometimes exposure to certain chemicals, such as insecticides and solvents, can impair taste. Avoid contact with these substances, and if you do come in contact with them and experience a problem with your sense of taste, see your doctor.

Take Care of Dental Problems

Gum disease can cause problems with taste, as can dentures and inflammation or infections in the mouth. Practice good oral hygiene, keep up to date with your dental appointments, and tell your dentist if you notice any problems with your sense of taste.

Don't Smoke

Smokers often report an improved sense of taste after quitting.

Section 44.6

Treatment for Taste Disorders

This section includes text excerpted from "Problems
with Taste," NIHSeniorHealth, National Institutes of
Health (NIH), January 2014.

Relief Is Possible

Although there is no treatment for any gradual loss of taste that
occurs with aging, relief from taste disorders is possible for many older
people. Depending on the cause of your problem with taste, your doctor
may be able to treat it or suggest ways to cope with it. Scientists are
studying how loss of taste occurs so that treatments can be developed.

Some patients regain their sense of taste when the condition or illness that is causing the loss of taste is over. For example, a middle ear
infection often affects taste temporarily. Often, correcting the general
medical problem can restore the sense of taste.

Check Your Medications

Often, a certain medication is the cause of a taste disorder, and
stopping or changing the medicine may help eliminate the problem.
If you take medications, ask your doctor if they can affect your sense
of taste. If so, ask if you can take other medications or safely reduce
the dose.

Do not stop taking your medications unless directed by your doctor.
Your doctor will work with you to get the medicines you need while
trying to reduce unwanted side effects.

If Your Diet Is Affected

Because your sense of taste may gradually decline, you may not
even notice the change. But your diet may change, and not for the
better. You may lose interest in food and eat less, but you may choose
foods that are high in fat and sugars. Or, you may eat more than you
should, hoping to get more flavor from every bite.

If you lose some or all of your sense of taste, there are things you can do to make your food taste better:

- Prepare foods with a variety of colors and textures

- Use aromatic herbs and hot spices to add more flavor; however avoid adding more sugar or salt to food

- If your diet permits, use small amounts of cheese, bacon bits, or butter on vegetables, as well as olive oil or toasted nuts

- Avoid combination dishes, such as casseroles, that can hide individual flavors and dilute taste.

If Your Sense of Taste Does Not Return

If you cannot regain your sense of taste, there are things you can do to ensure your safety. Take extra care to avoid food that may have spoiled. If you live with other people, ask them to smell and taste food to make sure it is fresh. People who live alone should discard food if there is a chance it is spoiled.

For those who wish to have additional help, there may be support groups in your area. These are often associated with smell and taste clinics in medical school hospitals. Some online bulletin boards also allow people with smell and taste disorders to share their experiences. Not all people with taste disorders will regain their sense of taste, but most can learn to live with it.

Chapter 45

Thrush

Candidiasis of the mouth and throat, also known as "thrush" or oropharyngeal candidiasis, is a fungal infection that occurs when there is overgrowth of a yeast called *Candida*. *Candida* yeasts normally live on the skin or mucous membranes in small amounts. However, if the environment inside the mouth or throat becomes imbalanced, the yeasts can multiply and cause symptoms. *Candida* overgrowth can also develop in the esophagus, and this is called *Candida* esophagitis or esophageal candidiasis.

Symptoms

Candida infections of the mouth and throat can manifest in a variety of ways. The most common symptom of oral thrush is white patches or plaques on the tongue and other oral mucous membranes. Other symptoms include:

- Redness or soreness in the affected areas

- Difficulty swallowing

- Cracking at the corners of the mouth (angular cheilitis)

It is important to see your doctor if you have any of these symptoms.

This chapter includes text excerpted from "Oropharyngeal/Esophageal Candidiasis ("Thrush")," Centers for Disease Control and Prevention (CDC), February 13, 2014.

Risk and Prevention

Who Gets Oral Candidiasis?

Candida infections of the mouth and throat are uncommon among adults who are otherwise healthy. Oral thrush occurs most frequently among babies less than one month old, the elderly, and groups of people with weakened immune systems. Other factors associated with oral and esophageal candidiasis include:

- HIV/AIDS
- Cancer treatments
- Organ transplantation
- Diabetes
- Corticosteroid use
- Dentures
- Broad-spectrum antibiotic use

How Can I Prevent Oral Candidiasis?

Good oral hygiene practices may help to prevent oral thrush in people with weakened immune systems. Some studies have shown that chlorhexidine (CHX) mouthwash can help to prevent oral candidiasis in people undergoing cancer treatment. People who use inhaled corticosteroids may be able to reduce the risk of developing thrush by washing out the mouth with water or mouthwash after using an inhaler.

Sources

Candida species are normal inhabitants of the mouth, throat, and the rest of the gastrointestinal tract. Usually, *Candida* yeasts live in and on the body in small amounts and do not cause any harm. However, the use of certain medications or a weakening of the immune system can cause *Candida* to multiply, which may cause symptoms of infection.

Diagnosis and Testing

A healthcare provider diagnoses the infection based on your symptoms, and by taking a scraping of the affected areas to examine under a microscope. A culture may also be performed; however, because

Candida organisms are normal inhabitants of the human mouth, a positive culture by itself does not make the diagnosis.

Treatment and Outcomes

Candida infections of the mouth and throat must be treated with prescription antifungal medication. The type and duration of treatment depends on the severity of the infection and patient-specific factors such as age and immune status. Untreated infections can lead to a more serious form of invasive candidiasis.

Oral candidiasis usually responds to topical treatments such as clotrimazole troches and nystatin suspension (nystatin "swish and swallow"). Systemic antifungal medication such as fluconazole or itraconazole may be necessary for oropharyngeal infections that do not respond to these treatments.

Candida esophagitis is typically treated with oral or intravenous fluconazole or oral itraconazole. For severe or azole-resistant esophageal candidiasis, treatment with amphotericin B may be necessary.

Statistics

The infection is not very common in the general population. It is estimated that between 5% and 7% of babies less than one month old will develop oral candidiasis. The prevalence of oral candidiasis among AIDS patients is estimated to be between 9% and 31%, and studies have documented clinical evidence of oral candidiasis in nearly 20% of cancer patients.

Chapter 46

Tongue Tie (Ankyloglossia)

What Is Ankyloglossia?

Ankyloglossia is a congenital condition characterized by an abnormally short, thickened, or tight lingual frenulum, or an anterior attachment of the lingual frenulum, that restricts mobility of the tongue. It variably causes reduced anterior tongue mobility and has been associated with functional limitations in breastfeeding; swallowing; articulation; orthodontic problems, including malocclusion, open bite, and separation of lower incisors; mechanical problems related to oral clearance; and psychological stress. One review including studies of infants, children, and adults reported rates of ankyloglossia ranging from 0.1 to 10.7 percent, but definitive incidence and prevalence statistics are elusive due to an absence of a criterion standard or clinically practical diagnostic criteria.

Difficulties of Ankyloglossia

Recognition of potential benefits of breastfeeding in recent years has resulted in a renewed interest in the functional sequelae of ankyloglossia. In infants with anterior or posterior ankyloglossia, there is a reported 25- to 80-percent incidence of breastfeeding difficulties,

This chapter includes text excerpted from "Treatments for Ankyloglossia and Ankyloglossia with Concomitant Lip-Tie," Agency for Healthcare Research and Quality (AHRQ), U.S. Department of Health and Human Services (HHS), May 4, 2015.

including failure to thrive, maternal nipple damage, maternal breast pain, poor milk supply, maternal breast engorgement, and refusing the breast. Ineffective latch is hypothesized to underlie these problems. Mechanistically, infants with restrictive ankyloglossia cannot extend their tongues over the lower gumline to form a proper seal and therefore use their jaws to keep the breast in the mouth for breastfeeding. Adequate tongue mobility is required for breastfeeding, and infants with ankyloglossia often cannot overcome their deficiency with conservative measures such as positioning and latching techniques, thereby requiring surgical correction.

Nonetheless, consensus on ankyloglossia's role in breastfeeding difficulties is lacking. A minority of surveyed pediatricians (10%) and otolaryngologists (30%) believe it commonly affects feeding, while 69 percent of lactation consultants feel that it frequently causes breastfeeding problems.

Treatment

The U.K. National Health Service and the Canadian Paediatric Society recommend treatment only if it interferes with breastfeeding. A standard definition of "interference" with breastfeeding is not provided, leaving room for interpretation and variation in treatment thresholds. The absence of data on the natural history of untreated ankyloglossia further promulgates uncertainty. Some propose that a short frenulum elongates spontaneously due to progressive stretching and thinning of the frenulum with age and use. However, there are no prospective longitudinal data on the congenitally short lingual frenulum. Without this information it is difficult to inform parents fully about the long-term implications of ankyloglossia, thereby complicating the decision-making process.

Research

Although most ankyloglossia research is focused on the infant and breastfeeding issues, concerns beyond infancy include speech-related issues, such as difficulty with articulation, and social concerns related to limited tongue mobility. Individuals with untreated ankyloglossia may experience difficulty with oral mechanism, particularly in relation to licking ice cream, kissing, drooling, playing wind instruments, and licking the lips. Self-esteem or psychological issues may also be a concern for affected older patients.

Part Six

Health Conditions That Affect Oral Health

Chapter 47

Cancer Treatment and Oral Complications

Chapter Contents

Section 47.1

Three Good Reasons to See a Dentist before Cancer Treatment

This section includes text excerpted from "Three Good Reasons to See a Dentist before Cancer Treatment," National Institute of Dental and Craniofacial Research (NIDCR), September 2015.

1. **Feel better**

    Cancer treatment can cause side effects in your mouth. A dental checkup before treatment starts can help prevent painful mouth problems.

2. **Save teeth and bones**

    A dentist will help protect your mouth, teeth, and jaw bones from damage caused by head and neck radiation and chemotherapy. Children also need special protection for their growing teeth and facial bones.

3. **Fight cancer**

    Serious side effects in the mouth can delay, or even stop, cancer treatment. To fight cancer best, your cancer care team should include a dentist

Protect Your Mouth during Cancer Treatment

Table 47.1. Protect Your Mouth

Brush gently, brush often	• Brush your teeth—and your tongue—gently with an extra-soft toothbrush. • Soften the bristles in warm water if your mouth is very sore. • Brush after every meal and at bedtime.
Floss gently— do it daily	• Floss once a day to remove plaque. • Avoid areas of your gums that are bleeding or sore, but keep flossing your other teeth.
Keep your mouth moist	• Rinse often with water. • Don't use mouthwashes that contain alcohol. • Use a saliva substitute to help moisten your mouth.

Table 47.1. Continued

Eat and drink with care	• Choose soft, easy-to-chew foods. • Protect your mouth from spicy, sour, or crunchy foods. Choose lukewarm foods and drinks instead of hot or icy-cold ones. • Avoid alcoholic drinks.
Stop using tobacco	• Ask your cancer care team to help you stop smoking or chewing tobacco. People who quit smoking or chewing tobacco have fewer mouth problems.

Tips to Help You Care for Mouth Problems

• **Sore Mouth, Sore Throat**

To help keep your mouth clean, rinse often with ¼ teaspoon of salt and ¼ teaspoon of baking soda in 1 quart (4 cups) of warm water. Follow with a plain water rinse. Ask your cancer care team about medicines that can help with the pain.

• **Dry Mouth**

Rinse your mouth often with water, use sugar-free gum or candy, and talk to your dentist about saliva substitutes.

• **Infections**

Call your cancer care team right away if you see a sore, swelling, bleeding, or a sticky, white film in your mouth.

• **Eating Problems**

Your cancer care team can help by giving you medicines to numb the pain from mouth sores and showing you how to choose foods that are easy to swallow.

• **Bleeding**

If your gums bleed or hurt, avoid flossing the areas that are bleeding or sore, but keep flossing other teeth. Soften the bristles of your toothbrush in warm water.

• **Stiffness in Chewing Muscles**

Three times a day, open and close your mouth as far as you can without pain. Repeat 20 times.

• **Vomiting**

Rinse your mouth after vomiting with 1/4 teaspoon of baking soda in 1 cup of warm water.

- **Cavities**

  Brush your teeth after meals and before bedtime. Your dentist might have you put fluoride gel on your teeth to help prevent cavities.

When Should You Call Your Cancer Care Team about Mouth Problems?

Take a moment each day to check how your mouth looks and feels. Call your cancer care team when:

- you first notice a mouth problem.

- an old problem gets worse.

- you notice any changes you're not sure about.

Section 47.2

Chemotherapy and Your Mouth

This section includes text excerpted from "Chemotherapy and Your Mouth," National Institute of Dental and Craniofacial Research (NIDCR), August 2013.

Are You Being Treated With Chemotherapy for Cancer?

If so, this section can help you. While chemotherapy helps treat cancer, it can also cause other things to happen in your body called side effects. **Some of these problems affect the mouth and could cause you to delay or stop treatment.** This section will tell you ways to help prevent mouth problems so you'll get the most from your cancer treatment.

To help prevent serious problems, see a dentist ideally 1 month before starting chemotherapy.

How Does Chemotherapy Affect the Mouth?

Chemotherapy is the use of drugs to treat cancer. These drugs kill cancer cells, but they may also harm normal cells, including cells in the mouth. Side effects include problems with your teeth and gums; the soft, moist lining of your mouth; and the glands that make saliva (spit).

It's important to know that side effects in the mouth can be serious.

- The side effects can hurt and make it hard to eat, talk, and swallow.

- You are more likely to get an infection, which can be dangerous when you are receiving cancer treatment.

- If the side effects are bad, you may not be able to keep up with your cancer treatment. Your doctor may need to cut back on your cancer treatment or may even stop it.

What Mouth Problems Does Chemotherapy Cause?

You may have certain side effects in your mouth from chemotherapy. Another person may have different problems. The problems depend on the chemotherapy drugs and how your body reacts to them. You may have these problems only during treatment or for a short time after treatment ends.

- Painful mouth and gums.
- Dry mouth.
- Burning, peeling, or swelling tongue.
- Infection.
- Change in taste.

Why Should I See a Dentist?

You may be surprised that your dentist is important in your cancer treatment. If you go to the dentist before chemotherapy begins, you can help prevent serious mouth problems. Side effects often happen because a person's mouth is not healthy before chemotherapy starts. Not all mouth problems can be avoided but the fewer side effects you have, the more likcly you will stay on your cancer treatment schedule. It's important for your dentist and cancer doctor to talk to each other about your cancer treatment. Be sure to give your dentist your cancer doctor's phone number.

When Should I See a Dentist?

You need to see the dentist one month, if possible, before chemotherapy begins. If you have already started chemotherapy and didn't go to a dentist, see one as soon as possible.

What Will the Dentist and Dental Hygienist Do?

- Check and clean your teeth.
- Take X-rays.
- Take care of mouth problems.
- Show you how to take care of your mouth to prevent side effects.

What Can I Do To Keep My Mouth Healthy?

You can do a lot to keep your mouth healthy during chemotherapy. The first step is to see a dentist before you start cancer treatment. Once your treatment starts, it's important to look in your mouth every day for sores or other changes. These tips can help prevent and treat a sore mouth:

Keep your mouth moist.

- Drink a lot of water.
- Suck ice chips.
- Use sugarless gum or sugar-free hard candy.
- Use a saliva substitute to help moisten your mouth.

Clean your mouth, tongue, and gums.

- Brush your teeth, gums, and tongue with an extra-soft toothbrush after every meal and at bedtime. If brushing hurts, soften the bristles in warm water.
- Use a fluoride toothpaste.
- Don't use mouthwashes with alcohol in them. Dental floss, a tube of tooth paste, and a tooth brush.
- Floss your teeth gently every day. If your gums bleed and hurt, avoid the areas that are bleeding or sore, but keep flossing your other teeth.
- Rinse your mouth several times a day with a solution of ¼ teaspoon of salt or 1 teaspoon of baking soda in 1 cup (8 ounces) of warm water. Follow with a plain water rinse.
- Dentures that don't fit well can cause problems. Talk to your cancer doctor or dentist about your dentures.

If your mouth is sore, watch what you eat and drink.

- Choose foods that are good for you and easy to chew and swallow.

- Take small bites of food, chew slowly, and sip liquids with your meals.

- Eat soft, moist foods such as cooked cereals, mashed potatoes, and scrambled eggs.

- If you have trouble swallowing, soften your food with gravy, sauces, broth, yogurt, or other liquids.

Call your doctor or nurse when your mouth hurts.

- Work with them to find medicines to help control the pain.

- If the pain continues, talk to your cancer doctor about stronger medicines.

Remember to stay away from

- Soda, juice, taco chips, and toothpicks

- Sharp, crunchy foods, like taco chips, that could scrape or cut your mouth.

- Foods that are hot, spicy, or high in acid, like citrus fruits and juices, which can irritate your mouth.

- Sugary foods, like candy or soda, that could cause cavities.

- Toothpicks, because they can cut your mouth.

- All tobacco products.

- Alcoholic drinks.

Section 47.3

Head and Neck Radiation Treatment and Your Mouth

This section includes text excerpted from "Head and Neck Radiation Treatment and Your Mouth," National Institute of Dental and Craniofacial Research (NIDCR), April 2013.

Are You Being Treated with Radiation for Cancer in Your Head or Neck?

While head and neck radiation helps treat cancer, it can also cause other things to happen in your mouth called side effects. **Some of these problems could cause you to delay or stop treatment.**

This section will tell you ways to help prevent mouth problems so you'll get the most from your cancer treatment. **To help prevent serious problems, see a dentist ideally one month before starting radiation.**

How Does Head and Neck Radiation Affect the Mouth?

Doctors use head and neck radiation to treat cancer because it kills cancer cells. But radiation to the head and neck can harm normal cells, including cells in the mouth. Side effects include problems with your teeth and gums; the soft, moist lining of your mouth; glands that make saliva (spit); and jaw bones.

It's important to know that side effects in the mouth can be serious.

- The side effects can hurt and make it hard to eat, talk, and swallow.

- You are more likely to get an infection, which can be dangerous when you are receiving cancer treatment.

- If the side effects are bad, you may not be able to keep up with your cancer treatment. Your doctor may need to cut back on your cancer treatment or may even stop it.

What Mouth Problems Does Head and Neck Radiation Cause?

You may have certain side effects in your mouth from head and neck radiation. Another person may have different problems. Some problems go away after treatment. Others last a long time, while some may never go away.

- Dry mouth
- A lot of cavities
- Loss of taste
- Sore mouth and gums
- Infections
- Jaw stiffness
- Jaw bone changes

Why Should I See a Dentist?

You may be surprised that your dentist is important in your cancer treatment. If you go to the dentist before head and neck radiation begins, you can help prevent serious mouth problems. Side effects often happen because a person's mouth is not healthy before radiation starts. Not all mouth problems can be avoided but the fewer side effects you have, the more likely you will stay on your cancer treatment schedule.

It's important for your dentist and cancer doctor to talk to each other before your radiation treatment begins. Be sure to give your dentist your cancer doctor's phone number.

When Should I See a Dentist?

You need to see the dentist 1 month, if possible, before your first radiation treatment. If you have already started radiation and didn't go to a dentist, see one as soon as possible.

What Will the Dentist and Dental Hygienist Do?

- Check and clean your teeth.
- Take X-rays.
- Take care of mouth problems.

- Show you how to take care of your mouth to prevent side effects.

- Show you how to prevent and treat jaw stiffness by exercising the jaw muscles three times a day. Open and close the mouth as far as possible (without causing pain) 20 times.

What Can I Do to Keep My Mouth Healthy?

You can do a lot to keep your mouth healthy during chemotherapy. The first step is to **see a dentist before you start cancer treatment.** Once your treatment starts, it's important to **look in your mouth every day** for sores or other changes. These tips can help prevent and treat a sore mouth:

Keep Your Mouth Moist

- Drink a lot of water.

- Suck ice chips.

- Use sugarless gum or sugar-free hard candy.

- Use a saliva substitute to help moisten your mouth.

Clean Your Mouth, Tongue, and Gums.

- Brush your teeth, gums, and tongue with an extra-soft toothbrush after every meal and at bedtime. If it hurts, soften the bristles in warm water.

- Use a fluoride toothpaste.

- Use the special fluoride gel that your dentist prescribes.

- Don't use mouthwashes with alcohol in them.

- Floss your teeth gently every day. If your gums bleed and hurt, avoid the areas that are bleeding or sore, but keep flossing your other teeth.

- Rinse your mouth several times a day with a solution of 1/4 teaspoon each of baking soda and salt in one quart of warm water. Follow with a plain water rinse.

- Dentures that don't fit well can cause problems. Talk to your cancer doctor or dentist about your dentures.

If Your Mouth Is Sore, Watch What You Eat and Drink

- Choose foods that are good for you and easy to chew and swallow.

- Take small bites of food, chew slowly, and sip liquids with your meals.

- Eat soft, moist foods such as cooked cereals, mashed potatoes, and scrambled eggs.

- If you have trouble swallowing, soften your food with gravy, sauces, broth, yogurt, or other liquids.

Call Your Doctor or Nurse When Your Mouth Hurts

- Work with them to find medicines to help control the pain.

- If the pain continues, talk to your cancer doctor about stronger medicines.

Remember to Stay Away from

- Sharp, crunchy foods, like taco chips, that could scrape or cut your mouth.

- Foods that are hot, spicy, or high in acid, like citrus fruits and juices, which can irritate your mouth.

- Sugary foods, like candy or soda, that could cause cavities.

- Toothpicks, because they can cut your mouth.

- All tobacco products.

- Alcoholic drinks.

Do Children Get Mouth Problems Too?

Head and neck radiation causes other side effects in children, depending on the child's age.

Problems with teeth are the most common. Permanent teeth may be slow to come in and may look different from normal teeth. Teeth may fall out. The dentist will check your child's jaws for any growth problems.

Before radiation begins, take your child to a dentist. The dentist will check your child's mouth carefully and pull loose teeth or those that may become loose during treatment. Ask the dentist or hygienist what you can do to help your child with mouth care.

Remember

- Visit your dentist before your head and neck radiation treatment starts.

- Take good care of your mouth during treatment.

- Talk to your dentist about using fluoride gel to help prevent the cavities that head and neck radiation causes.

- Talk regularly with your cancer doctor and dentist about any mouth problems you have during and after head and neck radiation treatment.

Section 47.4

What the Oncology Team Can Do

This section includes text excerpted from "Oral Complications of Cancer Treatment: What the Oncology Team Can Do," National Institute of Dental and Craniofacial Research (NIDCR), August 1, 2014.

Radiation to the head and neck and chemotherapy for any malignancy can cause a range of oral side effects. For some patients, these complications may become dose-limiting and slow—or even halt—cancer treatment. Preventing and managing oral complications help support optimal cancer therapy, enhancing both patient survival and quality of life.

Who Has Oral Complications?

Oral side effects occur in virtually all patients receiving radiation for head and neck malignancies, in approximately 80 percent of transplant recipients, and in about 40 percent of patients receiving primary chemotherapy. Risk for oral complications varies with the treatment regimen. Patients administered minimally myelosuppressive or non myelosuppressive therapy are at low risk. As chemotherapy becomes more aggressive, the likelihood of oral complications increases. Also at high risk are patients undergoing head and neck radiation for oral and pharyngeal cancer.

Most oral complications resolve when cancer treatment ends and the patient's overall condition improves. Others, such as xerostomia, may persist for years. Unfortunately, patients do not always receive medically necessary dental care that could help avert or minimize oral complications. Ensuring that your patients receive timely oral care helps them maintain the prescribed cancer regimen and complete treatment.

By adding oral care to the pretreatment regimen, you can:

- Prevent, eliminate or control oral pain.

- Prevent oral infections that could lead to serious systemic infections.

- Optimize nutritional support.

- Preserve or improve oral health.

- Prevent or reduce the incidence of bone necrosis in patients receiving radiation therapy to the head and neck.

- Improve the quality of life.

- Decrease the cost of care.

- Improve the likelihood that the patient will successfully complete planned cancer treatment.

Oral Complications of Cancer Treatment

General

- Oral mucositis/stomatitis

- Xerostomia/salivary gland dysfunction

- Pain

- Infection

- Xerostomia-associated cavities

- Taste alterations

- Nutritional compromise

- Functional disabilities
- Abnormal dental development in children

Treatment-specific

Chemotherapy

- Neurotoxicity
- Bleeding

Radiation therapy

- Radiation caries
- Trismus/tissue fibrosis
- Osteonecrosis

Minimizing Oral Complications of Cancer Therapy

- Consider use of palifermin for patients with hematologic malignancies receiving chemotherapy/radiation and autologous stem cell transplantation.
- Utilize salivary gland-sparing radiation techniques.
- Administer a radioprotectant, such as amifostine, to reduce risk of xerostomia in head and neck cancer patients.
- Encourage patients to maintain the oral hygiene regimen recommended by the dentist.
- Work with the dentist to prevent and control infections with appropriate treatment before, during, and after cancer therapy.
- Emphasize the importance of maintaining good nutrition.

Oral Evaluation before Cancer Treatment Makes a Difference

A pretreatment oral evaluation can identify potential problems and help educate the patient about the importance of good oral care. This evaluation can be conducted by a knowledgeable dentist in the community or by a hospital-based dental team. Ideally, the evaluation should be performed at least 1 month before cancer treatment starts to permit adequate healing from any required invasive procedures. The evaluation includes a thorough examination of hard and soft tissues, as well as radiographs to detect trauma and possible sources of infection. Before cancer treatment begins, the dentist will take the following steps:

- Identify and treat existing infections, problem teeth, and tissue injury or trauma.

- Stabilize or eliminate potential sites of infection.

- Remove orthodontic bands if highly stomatotoxic chemotherapy is planned or if the bands will be in the radiation field.

- Perform oral prophylaxis if indicated.

- Evaluate dentures and appliances for comfort and fit.

- Perform oral surgery at least 2 weeks prior to the initiation of radiation therapy to allow healing, and at least 7–10 days before myelosuppressive chemotherapy begins.

- Extract teeth that may pose a future problem to prevent extraction-induced osteonecrosis in adults receiving head and neck radiation.

- Consider extracting highly mobile primary teeth in children, and teeth that are expected to exfoliate during treatment.

- Instruct patients on oral hygiene, use of fluoride gel, nutrition, and the need to avoid tobacco and alcohol.

During the examination, the patient will also learn a home care regimen to protect mouth tissues and minimize oral complications. The dentist or dental hygienist will instruct the patient on special brushing and flossing techniques, mouth rinses, and other approaches to keep the mouth as moist and clean as possible to reduce the risk of infection and pain.

Oral Care during Treatment

Regular oral assessment and care are necessary during cancer therapy. Planning and communication between the oncology and dental teams can minimize the risk of oral complications and maximize the efficacy of dental and supportive care. Specific oral health considerations to remember when treating patients with chemotherapy or radiation include the following:

Radiation Therapy

Treat infections and ulcerations. Ulcerations and dry, friable tissues are prone to trauma and infection. Culture suspected infections and work with the dentist to manage the condition.

Provide dietary counseling. Instruct the patient on the importance of healthy eating to maintain nutritional status, emphasizing the need to avoid foods that irritate sore tissues or cause dental decay.

Teach exercises to reduce trismus. Fibrosis may develop if the chewing muscles are in the direct field of radiation. Work with the dentist to teach patients how to exercise and stretch these muscles properly.

Chemotherapy

Consider oral causes of fever. Fever of unknown origin may be related to an oral infection; dental consultation may be appropriate.

Schedule dental appointments carefully. Have the patient schedule appointments for times when blood counts will be at safe levels. If oral surgery is required, it should be performed at least 7–10 days before the patient receives myelosuppressive chemotherapy.

Determine hematologic status. Conduct blood work 24 hours before dental treatment to determine whether the patient's platelet count, clotting factors, and absolute neutrophil count are sufficient to prevent hemorrhage and infection.

Evaluate need for prophylactic antibiotic treatment. If the patient has a central venous catheter, determine if antibiotic prophylaxis is needed before dental treatment.

Follow-Up Oral Care

Once all complications of chemotherapy have resolved and blood counts have recovered, most patients may resume their normal dental care schedule. It is essential that the dentist know the patient's hematologic status before initiating any dental treatment or surgery. Advise the dentist if a patient has received intravenous bisphosphonate therapy due to its association with osteonecrosis of the jaw.

Once radiation therapy has been completed and acute oral complications have abated, the patient should be evaluated by a dentist every 4 to 8 weeks for the first 6 months. Thereafter, the dentist can determine a schedule based on the needs of the individual patient.

Long-Term Problems Following Head and Neck Radiation Therapy

Radiation therapy to the head and neck can cause oral complications that continue or emerge long after treatment has ended. Although patients may no longer be under an oncologist's care at that time, what they learn about oral health during their treatment will affect how they deal with subsequent complications. Patients receiving radiation therapy need to know about its risks:

- Radiation treatment carries a lifelong risk of osteonecrosis, xerostomia, and dental cavities.

- Because of the risk of osteonecrosis, people who have received radiation should avoid invasive surgical procedures (including extractions) that involve irradiated bone.

- Radiation to the head and neck may permanently reduce the quantity and quality of normal saliva, so ongoing oral care is crucial to optimize oral health. Daily fluoride tray application, good nutrition, and oral hygiene are especially important.

- Radiation may alter oral tissues, so dentures may need to be reconstructed after treatment is completed and the tissues have stabilized. Some people may not be able to wear dentures again.

- Craniofacial and dental structures may develop abnormally in younger children who receive high-dose radiation to those areas.

Helping Patients with Xerostomia

- Encourage patients to sip water often.

- Suggest using liquids to soften or thin foods.

- Recommend using sugarless gum or sugar-free hard candies to help stimulate saliva flow.

- Suggest using a commercial saliva substitute.

- Consider prescribing a saliva stimulant.

Helping Patients with Mouth Pain

- Prescribe topical anesthetics and systemic analgesics.

- Detect and treat oral infections early.

- Encourage patients to avoid eating irritating or rough-textured foods.

Hematopoietic Stem Cell Transplantation

Because of the pronounced immunosuppression that accompanies hematopoietic stem cell transplant procedures, patients have a high risk of developing acute oral complications, particularly mucositis, ulcerations, hemorrhage, infection, and xerostomia. Although these problems begin to resolve when hematologic status improves, immunosuppression may last for up to a year after the transplant, so the risk of complications continues. The oral cavity and salivary glands are also commonly involved in graft-versus-host disease in allograft recipients. Careful attention to oral care in the post-transplant period is important to the overall health of these patients.

Section 47.5

What the Dental Team Can Do

This section includes text excerpted from "Oral Complications of Cancer Treatment: What the Dental Team Can Do," National Institute of Dental and Craniofacial Research (NIDCR), July 14, 2015.

Oral Complications from Radiation

Oral complications from radiation to the head and neck or chemotherapy for any malignancy can compromise patients' health and quality of life, and affect their ability to complete planned cancer treatment. For some patients, the complications can be so debilitating that they may tolerate only lower doses of therapy, postpone scheduled treatments, or discontinue treatment entirely. Oral complications can also lead to serious systemic infections. Medically necessary oral care before, during, and after cancer treatment can prevent or reduce the incidence and severity of oral complications, enhancing both patient survival and quality of life.

Oral Complications Related to Cancer Treatment

Oral complications of cancer treatment arise in various forms and degrees of severity, depending on the individual and the cancer treatment. Chemotherapy often impairs the function of bone marrow, suppressing the formation of white blood cells, red blood cells, and platelets (myelosuppression). Some cancer treatments are described as stomatotoxic because they have toxic effects on the oral tissues. Following are lists of side effects common to both chemotherapy and radiation therapy, and complications specific to each type of treatment. You will need to consider the possibility of these complications each time you evaluate a patient with cancer.

Oral Complications Common to Both Chemotherapy and Radiation

- **Oral mucositis:** inflammation and ulceration of the mucous membranes; can increase the risk for pain, oral and systemic infection, and nutritional compromise.

- **Infection:** viral, bacterial, and fungal; results from myelosuppression, xerostomia, and/or damage to the mucosa from chemotherapy or radiotherapy.

- **Xerostomia/salivary gland dysfunction:** dryness of the mouth due to thickened, reduced, or absent salivary flow; increases the risk of infection and compromises speaking, chewing, and swallowing. Medications other than chemotherapy can also cause salivary gland dysfunction. Persistent dry mouth increases the risk for dental caries.

- **Functional disabilities:** impaired ability to eat, taste, swallow, and speak because of mucositis, dry mouth, trismus, and infection.

- **Taste alterations:** changes in taste perception of foods, ranging from unpleasant to tasteless.

- **Nutritional compromise:** poor nutrition from eating difficulties caused by mucositis, dry mouth, dysphagia, and loss of taste.

- **Abnormal dental development:** altered tooth development, craniofacial growth, or skeletal development in children secondary to radiotherapy and/or high doses of chemotherapy before age 9.

Other Complications of Chemotherapy

Neurotoxicity: persistent, deep aching and burning pain that mimics a toothache, but for which no dental or mucosal source can be found. This complication is a side effect of certain classes of drugs, such as the vinca alkaloids.

Bleeding: oral bleeding from the decreased platelets and clotting factors associated with the effects of therapy on bone marrow.

Other Complications of Radiation Therapy

Radiation caries: lifelong risk of rampant dental decay that may begin within 3 months of completing radiation treatment if changes in either the quality or quantity of saliva persist.

Trismus/tissue fibrosis: loss of elasticity of masticatory muscles that restricts normal ability to open the mouth.

Osteonecrosis: blood vessel compromise and necrosis of bone exposed to high-dose radiation therapy; results in decreased ability to heal if traumatized.

Radiation and Oral Complications

Oral complications occur in virtually all patients receiving radiation for head and neck malignancies, in approximately 80 percent of hematopoietic (blood-forming) stem cell transplant recipients, and in nearly 40 percent of patients receiving chemotherapy. Risk for oral complications can be classified as low or high:

Lower risk: Patients receiving minimally myelosuppressive or non myelosuppressive chemotherapy.

Higher risk: Patients receiving stomatotoxic chemotherapy resulting in prolonged myelosuppression, including patients undergoing hematopoietic stem cell transplantation; and patients undergoing head and neck radiation for oral, pharyngeal, and laryngeal cancer.

Some complications occur only during treatment; others, such as xerostomia, may persist for years. Unfortunately, patients with cancer do not always receive oral care until serious complications develop.

The Role of Pretreatment Oral Care

A thorough oral evaluation by a knowledgeable dentist before cancer treatment begins is important to the success of the regimen. Pretreatment oral care achieves the following:

- Reduces the risk and severity of oral complications.

- Allows for prompt identification and treatment of existing infections or other problems.

- Improves the likelihood that the patient will successfully complete planned cancer treatment.

- Prevents, eliminates, or reduces oral pain.

- Minimizes oral infections that could lead to potentially serious systemic infections.

- Prevents or minimizes complications that compromise nutrition.

- Prevents or reduces later incidence of bone necrosis.

- Preserves or improves oral health.

- Provides an opportunity for patient education about oral hygiene during cancer therapy.

- Improves the quality of life.

- Decreases the cost of care.

With a pretreatment oral evaluation, the dental team can identify and treat problems such as infection, fractured teeth or restorations, or periodontal disease that could contribute to oral complications when cancer therapy begins. The evaluation also establishes baseline data for comparing the patient's status in subsequent examinations.

Before the exam, you will need to obtain the patient's cancer diagnosis and treatment plan, medical history, and dental history. **Open communication with the patient's oncologist is essential to ensure that each provider has the information necessary to deliver the best possible care.**

Evaluation

Ideally, a comprehensive oral evaluation should take place 1 month before cancer treatment starts to allow adequate time for recovery from any required invasive dental procedures. The pretreatment evaluation includes a thorough examination of hard and soft tissues, as well as appropriate radiographs to detect possible sources of infection and pathology. Also take the following steps before cancer treatment begins:

- Identify and treat existing infections, carious and other compromised teeth, and tissue injury or trauma.

- Stabilize or eliminate potential sites of infection.

- Extract teeth in the radiation field that are nonrestorable or may pose a future problem to prevent later extraction-induced osteonecrosis.

- Conduct a prosthodontic evaluation if indicated. If a removable prosthesis is worn, make sure that it is clean and well adapted to the tissue. Instruct the patient not to wear the prosthesis during treatment, if possible; or at the least, not to wear it at night.

- Perform oral prophylaxis if indicated.

- Time oral surgery to allow at least 2 weeks for healing before radiation therapy begins. For patients receiving radiation treatment, this is the best time to consider surgical procedures. Oral surgery should be performed at least 7 to 10 days before the patient receives myelosuppressive chemotherapy. Medical consultation is indicated before invasive procedures.

- Remove orthodontic bands and brackets if highly stomatotoxic chemotherapy is planned or if the appliances will be in the radiation field.

- Consider extracting highly mobile primary teeth in children, and teeth that are expected to exfoliate during treatment.

- Prescribe an individualized oral hygiene regimen to minimize oral complications. Patients undergoing head and neck radiation therapy should be instructed on the use of supplemental fluoride.

Supplemental Fluoride

Fluoride rinses are not adequate to prevent tooth demineralization. Instead, a high-potency fluoride gel, delivered via custom gel-applicator trays, is recommended. Several days before radiation therapy begins, patients should start a daily 10-minute application of a 1.1% neutral pH sodium fluoride gel or a 0.4% stannous fluoride (unflavored) gel. Patients with porcelain crowns or resin or glass ionomer restorations should use a neutral pH fluoride. Be sure that the trays cover all tooth structures without irritating the gingival or mucosal tissues.

For patients reluctant to use a tray, a high-potency fluoride gel should be brushed on the teeth following daily brushing and flossing. Either 1.1% neutral pH sodium or 0.4% stannous fluoride gel is recommended, based on the patient's type of dental restorations.

Patients with radiation-induced salivary gland dysfunction must continue lifelong daily fluoride applications.

Education

Patient education is an integral part of the pretreatment evaluation and should include a discussion of potential oral complications. It is very important that the dental team impress on the patient that optimal oral hygiene during treatment, adequate nutrition, and avoiding tobacco and alcohol can prevent or minimize oral complications. To ensure that the patient fully understands what is required, provide detailed instructions on specific oral care practices, such as how and when to brush and floss, how to recognize signs of complications, and other instructions appropriate for the individual. Patients should understand that good oral care during cancer treatment contributes to its success.

Advise Patients To

- Brush teeth, gums, and tongue gently with an extra-soft toothbrush and fluoride toothpaste after every meal and before bed. If brushing hurts, soften the bristles in warm water.

- Floss teeth gently every day. If gums are sore or bleeding, avoid those areas but keep flossing other teeth.

- Follow instructions for using fluoride gel.

- Avoid mouthwashes containing alcohol.

- Rinse the mouth with a baking soda and salt solution, followed by a plain water rinse several times a day. (Use 1/4 teaspoon each of baking soda and salt in 1 quart of warm water.) Omit salt during mucositis.

- Exercise the jaw muscles three times a day to prevent and treat jaw stiffness from radiation. Open and close the mouth as far as possible without causing pain; repeat 20 times.

- Avoid candy, gum, and soda unless they are sugar-free.

- Avoid spicy or acidic foods, toothpicks, tobacco products, and alcohol.

- Keep the appointment schedule recommended by the dentist.

Instructions for Patients Using Supplemental Fluoride

If Using a Tray

- Place a thin ribbon of fluoride gel in each tray.

- Place the trays on the teeth and leave in place for 10 minutes. If gel oozes out of the tray, you are using too much.

- After 10 minutes, remove the trays and spit out any excess gel. Do not rinse.

- Rinse the applicator trays with water.

- Do not eat or drink for 30 minutes.

If Using a Brush-On Method

- After brushing with toothpaste, rinse as usual.

- Place a thin ribbon of gel on the toothbrush.

- Brush for 2 to 3 minutes.

- Spit out any excess gel. Do not rinse.

- Do not eat or drink for 30 minutes.

Oral Care during Cancer Treatment

Careful monitoring of oral health is especially important during cancer therapy to prevent, detect, and treat complications as soon as possible. When treatment is necessary, consult the oncologist before any dental procedure, including dental prophylaxis.

- Examine the soft tissues for inflammation or infection and evaluate for plaque levels and dental caries.

- Review oral hygiene and oral care protocols; prescribe antimicrobial therapy as indicated.

- Provide recommendations for treating dry mouth and other complications:
  - Sip water frequently.
  - Suck ice chips or sugar-free candy.
  - Chew sugar-free gum.
  - Use a saliva substitute spray or gel or a prescribed saliva stimulant if appropriate.
  - Avoid glycerin swabs.
- Take precautions to protect against trauma.
- Provide topical anesthetics or analgesics for oral pain.

Other Factors to Remember

Schedule dental work carefully. If oral surgery is required, allow at least 7 to 10 days of healing before the patient receives myelosuppressive chemotherapy. Elective oral surgery should not be performed for the duration of radiation treatment.

Determine hematologic status. If the patient is receiving chemotherapy, have the oncology team conduct blood work 24 hours before dental treatment to determine whether the patient's platelet count, clotting factors, and absolute neutrophil count are sufficient to recommend oral treatment. Postpone oral surgery or other oral invasive procedures if:

- platelet count is less than 75,000/mm3 or abnormal clotting factors are present.
- absolute neutrophil count is less than 1,000/mm3 (or consider prophylactic antibiotics).

Consider oral causes of fever. Fever of unknown origin may be related to an oral infection. Remember that oral signs of infection or other complications may be altered by immunosuppression related to chemotherapy.

Evaluate need for antibiotic prophylaxis. If the patient has a central venous catheter, consult the oncologist to determine if antibiotics are needed before any dental treatment to prevent endocarditis.

Follow-Up Oral Care

Chemotherapy

Once all complications of chemotherapy have resolved, patients may be able to resume their normal dental care schedule. However, if immune function continues to be compromised, determine the patient's hematologic status before initiating any dental treatment or surgery. This is particularly important to remember for patients who have undergone stem cell transplantation. Ask if the patient has received intravenous bisphosphonate therapy.

Radiation Therapy

Once the patient has completed head and neck radiation therapy and acute oral complications have abated, evaluate the patient regularly (every 4 to 8 weeks, for example) for the first 6 months. Thereafter, you can determine a schedule based on the patient's needs. However, keep in mind that oral complications can continue or emerge long after radiation therapy has ended.

Points to Remember

- High-dose radiation treatment carries a lifelong risk of xerostomia, dental caries, and osteonecrosis.

- Because of the risk of osteonecrosis, principally in the mandible, patients should avoid invasive surgical procedures, including extractions that involve irradiated bone. If an invasive procedure is required, use of antibiotics and hyperbaric oxygen therapy before and after surgery should be considered.

- Lifelong daily fluoride application, good nutrition, and conscientious oral hygiene are especially important for patients with salivary gland dysfunction.

- Dentures may need to be reconstructed if treatment altered oral tissues. Some people can never wear dentures again because of friable tissues and xerostomia.

- Dentists should closely monitor children who have received radiation to craniofacial and dental structures for abnormal growth and development.

- Dentists should be mindful about the recurrence of malignancies in patients with oral and head and neck cancers, and thoroughly examine all oral mucosal tissues at recall appointments.

Special Considerations for Hematopoietic Stem Cell Transplant Patients

The intensive conditioning regimens of transplantation can result in pronounced immunosuppression, greatly increasing a patient's risk of mucositis, ulceration, hemorrhage, infection, and xerostomia. The complications begin to resolve when hematologic status improves. Although the complete blood count and differential may be normal, immunosuppression may last for up to a year after the transplant, along with the risk of infections. Also, the oral cavity and salivary glands are commonly involved in graft-versus-host disease in allograft recipients. This can result in mucosal inflammation, ulceration, and xerostomia, so continued monitoring is necessary. Careful attention to oral care in the immediate and long-term post-transplant period is important to patients' overall health.

Chapter 48

Celiac Disease and Dental Enamel Defects

What Is Celiac Disease?

Celiac disease is a digestive disorder that damages the small intestine. The disease is triggered by eating foods containing gluten. Gluten is a protein found naturally in wheat, barley, and rye, and is common in foods such as bread, pasta, cookies, and cakes. Many pre-packaged foods, lip balms and lipsticks, hair and skin products, toothpastes, vitamin and nutrient supplements, and, rarely, medicines, contain gluten.

Celiac disease can be very serious. The disease can cause long-lasting digestive problems and keep your body from getting all the nutrients it needs. Celiac disease can also affect the body outside the intestine.

Celiac disease is different from gluten sensitivity or wheat intolerance. If you have gluten sensitivity, you may have symptoms similar to those of celiac disease, such as abdominal pain and tiredness. Unlike celiac disease, gluten sensitivity does not damage the small intestine.

This chapter contains text excerpted from the following sources: Text beginning with the heading "What Is Celiac Disease?" is excerpted from "Definition and Facts for Celiac Disease," National Institute of Diabetes and Digestive and Kidney Diseases (NIDDK), June 16, 2016; Text beginning with the heading "Dental Enamel Defects and Celiac Disease" is excerpted from "Dental Enamel Defects and Celiac Disease," National Institute of Diabetes and Digestive and Kidney Diseases (NIDDK), September 2014.

Celiac disease is also different from a wheat allergy. In both cases, your body's immune system reacts to wheat. However, some symptoms in wheat allergies, such as having itchy eyes or a hard time breathing, are different from celiac disease. Wheat allergies also do not cause long-term damage to the small intestine.

How Common Is Celiac Disease?

As many as one in 141 Americans has celiac disease, although most don't know it.

Who Is More Likely to Develop Celiac Disease?

Although celiac disease affects children and adults in all parts of the world, the disease is more common in Caucasians and more often diagnosed in females. You are more likely to develop celiac disease if someone in your family has the disease. Celiac disease also is more common among people with certain other diseases, such as Down syndrome, Turner syndrome, and type 1 diabetes.

Dental Enamel Defects and Celiac Disease

Celiac disease manifestations can extend beyond the classic gastro-intestinal problems, affecting any organ or body system. One manifes-tation—dental enamel defects—can help dentists and other healthcare providers identify people who may have celiac disease and refer them to a gastroenterologist. For some people with celiac disease, a dental visit, rather than a trip to the gastroenterologist, was the first step toward discovering their condition.

Not all dental enamel defects are caused by celiac disease, although the problem is fairly common among people with the condition, par-ticularly children, according to Alessio Fasano, M.D., medical direc-tor at the Massachusetts General Hospital for Celiac Research and Treatment. And dental enamel defects might be the only presenting manifestations of celiac disease.

Dental enamel problems stemming from celiac disease involve per-manent dentition and include tooth discoloration—white, yellow, or brown spots on the teeth—poor enamel formation, pitting or banding of teeth, and mottled or translucent-looking teeth. The imperfections are symmetrical and often appear on the incisors and molars.

Tooth defects resulting from celiac disease are permanent and do not improve after adopting a gluten-free diet—the primary treatment for celiac disease. However, dentists may use bonding, veneers, and other cosmetic solutions to cover dental enamel defects in older children and adults.

Similar Symptoms, Different Problem

Tooth defects that result from celiac disease may resemble those caused by too much fluoride or a maternal or early childhood illness.

"Dentists mostly say it's from fluoride, that the mother took tetracycline, or that there was an illness early on," said Peter H.R. Green, M.D., director of the Celiac Disease Center at Columbia University. "Celiac disease isn't on the radar screen of dentists in this country. Dentists should be made aware of these manifestations to help them identify people and get them to see their doctors so they can exclude celiac disease."

Green just completed a U.S. study with his dental colleague, Ted Malahias, D.D.S., that demonstrates celiac disease is highly associated with dental enamel defects in childhood—most likely due to the onset of celiac disease during enamel formation. The study, which did not identify a similar association in adults, concluded that all physician education about celiac disease should include information about the significance of dental enamel defects.

Other Oral Symptoms

Checking a patient's mouth is something primary care physicians also can do to help identify people who might have celiac disease. While dental enamel defects are the most prominent, a number of other oral problems are related to celiac disease, according to Green. These include:

- recurrent aphthous stomatitis, or canker sores or ulcers that recur inside the mouth

- atrophic glossitis, a condition characterized by a red, smooth, shiny tongue

- dry mouth syndrome

- squamous cell carcinoma—a type of cancer—of the pharynx and mouth

Chapter 49

Diabetes and Oral Health

How Can Diabetes Affect My Mouth?

Too much glucose, also called sugar, in your blood from diabetes can cause pain, infection, and other problems in your mouth. Your mouth includes:

- your teeth

- your gums

- your jaw

- tissues such as your tongue, the roof and bottom of your mouth, and the inside of your cheeks

- Glucose is present in your saliva—the fluid in your mouth that makes it wet. When diabetes is not controlled, high glucose levels in your saliva help harmful bacteria grow. These bacteria combine with food to form a soft, sticky film called plaque. Plaque also comes from eating foods that contain sugars or starches. Some types of plaque cause tooth decay or cavities. Other types of plaque cause gum disease and bad breath.

This chapter includes text excerpted from "Diabetes, Gum Disease, and Other Dental Problems," National Institute of Diabetes and Digestive and Kidney Diseases (NIDDK), September 2014.

Gum disease can be more severe and take longer to heal if you have diabetes. In turn, having gum disease can make your blood glucose hard to control.

What Happens If I Have Plaque?

Plaque that is not removed hardens over time into tartar and collects above your gum line. Tartar makes it more difficult to brush and clean between your teeth. Your gums become red and swollen, and bleed easily—signs of unhealthy or inflamed gums, called gingivitis.

When gingivitis is not treated, it can advance to gum disease called periodontitis. In periodontitis, the gums pull away from the teeth and form spaces, called pockets, which slowly become infected. This infection can last a long time. Your body fights the bacteria as the plaque spreads and grows below the gum line. Both the bacteria and your body's response to this infection start to break down the bone and the tissue that hold the teeth in place. If periodontitis is not treated, the gums, bones, and tissue that support the teeth are destroyed. Teeth may become loose and might need to be removed. If you have periodontitis, your dentist may send you to a periodontist, an expert in treating gum disease.

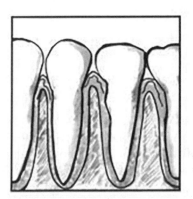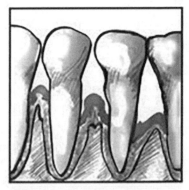

Figure 49.1. *Healthy Teeth and Periodontitis*

What Are the Most Common Mouth Problems from Diabetes?

The following table shows the most common mouth problems from diabetes.

Table 49.1. Common Mouth Problems from Diabetes

Problem	What It Is	Symptoms	Treatment
gingivitis	• unhealthy or inflamed gums	• red, swollen, and bleeding gums	• daily brushing and flossing • regular cleanings at the dentist
periodontitis	• gum disease, which can change from mild to severe	• red, swollen, and bleeding gums • gums that have pulled away from the teeth • long-lasting infection between the teeth and gums • bad breath that won't go away • permanent teeth that are loose or moving away from one another • changes in the way your teeth fit together when you bite • sometimes pus between the teeth and gums • changes in the fit of dentures, which are teeth you can remove	• deep cleaning at your dentist • medicine that your dentist prescribes • gum surgery in severe cases
thrush, called **candidiasis**	• the growth of a naturally occurring fungus that the body is unable to control	• sore, white—or sometimes red—patches on your gums, tongue, cheeks, or the roof of your mouth • patches that have turned into open sores	• medicine that your doctor or dentist prescribes to kill the fungus • cleaning dentures • removing dentures for part of the day or night, and soaking them in medicine that your doctor or dentist prescribes

Table 49.1. Continued

Problem	What It Is	Symptoms	Treatment
dry mouth, called **xerostomia**	• a lack of saliva in your mouth, which raises your risk for tooth decay and gum disease	• dry feeling in your mouth, often or all of the time • dry, rough tongue • pain in the mouth • cracked lips • mouth sores or infection • problems chewing, eating, swallowing, or talking	• taking medicine to keep your mouth wet that your doctor or dentist prescribes • rinsing with a fluoride mouth rinse to prevent cavities • using sugarless gum or mints to increase saliva flow • taking frequent sips of water • avoiding tobacco, caffeine, and alcoholic beverages • using a humidifier, a device that raises the level of moisture in your home, at night • avoiding spicy or salty foods that may cause pain in a dry mouth
oral burning	• a burning sensation inside the mouth caused by uncontrolled blood glucose levels	• burning feeling in the mouth • dry mouth • bitter taste • symptoms may worsen throughout the day	• seeing your doctor, who may change your diabetes medicine • once your blood glucose is under control, the oral burning will go away

More symptoms of a problem in your mouth are:

- dark spots or holes in your teeth
- pain in your mouth, face, or jaw that doesn't go away
- loose teeth
- pain when chewing
- a changed sense of taste or a bad taste in your mouth
- bad breath that doesn't go away when you brush your teeth

How Will I Know If I Have Mouth Problems from Diabetes?

Check your mouth for signs of problems from diabetes. If you notice any problems, see your dentist right away. Some of the first signs of gum disease are swollen, tender, or bleeding gums. Sometimes you won't have any signs of gum disease. You may not know you have it until you have serious damage. Your best defense is to see your dentist twice a year for a cleaning and checkup.

How Can I Prepare for a Visit to My Dentist?

Plan ahead. Talk with your doctor and dentist before the visit about the best way to take care of your blood glucose during dental work.

You may be taking a diabetes medicine that can cause low blood glucose, also called hypoglycemia. If you take insulin or other diabetes medicines, take them and eat as usual before visiting the dentist. You may need to bring your diabetes medicines and your snacks or meal with you to the dentist's office.

You may need to postpone any nonemergency dental work if your blood glucose is not under control. If you feel nervous about visiting the dentist, tell your dentist and the staff about your feelings. Your dentist can adapt the treatment to your needs. Don't let your nerves stop you from having regular checkups. Waiting too long to take care of your mouth may make things worse. If you feel nervous about visiting the dentist, tell your dentist and the staff about your feelings.

What If My Mouth Is Sore after My Dental Work?

A sore mouth is common after dental work. If this happens, you might not be able to eat or chew the foods you normally eat for several hours or days. For guidance on how to adjust your usual routine while your mouth is healing, ask your doctor:

- what foods and drinks you should have

- if you should change the time when you take your diabetes medicines

- if you should change the dose of your diabetes medicines

- how often you should check your blood glucose

How Does Smoking Affect My Mouth?

Smoking makes problems with your mouth worse. Smoking raises your chances of getting gum disease, oral and throat cancers, and oral fungal infections. Smoking also discolors your teeth and makes your breath smell bad.

Smoking and diabetes are a dangerous mix. Smoking raises your risk for many diabetes problems. If you quit smoking, you will lower your risk for heart attack, stroke, nerve disease, kidney disease, and amputation your cholesterol and blood pressure levels might improve your blood circulation will improve. If you smoke, stop smoking. Ask for help so that you don't have to do it alone. You can start by calling 1-800-QUITNOW or 1-800-784-8669.

How Can I Keep My Mouth Healthy?

You can keep your mouth healthy by taking these steps:

- Keep your blood glucose numbers as close to your target as possible. Your doctor will help you set your target blood glucose numbers and teach you what to do if your numbers are too high or too low.

- Eat healthy meals and follow the meal plan that you and your doctor or dietitian have worked out.

- Brush your teeth at least twice a day with fluoride toothpaste. Fluoride protects against tooth decay.

- Aim for brushing first thing in the morning, before going to bed, and after each meal and sugary or starchy snack.

- Use a soft toothbrush.

- Gently brush your teeth with the toothbrush angled towards the gum line.

- Use small, circular motions.

- Brush the front, back, and top of each tooth. Brush your tongue, too.

- Change your toothbrush every three months or sooner if the toothbrush looks worn or the bristles spread out. A new toothbrush removes more plaque.

- Drink water that contains added fluoride or ask your dentist about using a fluoride mouth rinse to prevent tooth decay.

- Ask your dentist about using an anti-plaque or anti-gingivitis mouth rinse to control plaque or prevent gum disease.

- Use dental floss to clean between your teeth at least once a day. Flossing helps prevent plaque from building up on your teeth. When flossing,

- slide the floss up and down and then curve it around the base of each tooth under the gums

- use clean sections of floss as you move from tooth to tooth

- Another way of removing plaque between teeth is to use a dental pick or brush—thin tools designed to clean between the teeth. You can buy these picks at drug stores or grocery stores.

- If you wear dentures, keep them clean and take them out at night. Have them adjusted if they become loose or uncomfortable.

- Call your dentist right away if you have any symptoms of mouth problems.

- See your dentist twice a year for a cleaning and checkup. Your dentist may suggest more visits if you need them.

- Follow your dentist's advice.

- If your dentist tells you about a problem, take care of it right away.

- Follow any steps or treatments from your dentist to keep your mouth healthy.

- Tell your dentist that you have diabetes.

- Tell your dentist about any changes in your health or medicines.

- Share the results of some of your diabetes blood tests, such as the A1C test or the fasting blood glucose test.

- Ask if you need antibiotics before and after dental treatment if your diabetes is uncontrolled.

- If you smoke, stop smoking.

Chapter 50

Disabilities and Oral Care

Chapter Contents

Section 50.1

Special Care in Oral Health

This section includes text excerpted from "Special Care in
Oral Health," National Institute of Dental and Craniofacial
Research (NIDCR), March 6, 2014.

What Is Special Care?

It is an approach to oral health management tailored to the individual needs of people with a variety of medical conditions or limitations that require more than routine delivery of oral care. Special care encompasses preventive, diagnostic, and treatment services.

A person with diabetes who is at increased risk of gum disease, a young child who needs dentures because of a genetic disorder, or a person with arthritis who cannot hold a toothbrush require special care. Standard treatment procedures can be adapted to fit most patients' needs and abilities. While some patients require more specialized care, most can be treated successfully in general dental practices.

Why Do Patients Need Special Care?

Some patients need routine oral healthcare, but have medical conditions or limitations that require delivery of care beyond the routine. The dental team, for example, may need to learn to transfer a patient with cerebral palsy from the wheelchair to the dental chair, to use some sign language to communicate with deaf patients, or to adapt oral hygiene devices so a patient can use them.

Other patients have medical and oral conditions that call for extraordinary care and require oral health professionals to have specialized knowledge. Surgical treatment of oral cancer or genetic craniofacial defects, such as cleft lip and palate, often require extensive reconstruction that involves many health specialists. Further, disorders such as ectodermal dysplasia and osteogenesis imperfecta directly affect tooth and facial development and demand specialized treatment.

In addition, many systemic diseases and certain medical treatments have oral health implications. Dental professionals may need to develop a treatment strategy for a patient who has received an organ transplant, determine the best anesthetic alternative for a patient who has heart disease, or develop an oral health plan for a patient who must undergo treatment for cancer.

Disability status also plays a role in special care and contributes to disparities in the oral health of affected Americans. The oral health of special care patients may be neglected because of a demanding disease, conditions such as developmental disabilities, or limited access to oral healthcare. The coordination of care and an understanding of special care issues in oral health are essential for all members of a patient's healthcare team, including medical and dental professionals and caregivers.

Section 50.2

Practical Oral Care for People with Autism

This section includes text excerpted from "Practical Oral Care for People with Autism," National Institute of Dental and Craniofacial Research (NIDCR), November 3, 2014.

Providing Oral Care to People with Autism

Providing oral care to people with autism requires adaptation of the skills you use every day. In fact, most people with mild or moderate forms of autism can be treated successfully in the general practice setting. This section will help you make a difference in the lives of people who need professional oral care.

Autism is a complex developmental disability that impairs communication and social, behavioral, and intellectual functioning. Some people with the disorder appear distant, aloof, or detached from other people or from their surroundings. Others do not react appropriately to common verbal and social cues, such as a parent's tone of voice or smile. Obsessive routines, repetitive behaviors, unpredictable body movements, and self-injurious behavior may all be symptoms that complicate dental care.

Autism varies widely in symptoms and severity, and some people have coexisting conditions such as intellectual disability or epilepsy. They can be among the most challenging of patients, but following the suggestions in this section can help make their dental treatment successful.

Making a difference in the oral health of a person with autism may go slowly at first, but determination can bring positive results and invaluable rewards.

Health Challenges in Autism and Strategies for Care

Before the appointment, obtain and review the patient's medical history. Consultation with physicians, family, and caregivers is essential to assembling an accurate medical history. Also, determine who can legally provide informed consent for treatment.

Communication problems and mental capabilities are central concerns when treating people with autism.

- Talk with the parent or caregiver to determine your patient's intellectual and functional abilities, and then communicate with the patient at a level he or she can understand.

- Use a "tell-show-do" approach to providing care. Start by explaining each procedure before it occurs. Take the time to show what you have explained, such as the instruments you will use and how they work. Demonstrations can encourage some patients to be more cooperative.

Behavior problems—which may include hyperactivity and quick frustration—can complicate oral healthcare for patients with autism. The invasive nature of oral care may trigger violent and self-injurious behavior such as temper tantrums or head banging.

- Plan a desensitization appointment to help the patient become familiar with the office, staff, and equipment through a step-by-step process. These steps may take several visits to accomplish.

- Have the patient sit alone in the dental chair to become familiar with the treatment setting. Some patients may refuse to sit in the chair and choose instead to sit on the operator's stool.

- Once your patient is seated, begin a cursory examination using your fingers.

- Next, use a toothbrush to brush the teeth and gain additional access to the patient's mouth. The familiarity of a toothbrush will help your patient feel comfortable and provide you with an opportunity to further examine the mouth.

- When the patient is prepared for treatment, make the appointment short and positive.

- Pay special attention to the treatment setting. Keep dental instruments out of sight and light out of your patient's eyes.

- Praise and reinforce good behavior after each step of a procedure. Ignore inappropriate behavior as much as you can.

- Try to gain cooperation in the least restrictive manner. Some patients' behavior may improve if they bring comfort items such as a stuffed animal or a blanket. Asking the caregiver to sit nearby or hold the patient's hand may be helpful as well.

- Use immobilization techniques only when absolutely necessary to protect the patient and staff during dental treatment—not as a convenience. There are no universal guidelines on immobilization that apply to all treatment settings. Before employing any kind of immobilization, it may help to consult available guidelines on federally funded care, your State department of mental health/disabilities, and your State Dental Practice Act. Guidelines on behavior management published by the American Academy of Pediatric Dentistry may also be useful. Obtain consent from your patient's legal guardian and choose the least restrictive technique that will allow you to provide care safely. Immobilization should not cause physical injury or undue discomfort.

- If all other strategies fail, pharmacological options are useful in managing some patients. Others need to be treated under general anesthesia. However, caution is necessary because some patients with developmental disabilities can have unpredictable reactions to medications.

People with autism often engage in perseveration, a continuous, meaningless repetition of words, phrases, or movements. Your patient may mimic the sound of the suction, for example, or repeat an instruction over and again. Avoid demonstrating dental equipment if it triggers perseveration, and note this in the patient's record.

Unusual responses to stimuli can create distractions and interrupt treatment. People with autism need consistency and can be especially sensitive to changes in their environment. They may exhibit unusual sensitivity to sensory stimuli such as sound, bright colors, and touch. Reactions vary: Some people with autism may overreact to noise and touch, while exposure to pain and heat may not provoke much reaction at all.

- Use the same staff, dental operatory, and appointment time to sustain familiarity. These details can help make dental treatment seem less threatening.

- Minimize the number of distractions. Try to reduce unnecessary sights, sounds, odors, or other stimuli that might be disruptive. Use an operatory that is somewhat secluded instead of one in the middle of a busy office. Also, consider lowering ambient light and asking the patient's caregiver whether soft music would help.

- Allow time for your patient to adjust and become desensitized to the noise of a dental setting. Some patients may be hypersensitive to the sound of dental instruments.

- Talk to the caregiver to get a sense of the patient's level of tolerance. People with autism differ in how they accept physical contact. Some are defensive and refuse any contact in or around the mouth, or cradling of the head or face. Others find such cradling comforting.

- Note your findings and experiences in the patient's chart.

Unusual and unpredictable body movements are sometimes observed in people with autism. These movements can jeopardize safety as well as your ability to deliver oral healthcare.

- Make sure the path from the reception area to the dental chair is clear.

- Observe the patient's movements and look for patterns. Try to anticipate the movements, either blending your movements with those of your patient or working around them.

Seizures may accompany autism but can usually be controlled with anticonvulsant medications. The mouth is always at risk during a seizure: Patients may chip teeth or bite the tongue or cheeks. People with controlled seizure disorders can easily be treated in the general dental office.

- Consult your patient's physician. Record information in the chart about the frequency of seizures and the medications used to control them. Determine before the appointment whether medications have been taken as directed. Know and avoid any factors that trigger your patient's seizures.

- Be prepared to manage a seizure. If one occurs during oral care, remove any instruments from the mouth and clear the area around the dental chair. Attaching dental floss to rubber dam clamps and mouth props when treatment begins can help you remove them quickly. Do not attempt to insert any objects between the teeth during a seizure.

- Stay with your patient, turn him or her to one side, and monitor the airway to reduce the risk of aspiration.

Record in the patient's chart strategies that were successful in providing care. Note your patient's preferences and other unique details that will facilitate treatment, such as music, comfort items, and flavor choices.

Oral Health Problems in Autism and Strategies for Care

People with autism experience few unusual oral health conditions. Although commonly used medications and damaging oral habits can cause problems, the rates of caries and periodontal disease in people with autism are comparable to those in the general population. Communication and behavioral problems pose the most significant challenges in providing oral care.

Damaging oral habits are common and include bruxism; tongue thrusting; self-injurious behavior such as picking at the gingiva or biting the lips; and pica—eating objects and substances such as gravel, cigarette butts, or pens. If a mouth guard can be tolerated, prescribe one for patients who have problems with self-injurious behavior or bruxism.

Dental caries risk increases in patients who have a preference for soft, sticky, or sweet foods; damaging oral habits; and difficulty brushing and flossing.

- Recommend preventive measures such as fluorides and sealants.

- Caution patients or their caregivers about medicines that reduce saliva or contain sugar. Suggest that patients drink water often, take sugar-free medicines when available, and rinse with water after taking any medicine.

399

- Advise caregivers to offer alternatives to cariogenic foods and beverages as incentives or rewards.

- Encourage independence in daily oral hygiene. Ask patients to show you how they brush, and follow up with specific recommendations. Perform hands-on demonstrations to show patients the best way to clean their teeth. If appropriate, show patients and caregivers how a modified toothbrush or floss holder might make oral hygiene easier.

- Some patients cannot brush and floss independently. Talk to caregivers about daily oral hygiene and do not assume that they know the basics. Use your experiences with each patient to demonstrate oral hygiene techniques and sitting or standing positions for the caregiver. Emphasize that a consistent approach to oral hygiene is important—caregivers should try to use the same location, timing, and positioning.

Periodontal disease occurs in people with autism in much the same way it does in persons without developmental disabilities.

- Some patients benefit from the daily use of an antimicrobial agent such as chlorhexidine.

- Stress the importance of conscientious oral hygiene and frequent prophylaxis.

Tooth eruption may be delayed due to phenytoin-induced gingival hyperplasia. Phenytoin is commonly prescribed for people with autism.

Trauma and injury to the mouth from falls or accidents occur in people with seizure disorders. Suggest a tooth saving kit for group homes. Emphasize to caregivers that traumas require immediate professional attention and explain the procedures to follow if a permanent tooth is knocked out. Also, instruct caregivers to locate any missing pieces of a fractured tooth, and explain that radiographs of the patient's chest may be necessary to determine whether any fragments have been aspirated.

Physical abuse often presents as oral trauma. Abuse is reported more frequently in people with developmental disabilities than in the general population. If you suspect that a child is being abused or neglected, State laws require that you call your Child Protective Services agency. Assistance is also available from the Childhelp® National Child Abuse Hotline at (800) 422-4453 or the Child Welfare Information Gateway.

Section 50.3

Practical Oral Care for People with Cerebral Palsy

This section includes text excerpted from "Practical Oral Care
for People with Cerebral Palsy," National Institute of Dental and
Craniofacial Research (NIDCR), August 1, 2014.

Providing Oral Care to People with Cerebral Palsy

Providing oral care to people with cerebral palsy requires adaptation of the skills you use every day. In fact, most people with mild or
moderate forms of cerebral palsy can be treated successfully in the
general practice setting. This section will help you make a difference
in the lives of people who need professional oral care.

Cerebral palsy is a complex group of motor abnormalities and functional impairments that affect muscle coordination. This developmental disability may be associated with uncontrolled body movements,
seizure disorders, balance-related abnormalities, sensory dysfunction,
and intellectual disability. For some, the disorder is mild, causing
movements to appear merely clumsy or awkward. These patients may
need little or no day-to-day supervision. Others, however, experience
such severe forms of cerebral palsy that they require a wheelchair and
a lifetime of personal care.

Cerebral palsy itself does not cause any unique oral abnormalities.
However, several conditions are more common or more severe in people
with cerebral palsy than in the general population.

Health Challenges in Cerebral Palsy and Strategies for Care

People with cerebral palsy may present with physical and mental
challenges that have implications for oral care. Before the appointment, obtain and review the patient's medical history. Consultation
with physicians, family, and caregivers is essential to assembling an
accurate medical history. Also, determine who can legally provide
informed consent for treatment.

401

The different types of cerebral palsy are classified according to associated motor impairments:

Spastic palsy presents with stiff or rigid muscles on one side of the body or in all four limbs, sometimes including the mouth, tongue, and pharynx. People with this form of cerebral palsy may have legs that turn inward and scissor as they walk, or arms that are flexed and positioned against their bodies. Many also have intellectual disability, seizures, and dysarthria (difficulty speaking).

Dyskinetic or athetoid palsy is characterized by hypotonia and slow, uncontrolled writhing movements. People with this type of cerebral palsy experience frequent changes in muscle tone in all areas of their bodies; muscles may be rigid during waking hours and normal during sleep. Dysarthria is also associated with this type.

Ataxic palsy is marked by problems with balance and depth perception, as well as an unsteady, wide-based gait. Hypotonia and tremors sometimes occur in people with this rare type of cerebral palsy.

Combined palsy reflects a combination of these types.

Everyone who has cerebral palsy has problems with movement and posture. Observe each patient, then tailor your care accordingly.

- Maintain clear paths for movement throughout the treatment setting. Keep instruments and equipment out of the patient's way.

- Some patients cannot be moved into the dental chair but instead must be treated in their wheelchairs. Some wheelchairs recline or are specially molded to fit people's bodies. Lock the wheels, then slip a sliding board (also called a transfer board) behind the patient's back to support the head and neck.

- If you need to transfer your patient from a wheelchair to the dental chair, ask about special preferences such as padding, pillows, or other things you can provide to ease the transition. The patient or caregiver can often explain how to make a smooth transfer.

Uncontrolled body movements are common in people with cerebral palsy. Their limbs move often, so providing oral care can be difficult. When patients with cerebral palsy attempt to move in order to help, their muscles often tense, increasing uncontrolled movements.

- Make the treatment environment calm and supportive. Try to help your patient relax. Relaxation will not stop uncontrolled body movements, but it may reduce their frequency or intensity.

- Place and maintain your patient in the center of the dental chair. Do not force arms and legs into unnatural positions, but allow the patient to settle into a position that is comfortable and will not interfere with dental treatment.

- Observe your patient's movements and look for patterns to help you anticipate direction and intensity. Trying to stop these movements may only intensify the involuntary response. Try instead to anticipate the movements, blending your movements with those of your patient or working around them.

- Softly cradle your patient's head during treatment. Be gentle and slow if you need to turn the patient's head.

- Exert gentle but firm pressure on your patient's arm or leg if it begins to shake.

- Try to keep appointments short, take frequent breaks, or consider prescribing muscle relaxants when long procedures are needed. People with cerebral palsy may need sedation, general anesthesia, or hospitalization if extensive dental treatment is required.

Primitive reflexes are common in many people with cerebral palsy and may complicate oral care. These reflexes often occur when the head is moved or the patient is startled, and efforts to control them may make them more intense. Three types of reflexes are most commonly observed during oral care.

Asymmetric tonic neck reflex: When a patient's head is turned, the arm and leg on that side stiffen and extend. The arm and leg on the opposite side flex.

Tonic labyrinthine reflex: If the neck is extended while a patient is lying on his or her back, the legs and arms also extend, and the back and neck arch.

Startle reflex: Any surprising stimuli, such as noises, lights, or a sudden movement on your part, can trigger uncontrolled, often forceful movements involving the whole body.

- Be empathic about your patient's concerns and frustrations.

- Minimize the number of distractions in the treatment setting. Movements, lights, sounds, or other stimuli can make it difficult for your patient to cooperate. Tell him or her about any such stimulus before it appears. For example, tell the patient before you move the dental chair.

Mental capabilities vary. Many people with cerebral palsy have mild or moderate intellectual disability, but only 25 percent have a severe form. Some have normal intelligence.

- Talk with the parent or caregiver to determine your patient's intellectual and functional abilities, then explain each procedure at a level the patient can understand. Allow extra time to explain oral health issues, instructions, or procedures.

- Use simple, concrete instructions and repeat them often to compensate for any short-term memory problems. Speak slowly and give only one direction at a time.

- Demonstrations can make patients more cooperative. For example, turn on the saliva ejector so the patient can hear it and feel it at the corner of the mouth. Then slowly introduce it inside the mouth, being careful not to trigger a gag reflex.

- Be consistent in all aspects of oral care. Use the same staff and dental operatory each time to help sustain familiarity. Consistency leads to improved cooperation.

- Listen actively, since communicating clearly is difficult for some—show your patient whether you understand. Be sensitive to the methods he or she uses to communicate, including gestures and verbal or nonverbal requests.

Seizures may accompany cerebral palsy, but can usually be controlled with anticonvulsant medications. The mouth is always at risk during a seizure: Patients may chip teeth or bite the tongue or cheeks. Patients with controlled seizure disorders can easily be treated in the general dental office.

- Consult your patient's physician. Record information in the chart about the frequency of seizures and the medications used to control them. Determine before the appointment whether medications have been taken as directed. Know and avoid any factors that trigger your patient's seizures.

- Be prepared to manage a seizure. If one occurs during oral care, remove any instruments from the mouth and clear the area around the dental chair. Attaching dental floss to rubber dam clamps and mouth props when treatment begins can help you remove them quickly. Do not attempt to insert any objects between the teeth during a seizure.

- Stay with your patient, turn him or her to one side, and monitor the airway to reduce the risk of aspiration.

Visual impairments affect a large number of people with cerebral palsy. The most common of these defects is strabismus, a condition in which the eyes are crossed or misaligned. People with cerebral palsy may develop visual motor skills, such as hand-eye coordination, later than other people.

- Determine the level of assistance your patient requires to move safely through the dental office.

- Use your patients' other senses to connect with them, establish trust, and make treatment a good experience. Tactile feedback, such as a warm handshake, can make your patients feel comfortable.

- Face your patients when you speak and keep them apprised of each upcoming step, especially when water will be used. Rely on clear, descriptive language to explain procedures and demonstrate how equipment might feel and sound. Provide written instructions in large print (16 point or larger).

Hearing loss and deafness can be accommodated with careful planning. Patients with a hearing problem may appear to be stubborn because of their seeming lack of response to a request.

- Patients may want to adjust their hearing aids or turn them off, since the sound of some instruments may cause auditory discomfort.

- If your patient reads lips, speak in a normal cadence and tone. If your patient uses a form of sign language, ask the interpreter to come to the appointment. Speak with this person in advance to discuss dental terms and your patient's needs.

- Visual feedback is helpful. Maintain eye contact with your patient. Before talking, eliminate background noise (turn off the radio and the suction). Sometimes people with a hearing loss simply need you to speak clearly in a slightly louder voice than normal. Remember to remove your facemask first or wear a clear face shield.

Dysarthria is common in people with cerebral palsy, due to problems involving the muscles that control speech and mastication.

- Be patient. Allow time for your patient to express himself or herself. Remember that many people with dysarthria have normal intelligence.

- Consult with the caregiver if you have difficulty understanding your patient's speech.

Gastroesophageal reflux sometimes affects people with cerebral palsy, including those who are tube-fed. Teeth may be sensitive or display signs of erosion. Consult your patient's physician about the management of reflux.

- Place patients in a slightly upright position for treatment.

- Talk with patients and caregivers about rinsing with plain water or a water and baking soda solution. Doing so at least four times a day can help mitigate the effects of gastric acid. Stress that using a fluoride gel, rinse, or toothpaste every day is essential.

Record in the patient's chart strategies that were successful in providing care. Note your patient's preferences and other unique details that will facilitate treatment, such as music, comfort items, and flavor choices.

Oral Health Problems in Cerebral Palsy and Strategies for Care

Cerebral palsy itself does not cause any unique oral abnormalities. However, several conditions are more common or more severe in people with cerebral palsy than in the general population.

Periodontal disease is common in people with cerebral palsy due to poor oral hygiene and complications of oral habits, physical abilities, and malocclusion. Another factor is the gingival hyperplasia caused by medications.

- Encourage independence in daily oral hygiene. Ask patients to show you how they brush, and follow up with specific recommendations on brushing methods or toothbrush adaptations. Involve your patients in hands-on demonstrations of brushing and flossing.

- Some patients cannot brush and floss independently because of impaired physical coordination or cognitive skills. Talk to caregivers about daily oral hygiene. Do not assume that all caregivers know the basics; demonstrate proper brushing and flossing techniques. A power toothbrush or a floss holder can simplify oral care. Also, use your experiences with each patient to demonstrate sitting or standing positions for the caregiver. Emphasize that a consistent approach to oral hygiene is important—caregivers should try to use the same location, timing, and positioning.

- Explain that some patients benefit from the daily use of an antimicrobial agent such as chlorhexidine. Recommend an appropriate delivery method based on your patient's abilities. Rinsing, for example, may not work for a patient with swallowing difficulties or one who cannot expectorate. Chlorhexidine applied using a spray bottle or toothbrush is equally efficacious.

- If use of particular medications has led to gingival hyperplasia, monitor for possible delayed tooth eruption and emphasize the importance of daily oral hygiene and frequent professional cleanings.

Dental caries is prevalent among people with cerebral palsy, primarily because of inadequate oral hygiene. Other risk factors include mouth breathing, the effects of medication, enamel hypoplasia, and food pouching.

- Caution patients or their caregivers about medicines that reduce saliva or contain sugar. Suggest that patients drink water often, take sugar-free medicines when available, and rinse with water after taking any medicine.

- Advise caregivers to offer alternatives to cariogenic foods and beverages as incentives or rewards.

- For people who pouch food, talk to caregivers about inspecting the mouth after each meal or dose of medicine. Remove food or medicine from the mouth by rinsing with water, sweeping the mouth with a finger wrapped in gauze, or using a disposable foam applicator swab.

- Recommend preventive measures such as fluorides and sealants.

Malocclusion in people with cerebral palsy usually involves more than just misaligned teeth—it is also a musculoskeletal problem. An open bite with protruding anterior teeth is common and is typically associated with tongue thrusting. The inability to close the lips because of an open bite also contributes to excessive drooling.

Unfortunately, correcting malocclusion is almost impossible in people with moderate or severe cerebral palsy. Orthodontic treatment may not be an option because of the risk of caries and enamel hypoplasia. However, a developmental disability in and of itself should not be perceived as a barrier to orthodontic treatment.

- The ability of the patient or the caregiver to maintain good daily oral hygiene is critical to the feasibility and success of orthodontic treatment.

- Inform caregivers of emergency procedures for accidents involving oral trauma, since protruding anterior teeth are more likely to be displaced, fractured, or avulsed.

Dysphagia, difficulty with swallowing, is often a problem in people with cerebral palsy. Food may stay in the mouth longer than usual, increasing the risk for caries. Additionally, the semi-soft foods caregivers may prepare for people with this problem tend to adhere to the teeth. Coughing, gagging, choking, and aspiration are other related concerns.

- Keep the breathing passages open by placing your patient in a slightly upright position with the head turned to one side during oral care.

- Use suction frequently or as tolerated by the patient. Use a rubber dam when indicated, but make sure you introduce it slowly, perhaps over a few appointments.

- Advise the caregiver to inspect the patient's mouth after eating and remove any residual food.

Drooling affects daily oral care as well as social interaction. Hypotonia contributes to drooling, as does an open bite and the inability to close the lips.

Bruxism is common in people with cerebral palsy, especially those with severe forms of the disorder. Bruxism can be intense and persistent and cause the teeth to wear prematurely. Before recommending mouth guards or bite splints, consider that gagging or swallowing problems may make them uncomfortable or unwearable.

Hyperactive bite and gag reflexes call for introducing instruments gently into the mouth. Consider using a mouth prop. A patient with a gagging problem benefits from an early morning appointment, before eating or drinking. Help minimize the gag reflex by placing your patient's chin in a neutral or downward position.

Trauma and injury to the mouth from falls or accidents occur in people with cerebral palsy. Suggest a tooth-saving kit for group homes. Emphasize to caregivers that traumas require immediate professional attention and explain the procedures to follow if a permanent tooth is knocked out. Also, instruct caregivers to locate any missing pieces of a fractured tooth, and explain that radiographs of the patient's chest may be necessary to determine whether any fragments have been aspirated.

Physical abuse often presents as oral trauma. Abuse is reported more frequently in people with developmental disabilities than in the general population. If you suspect that a child is being abused or neglected, State laws require that you call your Child Protective Services agency. Assistance is also available from the Childhelp® National Child Abuse Hotline at (800) 422-4453 or the Child Welfare Information Gateway.

Section 50.4

Practical Oral Care for People with Developmental Disabilities

This section includes text excerpted from "Continuing Education: Practical Oral Care for People with Developmental Disabilities," National Institute of Dental and Craniofacial Research (NIDCR), July 12, 2016.

Developmental Disabilities

Over the past three decades, a trend toward deinstitutionalization has brought people of all ages and levels of disability into the fabric of our communities. Today, approximately 80 percent of those with developmental disabilities are living in community-based group residences or at home with their families. People with disabilities and their caregivers now look to providers in the community for dental services.

Providing oral care to patients with developmental disabilities requires adaptation of the skills you use every day. In fact, most people with mild or moderate developmental disabilities can be treated successfully in the general practice setting. This section presents an overview of physical, mental, and behavioral challenges common in these patients and offers strategies for providing oral care.

Developmental disabilities such as autism, cerebral palsy, Down general faces syndrome, and intellectual disability are present during childhood or adolescence and last a lifetime. They affect the mind, the body, and the skills people use in everyday life: thinking, talking, and self-care. People with disabilities often need extra help to achieve and maintain good health. Oral health is no exception.

Health Challenges and Strategies for Care

Before the appointment, obtain and review the patient's medical history. Consultation with physicians, family, and caregivers is essential to assembling an accurate medical history. Also, determine who can legally provide informed consent for treatment.

Mental capabilities vary in people with developmental disabilities and influence how well they can follow directions in the operatory and at home.

- Determine each patient's mental capabilities and communication skills. Talk with caregivers about how the patient's abilities might affect oral healthcare. Be receptive to their thoughts and ideas on how to make the experience a success.

- Allow time to introduce concepts in language that patients can understand.

- Communicate respectfully with your patients and comfort those who resist dental care. Repeat instructions when necessary and involve your patients in hands-on demonstrations.

Behavior problems can complicate oral healthcare. Anxiety and fear about dental treatment can cause some patients to be uncooperative. Behaviors may range from fidgeting or temper tantrums to violent, self-injurious behavior such as head banging. This is challenging for everyone, but the following strategies can help reduce behavior problems:

- Set the stage for a successful visit by involving the entire dental team—from the receptionist's friendly greeting to the caring attitude of the dental assistant in the operatory.

- Arrange for a desensitizing appointment to help the patient become familiar with the office, staff, and equipment before treatment begins.

- Try to gain cooperation in the least restrictive manner. Some patients' behavior may improve if they bring comfort items such as a stuffed animal or a blanket. Asking the caregiver to sit nearby or hold the patient's hand may be helpful as well.

- Make appointments short whenever possible, providing only the treatment that the patient can tolerate. Praise and reinforce good behavior and try to end each appointment on a good note.

- Use immobilization techniques only when absolutely necessary to protect the patient and staff during dental treatment—not as a convenience. There are no universal guidelines on immobilization that apply to all treatment settings. Before employing any kind of immobilization, it may help to consult available guidelines on federally funded care, your State department of mental health/disabilities, and your State Dental Practice Act. Guidelines on behavior management published by the American Academy of Pediatric Dentistry may also be useful. Obtain consent from your patient's legal guardian and choose the least restrictive technique that will allow you to provide care safely. Immobilization should not cause physical injury or undue discomfort.

Mobility problems are a concern for many people with disabilities; some rely on a wheelchair or a walker to move around.

- Observe the physical impact a disability has and how a particular patient moves. Look for challenges such as uncontrolled body movements or concerns about posture.

- Maintain a clear path for movement throughout the treatment setting. Clinician standing behind a patient, cradling the patient's head while resting her hand around the patient's mandible. The clinician is using a transfer board.

- If you need to transfer your patient from a wheelchair to the dental chair, ask the patient or caregiver about special preferences such as padding, pillows, or other things you can provide. Often the patient or caregiver can explain how to make a smooth transfer.

- Certain patients cannot be moved into the dental chair but instead must be treated in their wheelchairs. Some wheelchairs recline or are specially molded to fit people's bodies. Lock the wheels, then slip a sliding board (also called a transfer board) behind the patient's back to support the head and neck.

Neuromuscular problems can affect the mouth. Some people with disabilities have persistently rigid or loose masticatory muscles. Others have drooling, gagging, and swallowing problems that complicate oral care.

- If a patient has a gagging problem, schedule an early morning appointment, before eating or drinking. Help minimize the gag reflex by placing your patient's chin in a neutral or downward position.

- If your patient has swallowing problems, tilt the head slightly to one side and place his or her body in a more upright position.

- If you use local anesthesia, be sure your patient does not chew the tongue or cheek. A short-lasting form of anesthesia may work well.

Uncontrolled body movements can jeopardize safety and your ability to deliver dental care. Pay special attention to the following:

- **Treatment setting:** Make the treatment setting calm and supportive. Place dental instruments behind the patient and carefully position other objects such as cords and the light above the dental chair.

- **Patient's position:** Determine in advance whether a patient will need to be treated in his or her wheelchair. If not, keep the patient in the center of the dental chair. Pillows can help maintain a comfortable position.

- **Your position:** Observe the patient's movements and look for patterns to help anticipate direction. Place yourself behind the patient and gently cradle the head to provide support. Rest your hand around the mandible.

Cardiac disorders, particularly mitral valve prolapse and heart valve damage, are common in people with developmental disabilities such as Down syndrome. Consult the patient's physician if you have questions about the medical history and the need for antibiotic prophylaxis.

Gastroesophageal reflux sometimes affects people with central nervous system disorders such as cerebral palsy. Teeth may be sensitive or display signs of erosion. Consult your patient's physician about the management of reflux.

- Place patients in a slightly upright position for treatment.

- Talk with patients and caregivers about rinsing with plain water or a water and baking soda solution. Doing so at least four times a day can help mitigate the effects of gastric acid. Stress that using a fluoride gel, rinse, or toothpaste every day is essential.

Seizures accompany many developmental disabilities. The mouth is always at risk during a seizure: Patients may chip teeth or bite the tongue or cheeks. Persons with controlled seizure disorders can easily be treated in the general dental office.

- Consult your patient's physician. Record information in the chart about the frequency of seizures and the medications used to control them. Determine before the appointment whether medications have been taken as directed. Know and avoid any factors that trigger your patient's seizures.

- Be prepared to manage a seizure. If one occurs during oral care, remove any instruments from the mouth and clear the area around the dental chair. Attaching dental floss to rubber dam clamps and mouth props when treatment begins can help you remove them quickly. Do not attempt to insert any objects between the teeth during a seizure.

- Stay with your patient, turn him or her to one side, and monitor the airway to reduce the risk of aspiration.

Visual impairments affect many people with developmental disabilities.

- Determine the level of assistance your patient requires to move safely through the office.

- Use your patients' other senses to connect with them, establish trust, and make treatment a good experience. Tactile feedback, such as a warm handshake, can make your patients feel comfortable.

- Face your patients when you speak and keep them apprised of each upcoming step, especially when water will be used. Rely on clear, descriptive language to explain procedures and demonstrate how equipment might feel and sound. Provide written instructions in large print (16 point or larger).

Hearing loss and deafness sometimes occur in people with developmental disabilities.

- Patients may want to adjust their hearing aids or turn them off, since the sound of some instruments may cause auditory discomfort.

- If your patient reads lips, speak in a normal cadence and tone. If your patient uses a form of sign language, ask the interpreter to come to the appointment. Speak with this person in advance to discuss dental terms and your patient's needs.

- Visual feedback is helpful. Maintain eye contact with your patient. Before talking, eliminate background noise (turn off the radio and the suction). Sometimes people with a hearing loss simply need you to speak clearly in a slightly louder voice than normal. Remember to remove your facemask first or wear a clear face shield.

Latex allergies can be a serious problem. People who have spina bifida or who have had frequent surgeries are especially prone to developing an allergic reaction or a sensitivity to latex. An allergic reaction can be life threatening.

- Ask patients and caregivers about the presence of a latex allergy before you begin treatment.

- Schedule appointments for your latex-allergic or sensitive patients at the beginning of the day when there are fewer airborne allergens circulating through the office.

- Use latex-free gloves and equipment and keep an emergency medical kit handy.

Oral Health Problems and Strategies for Care

People with developmental disabilities typically have more oral health problems than the general population. Focusing on each person's specific needs is the first step toward achieving better oral health.

Dental caries is common in people with developmental disabilities. In addition to discussing the problems associated with diet and oral hygiene, caution patients and caregivers about the cariogenic nature of prolonged bottle feeding and the adverse side effects of certain medications.

- Recommend preventive measures such as fluorides and sealants.

- Caution patients or their caregivers about medicines that reduce saliva or contain sugar. Suggest that patients drink water frequently, take sugar-free medicines when available, and rinse with water after taking any medicine.

- Advise caregivers to offer alternatives to cariogenic foods and beverages as incentives or rewards.

- Educate caregivers about preventing early childhood caries.

- Encourage independence in daily oral hygiene. Ask patients to show you how they brush, and follow up with specific recommendations. Perform hands-on demonstrations to show patients the best way to clean their teeth.

- If necessary, adapt a toothbrush to make it easier to hold. For example, place a tennis ball or bicycle grip on the handle, wrap the handle in tape, or bend the handle by softening it under hot water. Explain that floss holders and power toothbrushes are also helpful.

- Some patients cannot brush and floss independently. Talk to caregivers about daily oral hygiene and do not assume that they know the basics. Use your experiences with each patient to demonstrate oral care techniques and sitting or standing positions for the caregiver. Emphasize that a consistent approach to oral hygiene is important—caregivers should try to use the same location, timing, and positioning.

Periodontal disease occurs more often and at a younger age in people with developmental disabilities. Contributing factors include poor oral hygiene, damaging oral habits, and physical or mental disabilities. Gingival hyperplasia caused by medications such as some anticonvulsants, antihypertensives, and immunosuppressants also increases the risk for periodontal disease.

- Some patients benefit from the daily use of an antimicrobial agent such as chlorhexidine.

- Stress the importance of conscientious oral hygiene and frequent prophylaxis.

Malocclusion occurs in many people with developmental disabilities and may be associated with intraoral and perioral muscular abnormalities, delayed tooth eruption, underdevelopment of the maxilla, and oral habits such as bruxism and tongue thrusting. Malocclusion can make chewing and speaking difficult and increase the risk of periodontal disease, dental caries, and oral trauma. Orthodontic treatment may not be an option for many, but a developmental disability in and of itself should not be perceived as a barrier to orthodontic care. The ability of the patient or the caregiver to maintain good daily oral hygiene is critical to the feasibility and success of orthodontic treatment.

Damaging oral habits can be a problem for people with developmental disabilities. Some of the most common of these habits are bruxism, food pouching, mouth breathing, and tongue thrusting. Other oral habits include self-injurious behavior such as picking at the gingiva or biting the lips; rumination, where food is chewed, regurgitated, and swallowed again; and pica, eating objects and substances such as gravel, sand, cigarette butts, or pens.

- For people who pouch food, talk to caregivers about inspecting the mouth after each meal or dose of medicine. Remove food or medicine from the mouth by rinsing with water, sweeping the mouth with a finger wrapped in gauze, or using a disposable foam applicator swab.

- If a mouth guard can be tolerated, prescribe one for patients who have problems with self-injurious behavior or bruxism.

Oral malformations affect many people with developmental disabilities. Patients may present with enamel defects, high lip lines with dry gingiva, and variations in the number, size, and shape of teeth. Craniofacial anomalies such as facial asymmetry and hypoplasia of the midfacial region are also seen in this population. Identify any malformations and explain to the caregiver the implications for daily oral hygiene and future treatment planning.

Tooth eruption may be delayed in children with developmental disabilities. Eruption times are different for each child, and some children may not get their first primary tooth until they are 2 years old. Delays are often characteristic of certain disabilities such as Down syndrome. In other cases, eruption problems are attributable to the gingival hyperplasia that can result from medications such as phenytoin and cyclosporin. Dental examination by a child's first birthday and regularly thereafter can help identify atypical patterns of eruption.

Trauma and injury to the mouth from falls or accidents occur in people with seizure disorders or cerebral palsy. Suggest a tooth-saving kit for group homes. Emphasize to caregivers that traumas require immediate professional attention and explain the procedures to follow if a permanent tooth is knocked out. Also, instruct caregivers to locate any missing pieces of a fractured tooth, and explain that radiographs of the patient's chest may be necessary to determine whether any fragments have been aspirated.

Physical abuse often presents as oral trauma. Abuse is reported more frequently in people with developmental disabilities than in the general population. If you suspect that a child is being abused or neglected, State laws require that you call your Child Protective Services agency. Assistance is also available from the Childhelp® National Child Abuse Hotline at (800) 422-4453 or the Child Welfare Information Gateway.

Section 50.5

Practical Oral Care for People with Down Syndrome

This section includes text excerpted from "Practical Oral Care for People with Down Syndrome," National Institute of Dental and Craniofacial Research (NIDCR), November 3, 2014.

Down Syndrome

Down syndrome, a common genetic disorder, ranges in severity and is usually associated with medical and physical problems. For example, people with this developmental disability may have cardiac disorders, infectious diseases, hypotonia, and hearing loss. Additionally, most people with this disorder have mild or moderate intellectual disability, while a small percentage are severely affected. Developmental delays, such as in speech and language, are common.

Providing oral care to people with Down syndrome requires adaptation of the skills you use every day. In fact, most people with mild or moderate Down syndrome can be successfully treated in the general practice setting. This section will help you make a difference in the lives of people who need professional oral care.

Health Challenges in Down Syndrome and Strategies for Care

People with Down syndrome may present with mental and physical challenges that have implications for oral care. Before the appointment, obtain and review the patient's medical history. Consultation with physicians, family, and caregivers is essential to assembling an accurate medical history. Also, determine who can legally provide informed consent for treatment.

Intellectual disability. Although the mental capability of people with Down syndrome varies widely, many have mild or moderate intellectual disability that limits their ability to learn, communicate, and adapt to their environment. Language development is often delayed or impaired in people with Down syndrome; they understand more than they can verbalize. Also, ordinary activities of daily living and understanding the behavior of others as well as their own can present challenges.

- Listen actively, since speaking may be difficult for people with Down syndrome. Show your patient whether you understand.

- Talk with the parent or caregiver to determine your patient's intellectual and functional abilities, then explain each procedure at a level the patient can understand. Allow extra time to explain oral health issues or instructions and demonstrate the instruments you will use.

- Use simple, concrete instructions, and repeat them often to compensate for any short-term memory problems.

Behavior management is not usually a problem in people with Down syndrome because they tend to be warm and well behaved. Some can be stubborn or uncooperative, but most just need a little extra time and attention to feel comfortable. Gaining the patient's trust is the key to successful treatment.

- Talk to the caregiver or physician about techniques they have found to be effective in managing the patient's behavior. Share your ideas with them, and find out what motivates the patient. It may be that a new toothbrush at the end of each appointment is all it takes to ensure cooperation.

- Schedule patients with Down syndrome early in the day if possible. Early appointments can help ensure that everyone is alert and attentive and that waiting time is reduced.

- Set the stage for a successful visit by involving the entire dental team—from the receptionist's friendly greeting to the caring attitude of the dental assistant in the operatory.

- Provide oral care in an environment with few distractions. Try to reduce unnecessary sights, sounds, or other stimuli that might make it difficult for your patient to cooperate. Many people with Down syndrome, however, enjoy music and may be comforted by hearing it in the dental office during treatment.

- Plan a step-by-step evaluation, starting with seating the patient in the dental chair. If this is successful, perform an oral examination using only your fingers. If this, too, goes well, begin using dental instruments. Prophylaxis is the next step, followed by dental radiographs. Several visits may be needed to accomplish these tasks.

- Try to be consistent in all aspects of providing oral healthcare. Use the same staff, dental operatory, appointment times, and other details to help sustain familiarity. The more consistency you provide for your patients, the more likely that they will be cooperative.

- Comfort people who resist oral care and reward cooperative behavior with compliments throughout the appointment.

- Use immobilization techniques only when absolutely necessary to protect the patient and staff during dental treatment—not as a convenience. There are no universal guidelines on immobilization that apply to all treatment settings. Before employing any kind of immobilization, it may help to consult available guidelines on federally funded care, your State department of mental health/disabilities, and your State Dental Practice Act. Guidelines on behavior management published by the American Academy of Pediatric Dentistry may also be useful. Obtain consent from your patient's legal guardian and choose the least restrictive technique that will allow you to provide care safely. Immobilization should not cause physical injury or undue discomfort.

Medical conditions. Though their average life expectancy has risen to the mid-50s, people with Down syndrome are still at risk for problems in nearly every system in the body. Some problems are manifested in the mouth. For example, oral findings such as persistent gingival lesions, prolonged wound healing, or spontaneous gingival hemorrhaging may suggest an underlying medical condition and warrant consultation with the patient's physician.

Cardiac disorders are common in Down syndrome. In fact, mitral valve prolapse occurs in more than half of all adults with this developmental disability. Many others are at risk of developing valve dysfunction that leads to congestive heart failure, even if they have no known cardiac disease. Consult the patient's physician if you have questions about the medical history and the need for antibiotic prophylaxis.

Compromised immune systems lead to more frequent oral and systemic infections and a high incidence of periodontal disease in people with Down syndrome. Aphthous ulcers, oral Candida infections, and acute necrotizing ulcerative gingivitis are common. Chronic respiratory infections contribute to mouth breathing, xerostomia, and fissured lips and tongue.

- Treat acute necrotizing ulcerative gingivitis and other infections aggressively.

- Talk to patients and their caregivers about preventing oral infections with regular dental appointments and daily oral care.

- Stress the importance of using fluoride to prevent dental caries associated with xerostomia.

- Use lip balm during treatment to ease the strain on your patient's lips.

Hypotonia affects the muscles in various areas of the body, including the mouth and large skeletal muscles. When it involves the mouth, it leads to an imbalance of forces on the teeth and contributes to an open bite. If the muscles controlling facial expression and mastication are affected, problems with chewing, swallowing, drooling, and speaking can result. A related problem is atlantoaxial instability, a spinal defect that increases the mobility of the cervical vertebrae and often leads to an unsteady gait and neck pain.

- Maintain a clear path for movement throughout the treatment setting.

- Determine the best position for your patient in the dental chair and the safest way to move his or her body, especially the head and neck. Talk with the physician or caregiver about ways to protect the spinal cord. Use pillows to stabilize your patient and make him or her more comfortable.

Seizures sometimes occur in this population, especially among infants, but can usually be controlled with anticonvulsant medications. The mouth is always at risk during a seizure: Patients may chip teeth or bite the tongue or cheeks. People with controlled seizure disorders can easily be treated in the general dental office.

- Consult your patient's physician. Record information in the chart about the frequency of seizures and the medications used to control them. Determine before the appointment whether medications have been taken as directed. Know and avoid any factors that trigger your patient's seizures.

- Be prepared to manage a seizure. If one occurs during oral care, remove any instruments from the mouth and clear the area around the dental chair. Attaching dental floss to rubber dam clamps and mouth props when treatment begins can help you remove them quickly. Do not attempt to insert any objects between the teeth during a seizure.

- Stay with your patient, turn him or her to one side, and monitor the airway to reduce the risk of aspiration.

Hearing loss and deafness may further complicate poor communication skills, but these, too, can be accommodated with planning. Patients with a hearing problem may appear to be stubborn because of their seeming lack of response to a request.

- Patients may want to adjust their hearing aids or turn them off, since the sound of some instruments may cause auditory discomfort.

- If your patient reads lips, speak in a normal cadence and tone. If your patient uses a form of sign language, ask the interpreter to come to the appointment. Speak with this person in advance to discuss dental terms and your patient's needs.

- Visual feedback is helpful. Maintain eye contact with your patient. Before talking, eliminate background noise (turn off the radio and the suction). Sometimes people with a hearing loss simply need you to speak clearly in a slightly louder voice than normal. Remember to remove your facemask first or wear a clear face shield.

Visual impairments such as strabismus (crossed or misaligned eyes), glaucoma, and cataracts can affect people with Down syndrome.

Determine the level of assistance your patient requires to move safely through the dental office.

Use your patients' other senses to connect with them, establish trust, and make treatment a better experience. Tactile feedback, such as a warm handshake, can make your patients feel comfortable.

Face your patients when you speak and keep them apprised of each upcoming step, especially when water will be used. Rely on clear, descriptive language to explain procedures and demonstrate how equipment might feel and sound. Provide written instructions in large print (16 point or larger).

Oral Health Problems in Down Syndrome and Strategies for Care

People with Down syndrome have no unique oral health problems. However, some of the problems they have tend to be frequent and severe. Early professional treatment and daily care at home can mitigate their severity and allow people with Down syndrome to enjoy the benefits of a healthy mouth.

Periodontal disease is the most significant oral health problem in people with Down syndrome. Children experience rapid, destructive periodontal disease. Consequently, large numbers of them lose their permanent anterior teeth in their early teens. Contributing factors include poor oral hygiene, malocclusion, bruxism, conical-shaped tooth roots, and abnormal host response because of a compromised immune system.

- Some patients benefit from the daily use of an antimicrobial agent such as chlorhexidine. Recommend an appropriate delivery method based on your patient's abilities. Rinsing, for example, may not work for a person who has swallowing difficulties or one who cannot expectorate. Chlorhexidine applied using a spray bottle or toothbrush is equally efficacious.

- If use of particular medications has led to gingival hyperplasia, emphasize the importance of daily oral hygiene and frequent professional cleanings.

- Encourage independence in daily oral hygiene. Ask patients to show you how they brush, and follow up with specific recommendations on brushing methods or toothbrush adaptations. Involve patients in hands-on demonstrations of brushing and flossing.

- Some people with Down syndrome can brush and floss independently, but many need help. Talk to their caregivers about daily oral hygiene. Do not assume that all caregivers know the basics; demonstrate proper brushing and flossing techniques. A power toothbrush or a floss holder can simplify oral care. Also, use your experiences with each patient to demonstrate sitting or standing positions for the caregiver. Emphasize that a consistent approach to oral hygiene is important-caregivers should try to use the same location, timing, and positioning.

Dental caries. Children and young adults who have Down syndrome have fewer caries than people without this developmental disability. Several associated oral conditions may contribute to this fact: delayed eruption of primary and permanent teeth; missing permanent teeth; and small-sized teeth with wider spaces between them, which make it easier to remove plaque. Additionally, the diets of many children with Down syndrome are closely supervised to prevent obesity; this helps reduce consumption of cariogenic foods and beverages.

By contrast, some adults with Down syndrome are at an increased risk of caries due to xerostomia and cariogenic food choices. Also, hypotonia contributes to chewing problems and inefficient natural cleansing action, which allow food to remain on the teeth after eating.

- Advise patients taking medicines that cause xerostomia to drink water often. Suggest taking sugar-free medicines if available and rinsing with water after dosing.

- Recommend preventive measures such as topical fluoride and sealants. Suggest fluoride toothpaste, gel, or rinse, depending on your patient's needs and abilities.

- Emphasize non cariogenic foods and beverages as snacks. Advise caregivers to avoid using sweets as incentives or rewards.

Several **orofacial features** are characteristic of people with Down syndrome. The Illustration of a child with Down syndrome midfacial region may be underdeveloped, affecting the appearance of the lips, tongue, and palate.

- The maxilla, the bridge of the nose, and the bones of the midface region are smaller than in the general population, creating a prognathic occlusal relationship. Mouth breathing may occur because of smaller nasal passages, and the tongue may protrude because of a smaller midface region. People with Down syndrome often have a strong gag reflex due to placement of the tongue, as well as anxiety associated with any oral stimulation.

- The palate, although normal sized, may appear highly vaulted and narrow. This deceiving appearance is due to the unusual thickness of the sides of the hard palate. This thickness restricts the amount of space the tongue can occupy in the mouth and affects the ability to speak and chew.

- The lips may grow large and thick. Fissured lips may result from chronic mouth breathing. Additionally, hypotonia may cause the mouth to droop and the lower lip to protrude. Increased drooling, compounded by a chronically open mouth, contributes to angular cheilitis.

- The tongue also develops cracks and fissures with age; this condition can contribute to halitosis.

Malocclusion is found in most people with Down syndrome because of the delayed eruption of permanent teeth and the underdevelopment of the maxilla. A smaller maxilla contributes to an open bite, leading to poor positioning of teeth and increasing the likelihood of periodontal disease and dental caries.

- Orthodontia should be carefully considered in people with Down syndrome. Some may benefit, while others may not.

- In and of itself, Down syndrome is not a barrier to orthodontic care. The ability of the patient or caregiver to maintain good daily oral hygiene is critical to the feasibility and success of treatment.

Tooth anomalies are common in Down syndrome.

Congenitally missing teeth occur more often in people with Down syndrome than in the general population. Third molars, laterals, and mandibular second bicuspids are the most common missing teeth.

Delayed eruption of teeth, often following an abnormal sequence, affects some children with Down syndrome. Primary teeth may not appear until age 2, with complete dentition delayed until age 4 or 5. Primary teeth are then retained in some children until they are 14 or 15.

Irregularities in tooth formation, such as microdontia and malformed teeth, are also seen in people with Down syndrome. Crowns tend to be smaller, and roots are often small and conical, which can lead to tooth loss from periodontal disease. Severe illness or prolonged fevers can lead to hypoplasia and hypocalcification.

- Examine a child by his or her first birthday and regularly thereafter to help identify unusual tooth formation and patterns of eruption.

- Consider using a panoramic radiograph to determine whether teeth are congenitally missing. Patients often find this technique less threatening than individual films.

- Maintain primary teeth as long as possible. Consider placing space maintainers where teeth are missing.

Trauma and injury to the mouth from falls or accidents occur in people with Down syndrome. Suggest a tooth-saving kit for group homes. Emphasize to caregivers that traumas require immediate professional attention and explain the procedures to follow if a permanent tooth is knocked out. Also, instruct caregivers to locate any missing pieces of a fractured tooth, and explain that radiographs of the patient's chest may be necessary to determine whether any fragments have been aspirated.

Physical abuse often presents as oral trauma. Abuse is reported more frequently in people with developmental disabilities than in the general population. If you suspect that a child is being abused or neglected, State laws require that you call your Child Protective Services agency. Assistance is also available from the Childhelp® National Child Abuse Hotline at (800) 422-4453 or the Child Welfare Information Gateway.

Section 50.6

Practical Oral Care for People with Intellectual Disability

This section includes text excerpted from "Practical Oral Care for People with Intellectual Disability," National Institute of Dental and Craniofacial Research (NIDCR), November 3, 2014.

Intellectual Disability

Intellectual disability is a disorder of mental and adaptive functioning, meaning that people who are affected are challenged by the skills they use in everyday life. Intellectual disability is not a disease or a mental illness; it is a developmental disability that varies in severity and is usually associated with physical problems. While one person with intellectual disability may have slight difficulty thinking and communicating, another may face major challenges with basic self-care and physical mobility.

Providing oral care to people with intellectual disability requires adaptation of the skills you use every day. In fact, most people with mild or moderate intellectual disability can be treated successfully in the general practice setting. This section will help you make a difference in the lives of people who need professional oral care.

Health Challenges in Intellectual Disability and Strategies for Care

Many people with intellectual disability also have other conditions such as cerebral palsy, seizure or psychiatric disorders, attention deficit/hyperactivity disorder, or problems with vision, communication, and eating. Though language and communication problems are common in anyone with intellectual disability, motor skills are typically more affected when a person has coexisting conditions.

Before the appointment, obtain and review the patient's medical history. Consultation with physicians, family, and caregivers is essential to assembling an accurate medical history. Also, determine who can legally provide informed consent for treatment.

Mental challenges. People with intellectual disability learn slowly and often with difficulty. Ordinary activities of daily living, such as brushing teeth and getting dressed, and understanding the behavior of others as well as their own, can all present challenges to a person with intellectual disability.

- Set the stage for a successful visit by involving the entire dental team—from the receptionist's friendly greeting to the caring attitude of the dental assistant in the operatory. All should be aware of your patient's mental challenges.

- Reduce distractions in the operatory, such as unnecessary sights, sounds, or other stimuli, to compensate for the short attention spans commonly observed in people with intellectual disability.

- Talk with the parent or caregiver to determine your patient's intellectual and functional abilities, then explain each procedure at a level the patient can understand. Allow extra time to explain oral health issues or instructions and demonstrate the instruments you will use.

- Address your patient directly and with respect to establish a rapport. Even if the caregiver is in the room, direct all questions and comments to your patient.

- Use simple, concrete instructions and repeat them often to compensate for any short-term memory problems. Speak slowly and give only one direction at a time.

- Be consistent in all aspects of oral care, since long-term memory is usually unaffected. Use the same staff and dental operatory each time to help sustain familiarity. The more consistency you provide for your patients, the more likely they will cooperate.

- Listen actively, since communicating clearly is often difficult for people with intellectual disability. Show your patient whether you understand. Be sensitive to the methods he or she uses to communicate, including gestures and verbal or nonverbal requests.

Behavior challenges. While most people with intellectual disability do not pose significant behavior problems that complicate oral care, anxiety about dental treatment occurs frequently. People unfamiliar with a dental office and its equipment and instruments may exhibit fear. Some react to fear with uncooperative behavior, such as crying, wiggling, kicking, aggressive language, or anything that will help them avoid treatment. You can make oral healthcare a better experience by comforting your patients and acknowledging their anxiety.

- Talk to the caregiver or physician about techniques they have found to be effective in managing the patient's behavior.

- Schedule patients with intellectual disability early in the day if possible. Early appointments can help ensure that everyone is alert and attentive and that waiting time is reduced.

- Keep appointments short and postpone difficult procedures until after your patient is familiar with you and your staff.

- Allow extra time for your patients to get comfortable with you, your office, and the entire oral healthcare team. Invite patients and their families to visit your office before beginning treatment.

- Permit the parents or caregiver to come into the treatment setting to provide familiarity, help with communication, and offer a calming influence by holding your patient's hand during treatment. Some patients' behavior may improve if they bring comfort items such as a stuffed animal or blanket.

- Reward cooperative behavior with compliments throughout the appointment.

- Consider nitrous oxide/oxygen sedation to reduce anxiety and fear and improve cooperation. Obtain informed consent from the legal guardian before administering any kind of sedation.

- Use immobilization techniques only when absolutely necessary to protect the patient and staff during dental treatment—not as a convenience. There are no universal guidelines on immobilization that apply to all treatment settings. Before employing any kind of immobilization, it may help to consult available guidelines on federally funded care, your State department of mental health/disabilities, and your State Dental Practice Act. Guidelines on behavior management published by the American Academy of Pediatric Dentistry may also be useful. Obtain consent from your patient's legal guardian and choose the least restrictive technique that will allow you to provide care safely. Immobilization should not cause physical injury or undue discomfort.

People with intellectual disability often engage in perseveration, a continuous, meaningless repetition of words, phrases, or movements.

Your patient may mimic the sound of the suction, for example, or repeat an instruction over and again. Avoid demonstrating dental equipment if it triggers perseveration, and note this in the patient's record.

Physical challenges. Intellectual disability does not always include a specific physical trait, although many people have distinguishing features such as orofacial abnormalities, scoliosis, unsteady gait, or hypotonia due to coexisting conditions. Countering physical challenges requires attention to detail.

- Maintain clear paths for movement throughout the treatment setting. Keep instruments and equipment out of the patient's way.

- Place and maintain your patient in the center of the dental chair to minimize the risk of injury. Placing pillows on both sides of the patient can provide stability.

- If you need to transfer your patient from a wheelchair to the dental chair, ask the patient or caregiver about special preferences such as padding, pillows, or other things you can provide to ease the transition. The patient or caregiver can often explain how to make a smooth transfer.

- Some patients cannot be moved into the dental chair but instead must be treated in their wheelchairs. Some wheelchairs recline or are specially molded to fit people's bodies. Lock the wheels, then slip a sliding board (also called a transfer board) behind the patient's back to provide support for the head and neck during care.

Cerebral palsy occurs in one-fourth of those who have intellectual disability and tends to affect motor skills more than cognitive skills. Uncontrolled body movements and reflexes associated with cerebral palsy can make it difficult to provide care.

- Place and maintain your patient in the center of the dental chair. Do not force arms and legs into unnatural positions, but allow your patient to settle into a position that is comfortable and will not interfere with dental treatment.

- Observe your patient's movements and look for patterns to help you anticipate direction and intensity. Trying to stop these movements may only intensify the involuntary response. Try instead to anticipate the movements, blending your movements with those of your patient or working around them.

- Softly cradle your patient's head during treatment. Be gentle and slow if you need to turn the patient's head.

- Help minimize the gag reflex by placing your patient's chin in a neutral or downward position.

- Stay alert and work efficiently in short appointments.

- Exert gentle but firm pressure on your patient's arm or leg if it begins to shake.

- Take frequent breaks or consider prescribing muscle relaxants when long procedures are needed. People with cerebral palsy may need sedation, general anesthesia, or hospitalization if extensive dental treatment is required.

Cardiovascular anomalies such as heart murmurs and damaged heart valves occur frequently in people with intellectual disability, especially those with Down syndrome or multiple disabilities. Consult the patient's physician to determine if antibiotic prophylaxis is necessary for dental treatment.

Seizures are common in this population but can usually be controlled with anticonvulsant medications. The mouth is always at risk during a seizure: Patients may chip teeth or bite the tongue or cheeks. Persons with controlled seizure disorders can easily be treated in the general dental office.

- Consult your patient's physician. Record information in the chart about the frequency of seizures and the medications used to control them. Determine before the appointment whether medications have been taken as directed. Know and avoid any factors that trigger your patient's seizures.

- Be prepared to manage a seizure. If one occurs during oral care, remove any instruments from the mouth and clear the area around the dental chair. Attaching dental floss to rubber dam clamps and mouth props when treatment begins can help you remove them quickly. Do not attempt to insert any objects between the teeth during a seizure.

- Stay with your patient, turn him or her to one side, and monitor the airway to reduce the risk of aspiration.

Visual impairments, most commonly strabismus (crossed or misaligned eyes) and refractive errors, can be managed with careful planning.

- Determine the level of assistance your patient requires to move safely through the dental office.

- Use your patients' other senses to connect with them, establish trust, and make treatment a good experience. Tactile feedback, such as a warm handshake, can make your patients feel comfortable.

- Face your patients when you speak and keep them apprised of each upcoming step, especially when water will be used. Rely on clear, descriptive language to explain procedures and demonstrate how equipment might feel and sound. Provide written instructions in large print (16 point or larger).

Hearning loss and deafness can also be accommodated with careful planning. Patients with a hearing problem may appear to be stubborn because of their seeming lack of response to a request.

- Patients may want to adjust their hearing aids or turn them off, since the sound of some instruments may cause auditory discomfort.

- If your patient reads lips, speak in a normal cadence and tone. If your patient uses a form of sign language, ask the interpreter to come to the appointment. Speak with this person in advance to discuss dental terms and your patient's needs.

- Visual feedback is helpful. Maintain eye contact with your patient. Before talking, eliminate background noise (turn off the radio and the suction). Sometimes people with a hearing loss simply need you to speak clearly in a slightly louder voice than normal. Remember to remove your facemask first or wear a clear face shield.

Oral Health Problems in Intellectual Disability and Strategies for Care

In general, people with intellectual disability have poorer oral health and oral hygiene than those without this condition. Data indicate that people who have intellectual disability have more untreated caries and a higher prevalence of gingivitis and other periodontal diseases than the general population.

Periodontal disease. Medications, malocclusion, multiple disabilities, and poor oral hygiene combine to increase the risk of periodontal disease in people with intellectual disability.

- Encourage independence in daily oral hygiene. Ask patients to show you how they brush, and follow up with specific recommendations on brushing methods or toothbrush adaptations. Involve your patients in hands-on demonstrations of brushing and flossing.

- Some patients cannot brush and floss independently due to impaired physical coordination or cognitive skills. Talk to their caregivers about daily oral hygiene. Do not assume that all caregivers know the basics; demonstrate proper brushing and flossing techniques. A power toothbrush or a floss holder can simplify oral care. Also, use your experiences with each patient to demonstrate sitting or standing positions for the caregiver. Emphasize that a consistent approach to oral hygiene is important—caregivers should try to use the same location, timing, and positioning.

- Some patients benefit from the daily use of an antimicrobial agent such as chlorhexidine. Recommend an appropriate delivery method based on your patient's abilities. Rinsing, for example, may not work for a patient who has swallowing difficulties or one who cannot expectorate. Chlorhexidine applied using a spray bottle or toothbrush is equally efficacious.

- If use of particular medications has led to gingival hyperplasia, emphasize the importance of daily oral hygiene and frequent professional cleanings.

Dental caries. People with intellectual disability develop caries at the same rate as the general population. The prevalence of untreated dental caries, however, is higher among people with intellectual disability, particularly those living in noninstitutional settings.

- Emphasize non cariogenic foods and beverages as snacks. Advise caregivers to avoid using sweets as incentives or rewards.

- Advise patients taking medicines that cause xerostomia to drink water often. Suggest sugar-free medicine if available and stress the importance of rinsing with water after dosing.

- Recommend preventive measures such as fluorides and sealants.

Malocclusion. The prevalence of malocclusion in people with intellectual disability is similar to that found in the general population, except for those with coexisting conditions such as cerebral palsy or Down syndrome. A developmental disability in and of itself should not be perceived as a barrier to orthodontic treatment. The ability of the patient or caregiver to maintain good daily oral hygiene is critical to the feasibility and success of treatment.

Missing permanent teeth, delayed eruption, and enammel hypoplasia are more common in people with intellectual disability and coexisting conditions than in people with intellectual disability alone.

- Examine a child by his or her first birthday and regularly there-after to help identify unusual tooth formation and patterns of eruption.

- Consider using a panoramic radiograph to determine whether teeth are congenitally missing. Patients often find this technique less threatening than individual films.

- Take appropriate steps to reduce sensitivity and risk of caries in your patients with enamel hypoplasia.

Damaging oral habites are a problem for some people with intellectual disability. Common habits include bruxism; mouth breathing; tongue thrusting; self-injurious behavior such as picking at the gingiva or biting the lips; and pica, eating objects and substances such as gravel, cigarette butts, or pens. If a mouth guard can be tolerated, prescribe one for patients who have problems with self-injurious behavior or bruxism.

Trauma and injury to the mouth from falls or accidents occur in people with intellectual disability. Suggest a tooth-saving kit for group homes. Emphasize to caregivers that traumas require immediate professional attention and explain the procedures to follow if a permanent tooth is knocked out. Also, instruct caregivers to locate any missing pieces of a fractured tooth, and explain that radiographs of the patient's chest may be necessary to determine whether any fragments have been aspirated.

Physical abuse often presents as oral trauma. Abuse is reported more frequently in people with developmental disabilities than in the general population. If you suspect that a child is being abused or neglected, State laws require that you call your Child Protective Services agency. Assistance is also available from the Childhelp® National Child Abuse Hotline at (800) 422-4453 or the Child Welfare Information Gateway.

Section 50.7

Every Day Dental Care Guide for People with Developmental Disability

This section includes text excerpted from "Dental Care Every Day: A Caregiver's Guide," National Institute of Dental and Craniofacial Research (NIDCR), July 31, 2014.

Taking care of someone with a developmental disability requires patience and skill. As a caregiver, you know this as well as anyone does. You also know how challenging it is to help that person with dental care. It takes planning, time, and the ability to manage physical, mental, and behavioral problems. Dental care isn't always easy, but you can make it work for you and the person you help. This section will show you how to help someone brush, floss, and have a healthy mouth.

Everyone needs dental care every day. Brushing and flossing are crucial activities that affect our health. In fact, dental care is just as important to your client's health and daily routine as taking medications and getting physical exercise. A healthy mouth helps people eat well, avoid pain and tooth loss, and feel good about themselves.

Getting Started

Location. The bathroom isn't the only place to brush someone's teeth. For example, the kitchen or dining room may be more comfortable. Instead of standing next to a bathroom sink, allow the person to sit at a table. Place the toothbrush, toothpaste, floss, and a bowl and glass of water on the table within easy reach.

No matter what location you choose, make sure you have good light. You can't help someone brush unless you can see inside that person's mouth. Positioning your body lists ideas on how to sit or stand when you help someone brush and floss.

Behavior. Problem behavior can make dental care difficult. Try these ideas and see what works for you.

- At first, dental care can be frightening to some people. Try the "tell-show-do" approach to deal with this natural reaction.

Tell your client about each step before you do it. For example, explain how you'll help him or her brush and what it feels like. **Show** how you're going to do each step before you do it. Also, it might help to let your client hold and feel the toothbrush and floss. **Do** the steps in the same way that you've explained them.

- Give your client time to adjust to dental care. Be patient as that person learns to trust you working in and around his or her mouth.

- Use your voice and body to communicate that you care. Give positive feedback often to reinforce good behavior.

- Have a routine for dental care. Use the same technique at the same time and place every day. Many people with developmental disabilities accept dental care when it's familiar. A routine might soothe fears or help eliminate problem behavior.

- Be creative. Some caregivers allow their client to hold a favorite toy or special item for comfort. Others make dental care a game or play a person's favorite music. If none of these ideas helps, ask your client's dentist or dental hygienist for advice.

Three Steps to a Healthy Mouth

Like everyone else, people with developmental disabilities can have a healthy mouth if these three steps are followed:

- Brush every day
- Floss every day
- Visit a dentist regularly

Step 1. Brush Every Day

If the person you care for is unable to brush, these suggestions might be helpful.

- First, wash your hands and put on disposable gloves. Sit or stand where you can see all of the surfaces of the teeth.

- Be sure to use a regular or power toothbrush with soft bristles.

- Use a pea-size amount of toothpaste with fluoride, or none at all. Toothpaste bothers people who have swallowing problems. If this is the case for the person you care for, brush with water instead.

- Brush the front, back, and top of each tooth. Gently brush back and forth in short strokes.

- Gently brush the tongue after you brush the teeth.

- Help the person rinse with plain water. Give people who can't rinse a drink of water or consider sweeping the mouth with a finger wrapped in gauze.

Get a new toothbrush with soft bristles every 3 months, after a contagious illness, or when the bristles are worn.

If the person you care for can brush but needs some help, the following ideas might work for you. You may think of other creative ways to solve brushing problems based on your client's special needs.

Make the toothbrush easier to hold.

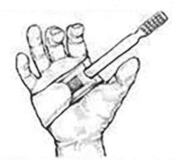

Figure 50.1. *Velcro Strap*

The same kind of Velcro® strap used to hold food utensils is helpful for some people.

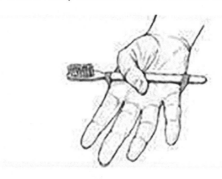

Figure 50.2. *Rubber Band and Toothbrush*

Others attach the brush to the hand with a wide elastic or rubber band. Make sure the band isn't too tight.

Make the toothbrush handle bigger.

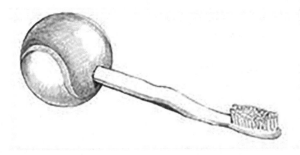

Figure 50.3. *Brushball*

You can also cut a small slit in the side of a tennis ball and slide it onto the handle of the toothbrush.

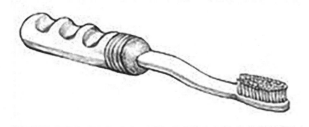

Figure 50.4. *Grip Brush*

You can buy a toothbrush with a large handle, or you can slide a bicycle grip onto the handle. Attaching foam tubing, available from home healthcare catalogs, is also helpful.

Try other toothbrush options.

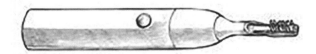

Figure 50.5. *Electric Brush*

A power toothbrush might make brushing easier. Take the time to help your client get used to one.

Guide the Toothbrush.

Help brush by placing your hand very gently over your client's hand and guiding the toothbrush. If that doesn't work, you may need to brush the teeth yourself.

Step 2. Floss Every Day

Flossing cleans between the teeth where a toothbrush can't reach. Many people with disabilities need a caregiver to help them floss. Flossing is a tough job that takes a lot of practice. Waxed, unwaxed, flavored, or plain floss all do the same thing. The person you care for might like one more than another, or a certain type might be easier to use.

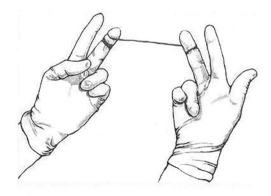

Figure 50.6. *Floss on Finger*

- Use a string of floss 18 inches long. Wrap that piece around the middle finger of each hand.

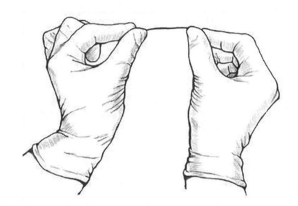

Figure 50.7. *Hold floss*

Grip the floss between the thumb and index finger of each hand.
Start with the lower front teeth, then floss the upper front teeth.
Next, work your way around to all the other teeth.

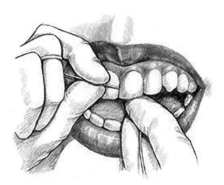

Figure 50.8. *Mouth Floss*

Work the floss gently between the teeth until it reaches the gumline. Curve the floss around each tooth and slip it under the gum.
Slide the floss up and down. Do this for both sides of every tooth, one
side at a time.

Adjust the floss a little as you move from tooth to tooth so the floss
is clean for each one.

Try a floss holder.

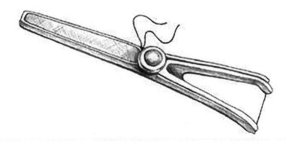

Figure 50.9. *Floss Holder*

*If you have trouble flossing, try using a floss holder instead of holding the floss with
your fingers.*

The dentist may prescribe a special rinse for your client. Fluoride
rinses can help prevent cavities. Chlorhexidine rinses fight germs that
cause gum disease. Follow the dentist's instructions and tell your client
not to swallow any of the rinse. Ask the dentist for creative ways to
use rinses for a client with swallowing problems.

439

Positioning Your Body: Where to Sit or Stand

Keeping people safe when you clean their mouth is important. Experts in providing dental care for people with developmental disabilities recommend the following positions for caregivers. If you work in a group home or related facility, get permission from your supervisor before trying any of these positions.

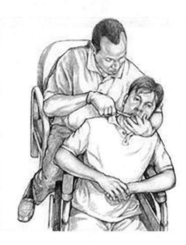

Figure 50.10. *Positioning Your Body: For a Person in a Wheelchair*

If the person you're helping is in a wheelchair, sit behind it. Lock the wheels, then tilt the chair into your lap.

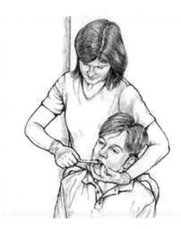

Figure 50.11. *Positioning Your Body: For a Person Standing Behind*

Stand behind the person or lean against a wall for additional support. Use your arm to hold the person's head gently against your body.

Step 3. Visit a Dentist Regularly

Your client should have regular dental appointments. Professional cleanings are just as important as brushing and flossing every day. Regular examinations can identify problems before they cause unnecessary pain.

As is the case with dental care at home, it may take time for the person you care for to become comfortable at the dental office. A "get acquainted" visit with no treatment provided might help: The person can meet the dental team, sit in the dental chair if he or she wishes, and receive instructions on how to brush and floss. Such a visit can go a long way toward making dental appointments easier.

Prepare for Every Dental Visit: Your Role

Be prepared for every appointment. You're an important source of information for the dentist. If you have questions about what the dentist will need to know, call the office before the appointment.

- **Know the person's dental history.** Keep a record of what happens at each visit. Talk to the dentist about what occurred at the last appointment. Remind the dental team of what worked and what didn't.

- **Bring a complete medical history.** The dentist needs each patient's medical history before treatment can begin. Bring a list of all the medications the person you care for is taking and all known allergies.

- **Bring all insurance, billing, and legal information.** Know who is responsible for payment. The dentist may need permission, or legal consent, before treatment can begin. Know who can legally give consent.

- **Be on time.**

Remember...

Brushing and flossing every day and seeing the dentist regularly can make a big difference in the quality of life of the person you care for. If you have questions or need more information, talk to a dentist.

Chapter 51

Heart Disease and Oral Health

Studies have shown that oral health affects far more than just a person's smile. In fact, it has an impact on many aspects of a person's overall health, including their risk of developing heart disease. More than 80% of Americans have some form of periodontal (gum) disease, which is generally related to infrequent brushing of teeth and failure to visit a dentist regularly. Research suggests that those with moderate or advanced forms of gum disease may face a risk of cardiovascular illness that is up to 70% higher than people who practice good oral hygiene and brush their teeth at least twice per day.

Scientists believe that the connection between oral health and heart disease centers around bacteria. Periodontal disease is caused by bacteria in the mouth. When these bacteria enter the bloodstream—through a sore in the mouth, for instance, or a gap around a tooth—they may become incorporated into the buildup of fatty deposits or plaques in the lining of artery walls. These plaque deposits can restrict the flow of blood through arteries, leading to serious health problems such as blood clots or atherosclerosis. Bacteria from the mouth may also travel through the bloodstream and attach to damaged areas of the heart, resulting in an infection of the heart lining called endocarditis.

"Heart Disease and Oral Health," © 2017 Omnigraphics. Reviewed September 2016.

Finally, gum disease bacteria may stimulate the liver and the immune system in ways that produce inflammation. Inflammation causes further narrowing of the blood vessels, which can lead to a heart attack or stroke.

Oral Health Symptoms Linked to Cardiovascular Risk

The risk of developing heart disease is highest for people with advanced periodontal disease or chronic gum conditions such as gingivitis. When these oral health conditions are undiagnosed or untreated, they may cause some of the following symptoms:

- gums that are red, swollen, or tender
- gums that bleed frequently while eating, brushing, or flossing
- gums that appear to be pulling away from teeth
- bad breath (halitosis) that occurs frequently
- a bad taste in the mouth
- pus or other signs of infection in the mouth
- teeth that are loose or appear to be moving away from other teeth
- changes in the alignment of teeth or bite

Practicing good oral hygiene, such as brushing the teeth at least twice per day and visiting a dentist regularly for examinations and professional cleanings, is the best method of preventing periodontal disease. Although good oral health does not necessarily prevent the development of cardiovascular disease, it can lead to improvements in overall health.

Heart Disease and Dental Treatment

The link between oral health and cardiovascular disease means that some forms of dental care and treatment may pose risks for people with pre-existing heart and artery conditions. To reduce the risk of endocarditis from bacteria entering the bloodstream, the American Heart Association (AHA) recommends that people with certain heart conditions take antibiotics before undergoing dental procedures that involve incisions in the gums or manipulation of the tissues surroundings the root of a tooth. Antibiotics are not necessary for routine dental procedures like X-rays, anesthetic injections, adjustment of orthodontic appliances, placement of dentures, or bleeding from injuries to the lips or mouth. Some of the heart conditions that increase the risk of infection from dental procedures include the following:

- artificial heart valves

- heart transplants

- a past history of endocarditis

- a heart defect that was not repaired or was repaired with a prosthetic material or device

- cyanotic heart disease that was not repaired or partially repaired

In addition to these conditions that require pre-treatment with antibiotics, other cardiovascular conditions may affect dental treatment in other ways. For instance, some medications that are commonly prescribed to treat high blood pressure, high cholesterol, or angina may have oral effects that the dentist must take into consideration. Blood-thinning medications may cause excessive bleeding following oral surgery, while calcium channel blockers may cause gum overgrowth that requires dental intervention.

Some medications prescribed to treat high cholesterol may make patients feel faint when they arise from a reclining dental chair, while some drugs used to treat high blood pressure can cause dry mouth or an altered sense of taste. Electromagnetic devices used in a dentist's office could potentially interfere with a pacemaker.

Because of the many points of interaction between oral health and cardiovascular health, patients with any type of condition affecting the heart or arteries should inform their dentist prior to undergoing treatment. In addition, they should provide their dentist with a complete and up-to-date list of all the medications they take, including prescription drugs, over-the-counter medicines, vitamins, and supplements.

References

1. "Cardiovascular Diseases," Colgate Oral Health Center, 2016.

2. "How May Dental Health Be Linked to Cardiovascular Disease?" SimplyHealth, 2012.

Chapter 52

Immune System Disorders and Oral Health

Chapter Contents

Section 52.1

Latex Allergy and Dental Treatment

This section includes text excerpted from "Infection Control," Centers for Disease Control and Prevention (CDC), July 10, 2013.

What Is Contact Dermatitis?

Occupationally related contact dermatitis can develop from frequent and repeated use of hand hygiene products, exposure to chemicals, and glove use. Contact dermatitis is classified as either irritant or allergic. Irritant contact dermatitis is common, nonallergic, and develops as dry, itchy, irritated areas on the skin around the area of contact. By comparison, allergic contact dermatitis (type IV hypersensitivity) can result from exposure to accelerators and other chemicals used in the manufacture of rubber gloves as well as from exposure to other chemicals found in the dental practice setting. Allergic contact dermatitis often manifests as a rash beginning hours after contact and, like irritant dermatitis, is usually confined to the areas of contact.

What Is Latex Allergy?

Latex allergy (type I hypersensitivity to latex proteins) can be a more serious systemic allergic reaction. It usually begins within minutes of exposure but can sometimes occur hours later. It produces varied symptoms, which commonly include runny nose, sneezing, itchy eyes, scratchy throat, hives, and itchy burning sensations. However, it can involve more severe symptoms including asthma marked by difficult breathing, coughing spells, and wheezing; cardiovascular and gastrointestinal ailments; and in rare cases, anaphylaxis and death.

What Are the Categories of Glove-Associated Skin Reactions?

Table 52.1. Glove-Associated Skin Reactions

	Irritant Contact Dermatitis	Allergic Contact Dermatitis (Type IV [delayed] Hypersensitivity)	Latex Allergy (Type I [immediate] Hypersensitivity or NRL*_ protein allergy)
Causative Agents	Toxic chemicals (e.g., biocides, detergents); excessive perspiration; irritating chemicals used in hand products and in glove manufacture	Accelerators and other chemicals used in glove manufacture; sterilants and disinfectants (e.g., glutaraldehyde); bonding agents (e.g., methracrylates); local anesthetics	Latex proteins from *Hevea brasiliensis* (rubber tree)
Reactions	Skin reactions usually confined to the area of contact	Skin reactions usually confined to the area of contact	Skin and systemic reactions can occur as soon as 2–3 minutes, or as long as several hours after skin or mucous membrane contact with the protein allergens
	Acute: Red, dry, itchy irritated areas	**Acute:** Itchy, red rash, small blisters	**Acute:** Hives, swelling, runny nose, nausea, abdominal cramps, dizziness, low blood pressure, bronchospasm, anaphylaxis (shock)
	Chronic: Dry, thickened skin, crusting, deep painful cracking, scabbing sores, peeling	**Chronic:** Dry thickened skin, crusting, scabbing sores, vesicles, peeling (appears 4–96 hours after exposure)	**Chronic:** As above, increased potential for extensive, more severe reaction

Table 52.1. Continued

	Irritant Contact Dermatitis	Allergic Contact Dermatitis (Type IV [delayed] Hypersensitivity)	Latex Allergy (Type I [immediate] Hypersensitivity or NRL*_ protein allergy)
Diagnosis	By medical history, symptoms, and exclusion of Type IV and Type I hypersensitivity Not an allergic reaction	By medical history, symptoms, and skin patch test	By medical history, symptoms, and skin-prick or blood test
	* NRL=natural rubber latex		

Dental healthcare personnel experiencing contact dermatitis or latex allergy symptoms should seek a definitive diagnosis by an experienced healthcare professional (e.g., dermatologist, allergist) to determine the specific etiology and appropriate treatment for their condition, as well as to determine what work restrictions or accommodations may be necessary.

Why Are Powder-Free Gloves Recommended?

Proteins responsible for latex allergies are attached to glove powder. When powdered gloves are worn, more latex protein reaches the skin. Also, when gloves are put on or removed, particles of latex protein powder become aerosolized and can be inhaled, contacting mucous membranes. As a result, allergic dental healthcare personnel and patients can experience symptoms related to cutaneous, respiratory, and conjunctival exposure. Dental healthcare personnel can become sensitized to latex proteins after repeated exposure. Work areas where only powder-free, low-allergen (i.e., reduced-protein) gloves are used show low or undetectable amounts of allergy-causing proteins.

What Are Some Considerations for Providing Dental Treatment to Patients with Latex Allergy?

Patients with a latex allergy should not have direct contact with latex-containing materials and should be treated in a "latex safe" environment. Such patients also may be allergic to the chemicals used in manufacturing natural rubber latex gloves, as well as to metals, plastics, or other materials used to provide dental care. By obtaining thorough patient health histories and preventing patients from having contact with potential allergens, dental healthcare professionals can minimize the possibility of patients having adverse reactions. Considerations in providing safe treatment for patients with possible or documented latex allergy include (but are not limited to) the following:

- Screen all patients for latex allergy (e.g., obtain their health history, provide medical consultation when latex allergy is suspected).

- Be aware of some common predisposing conditions (e.g., spina bifida, urogenital anomalies, or allergies to avocados, kiwis, nuts, or bananas).

- Be familiar with the different types of hypersensitivity—immediate and delayed—and the risks that these pose for patients and staff.

- Consider sources of latex other than gloves. Dental patients with a history of latex allergy may be at risk from a variety of dental products including, but not limited to, prophylaxis cups, rubber dams, and orthodontic elastics.

- Provide an alternative treatment area free of materials containing latex. Ensure a latex-safe environment or one in which no personnel use latex gloves and no patient contact occurs with other latex devices, materials, and products.

- Remove all latex-containing products from the patient's vicinity. Adequately cover/isolate any latex-containing devices that cannot be removed from the treatment environment.

- Be aware that latent allergens in the ambient air can cause respiratory and or anaphylactic symptoms in people with latex hypersensitivity. Therefore, to minimize inadvertent exposure to airborne latex particles among patients with latex allergy, try to give them the first appointments of the day.

- Frequently clean all working areas contaminated with latex powder/dust.

- Frequently change ventilation filters and vacuum bags used in latex-contaminated areas.

- Have latex-free kits (e.g., dental treatment and emergency kits) available at all times.

- Be aware that allergic reactions can be provoked from indirect contact as well as direct contact (e.g., being touched by someone who has worn latex gloves). Hand hygiene, therefore, is essential.

- Communicate latex allergy procedures (e.g., verbal instructions, written protocols, posted signs) to other personnel to prevent them from bringing latex-containing materials into the treatment area.

- If latex-related complications occur during or after the procedure, manage the reaction and seek emergency assistance as indicated. Follow current medical emergency response recommendations for management of anaphylaxis.

Section 52.2

Mouth Problems with HIV

This section contains text excerpted from the following sources: Text beginning with the heading "Your Mouth, Your Health" is excerpted from "Oral Health Issues," AIDS.gov, U.S. Department of Health and Human Services (HHS), July 5, 2014; Text beginning with the heading "Mouth Problems Can Be Painful, Annoying, and Lead to Other Problems" is excerpted from "Mouth Problems and HIV," National Institute of Dental and Craniofacial Research (NIDCR), August 1, 2014.

Your Mouth, Your Health

When you are focused on your overall health and well-being—and especially when you are dealing with a chronic health condition like HIV—it can be easy to overlook dental issues and oral healthcare.

But good dental hygiene is an important part of managing your HIV disease. If you wait until you are having problems with your teeth and gums to see a dentist, you can end up with an infection, pain, and/or tooth loss.

Poor oral health can even lead to malnutrition. If you can't chew or swallow because your mouth hurts, you may not eat enough to keep yourself healthy. This also can affect how your body absorbs your HIV medication. In addition, any infection can stimulate the virus to grow, resulting in loss of viral suppression and higher viral loads.

HIV and Oral Health

Your mouth may be the first part of your body to show signs of HIV infection. Oral opportunistic infections, such as candidiasis (thrush), are sometimes the first indicator that your immune system is not working properly—and oral health can be an important indicator of how HIV is affecting your body.

Anyone can have oral health problems, but HIV disease can make you more susceptible to:

- Oral warts, which can also progress to oral cancer
- Fever blisters
- *Oral hairy leukoplakia*
- Thrush
- Canker sores
- Cavities
- Gum disease (periodontitis and gingivitis)

In addition, bacterial infections that begin in the mouth, such as tooth decay, can become more serious and, if not treated, spread into your bloodstream and harm your heart and other organs. This is particularly dangerous for people living with HIV/AIDS who may have compromised immune systems.

People with HIV/AIDS may also experience dry mouth, which increases the risk of tooth decay and can make chewing, eating, swallowing, and even talking difficult. Some HIV medications can cause dry mouth.

The best ways to avoid these problems include:

- See your dentist regularly for cleanings and ask about the best way to care for your mouth and teeth.
- Brush your teeth at least twice a day. (After every meal is better!)
- Floss every day. Flossing cleans parts of your teeth that your toothbrush can't reach.
- Take all your HIV medications on schedule—this will protect your immune system and prevent oral opportunistic infections.
- Let your doctor know if your HIV meds are causing you to have dry mouth. There are remedies.
- Examine your mouth often and tell your primary care provider if you notice any unusual changes in the way your mouth looks or feels.

• If you do not have a dentist, ask your regular clinic or provider to refer you to one.

I Have Never Had Problems with My Teeth, Why Do I Need to See a Dentist?

People with HIV are more prone to some conditions which can cause serious dental problems. In addition, any infection can result in your virus starting to replicate and increasing your viral load. So to prevent complications, you should see your dental provider regularly for check-ups and cleanings.

Do I Need to Tell the Dentist That I Have HIV?

Yes, it is important that you tell your dentist that you have HIV. That's not because your dentist will need to take additional precautions—all healthcare professionals use "universal precautions" to prevent the transmission of bloodborne disease to patients and vice versa. However, he or she will know to look for particular oral health problems that you might be at risk for.

Mouth Problems Can Be Painful, Annoying, and Lead to Other Problems

You may be told that oral problems are minor compared to other things you have to deal with. But you know that they can cause discomfort and embarrassment and really affect how you feel about yourself. Oral problems can also lead to trouble with eating. If mouth pain or tenderness makes it difficult to chew and swallow, or if you can't taste food as well as you used to, you may not eat enough. And, your doctor may tell you to eat more than normal so your body has enough energy to deal with HIV.

Mouth Problems Can Be Treated

The most common oral problems linked with HIV can be treated. So talk with your doctor or dentist about what treatment might work for you.

Remember, with the right treatment, your mouth can feel better. And that's an important step toward living well, not just longer, with HIV.

Table 52.2. Mouth Problems and Treatment

Description	It Could Be:	What and Where?	Painful?	Contagious?	Treatment
Red sores *ulcers*	Aphthous ulcers. Also known as Canker Sores	Red sores that might also have a yellow-gray film on top. They are usually on the moveable parts of the mouth such as the tongue or inside of the cheeks and lips.	Yes	No	Mild cases—Over-the-counter cream or prescription mouthwash that contains corticosteroids; More severe cases—corticosteroids in a pill form
	OR				
	Herpes A viral infection	Red sores usually on the roof of the mouth. They are sometimes on the outside of the lips, where they are called fever blisters.	Sometimes	Yes	Prescription pill can reduce healing time and frequency of outbreaks.
White hairlike growth	Hairy Leukoplakia caused by the Epstein-Barr virus	White patches that do not wipe away; sometimes very thick and "hairlike." Usually appear on the side of the tongue or sometimes inside the cheeks and lower lip.	Not usually	No	Mild cases—not usually required; More severe cases—a prescription pill that may reduce severity of symptoms. In some severe cases, a pain reliever might also be required.

Table 52.2. Continued

Description	It Could Be:	What and Where?	Painful?	Contagious?	Treatment
White creamy or bumpy patches like cottage cheese	Candidiasis, a fungal (yeast) infection—Also known as thrush	White or yellowish patches (or can sometimes be red). If wiped away, there will be redness or bleeding underneath. They can appear anywhere in the mouth.	Sometimes, a burning feeling	No	Mild cases—prescription antifungal lozenge or mouthwash; More severe cases—prescription antifungal pills.
Warts		Small, white, gray, or pinkish rough bumps that look like cauliflower. They can appear inside the lips and on other parts of the mouth.	Not usually	Possibly	Inside the mouth—a doctor can remove them surgically or use "cryosurgery"—a way of freezing them off; On the lips—a prescription cream that will wear away the wart. Warts can return after treatment.

If You Have Dry Mouth

Dry mouth happens when you do not have enough saliva, or spit, to keep your mouth wet. Saliva helps you chew and digest food, protects teeth from decay, and prevents infections by controlling bacteria and fungi in the mouth. Without enough saliva you could develop tooth decay or other infections and might have trouble chewing and swallowing. Your mouth might also feel sticky, dry and have a burning feeling. And you may have cracked, chapped lips.

To help with a dry mouth, try these things:

- Sip water or sugarless drinks often
- Chew sugarless gum or suck on sugarless hard candy
- Avoid tobacco
- Avoid alcohol
- Avoid salty foods
- Use a humidifier at night

Talk to your doctor or dentist about prescribing artificial saliva, which may help keep your mouth moist.

Chapter 53

Meth (Methamphetamine) Mouth

What Is Methamphetamine (Meth)?

Also known as: "Meth," "Speed," "chalk," and "tina"; or for crystal meth, "ice," "crank," "glass," "fire," and "go fast"

Methamphetamine—known as "meth"—is a very addictive stimulant drug. Stimulants are a class of drugs that can boost mood, increase feelings of well-being, increase energy, and make you more alert—but they also have dangerous effects like raising heart rate and blood pressure.

Methamphetamine is a manmade, white, bitter-tasting powder. Sometimes it's made into a white pill or a shiny, white or clear rock called a crystal. Most of the meth used in the United States comes from "superlabs"—big illegal laboratories that make the drug in large quantities. But it is also made in small labs using cheap, over-the-counter ingredients such as pseudoephedrine, which is common in cold medicines. Other chemicals, some of them toxic, are also involved in making methamphetamine.

This chapter contains text excerpted from the following sources: Text beginning with the heading "What Is Methamphetamine (Meth)?" is excerpted from "Methamphetamine (Meth)," NIDA for Teens, National Institutes of Health (NIH), July 5, 2016; Text under the heading "Recent Findings" is excerpted from "Meth Mouth: Some Ugly Numbers," NIDA for Teens, National Institutes of Health (NIH), August 10, 2016.

459

Methamphetamine is classified as a Schedule II drug, meaning it has high potential for abuse and is available only through a prescription that cannot be refilled. It is prescribed by a doctor in rare cases to treat attention deficit hyperactivity disorder and other conditions. In these cases, the dose is much lower than what is typically used for the purpose of getting high.

How Is Methamphetamine Used?

Methamphetamine is swallowed, snorted, injected with a needle, or smoked. "Crystal meth" is a large, usually clear crystal that is smoked in a glass pipe. Smoking or injecting the drug delivers it very quickly to the brain, where it produces an immediate and intense high. Because the feeling doesn't last long, users often take the drug repeatedly, in a "binge and crash" pattern.

How Does Methamphetamine Affect the Brain?

Methamphetamine causes a release of the neurotransmitter dopamine in the brain. The release of small amounts of dopamine makes a person feel pleasure when they do things like listen to music, play video games, or eat tasty food. Methamphetamine's ability to release dopamine very quickly in the brain produces the feelings of extreme pleasure, sometimes referred to as a "rush" or "flash," that many users experience. After the effects have worn off, the brain has less dopamine, which can lead to depression.

Regular use of methamphetamine causes chemical and molecular changes in the brain. The activity of the dopamine system changes, causing problems with movement and thinking. Some of these changes remain long after methamphetamine use has stopped. Although, some may reverse after a person is off the drug for a long period of time, perhaps more than a year, methamphetamine may destroy nerve cells that produce dopamine and another neurotransmitter called serotonin.

What Are the Other Effects of Methamphetamine?

The release of dopamine in the brain causes several physical effects, similar to those of other stimulants like cocaine. These include:

- Feeling very awake and active
- Fast heart rate and irregular heartbeat
- Higher blood pressure

- Higher body temperature
- Increased risk for HIV/AIDS or hepatitis (a liver disease) from unsafe sex and shared needles

Effects of Long-Term Use

Continued methamphetamine use may cause effects that last for a long time, even after a person quits using the drug. These effects include:

- Anxiety and confusion
- Problems sleeping
- Mood swings
- Violent behavior
- Psychosis (hearing, seeing, or feeling things that are not there)
- Skin sores caused by scratching
- Severe weight loss
- Severe dental problems, known as "meth mouth"
- Problems with thinking, emotion, and memory

Recent Findings

Using meth can have a lot of really unpleasant effects on the body. One of those effects is "meth mouth," where a meth user's teeth become broken, stained, and rotten, and may eventually fall out.

Well, the news about meth mouth got even worse recently: Turns out it happens to meth users a lot more often than was previously known.

Researchers examined 571 meth users and found that:

- 96 percent of them had cavities (a cavity is a hole or other damage to the outside layers of a tooth—but you probably knew that).

- Adults who said they used meth "moderately" or "heavily" were twice as likely to have untreated cavities as "light" users— "light" users had used the drug for less than 10 days over the previous month. (If a cavity goes untreated, it grows larger and larger, it can cause a really bad toothache, the cavity can become infected, and the tooth may have to be removed.)

- 58 percent of the meth users had untreated tooth decay, compared with 27 percent of the general population in the United States.

- Only 23 percent kept all of their natural teeth, compared to 48 percent of the general population in the United States. That's a lot of additional tooth loss for the people who used meth.

- A significant number of meth users (40 percent) said they were often self-conscious or embarrassed because of the condition of their teeth or dentures.

Chapter 54

Organ Transplantation and Oral Health Management

Dental Management of the Organ Transplant or Stem Cell Transplant Patient

Organ and stem cell transplant patients are at increased risk for serious oral health problems. A weakened medical condition and the side effects of transplant medications can lead to infections, dry mouth, ulcers, gum overgrowth, and other oral complications that can also affect overall health.

Managing Oral Health before Transplantation

Before treating a prospective transplant recipient, obtain and review the patient's medical and dental histories, perform a noninvasive

This chapter contains text excerpted from the following sources: Text beginning with the heading "How Does Transplantation Affect Oral Health?" is excerpted from "Organ and Stem Cell Transplantation and Oral Health," National Institute of Dental and Craniofacial Research (NIDCR), October 23, 2014; Text beginning with the heading "Patient Population" is excerpted from "Dental Management of the Organ or Stem Cell Transplant Patient," National Institute of Dental and Craniofacial Research (NIDCR), August 11, 2016; Text beginning with the heading "Tips for Dental Management of the Organ or Stem Cell Transplant Patient" is excerpted from "Organ or Stem Cell Transplant and Your Mouth," National Institute of Dental and Craniofacial Research (NIDCR), July 20, 2016.

initial oral examination (without periodontal probing), and obtain radiographs. After the examination, discuss with your patient's physician the current status of your patient's overall health and immune system. Decisions about the timing of treatment, the need for antibiotic prophylaxis, precautions to prevent excessive bleeding, and the appropriate medication and dosage should be considered during your discussion.

Whether a patient can tolerate dental treatment is a crucial concern. For some patients, it will be safer to undergo extensive dental treatment after their overall health improves after transplantation.

Preparing for Dental Treatment before Transplantation

Before starting your patient's dental treatment before transplantation, consider several factors:

- **Antibiotic prophylaxis:** Consult with the patient's physician to determine whether antibiotic prophylaxis is required to prevent systemic infection from invasive dental procedures. Unless advised otherwise by the physician, the American Heart Association's standard regimen to prevent endocarditis is an accepted option.

- **Oral infection:** If the patient presents with an active oral infection, such as a purulent periodontal infection or an abscessed tooth, antibiotics should be given to the patient before and after dental treatment to prevent systemic infection. Confirm the choice of antibiotic with the patient's physician. Before transplantation, the active oral infection must be eliminated.

- **Excessive bleeding:** Several factors can cause bleeding problems in transplant candidates, such as the disease itself or medications. For example, patients may have a decreased platelet count or be on anticoagulant medications. Patients with end-stage liver disease may have excessive bleeding because the liver is no longer producing sufficient amounts of clotting factors. Before treatment, assess the patient's bleeding potential with the appropriate laboratory tests and take precautions to limit bleeding.

  - Consult with your patient's physician about whether antifibrinolytic drugs, vitamin K, fresh frozen plasma, or other interventions are appropriate for critical dental procedures. The physician also may decide to temporarily decrease the patient's level of anticoagulation before extensive dental surgeries. Because of bleeding risk, some patients are suitable for surgery only in a hospital setting or dental offices designed to handle emergency medical situations.

- Use aggressive suctioning techniques when performing extractions or other invasive procedures to prevent your patient from swallowing blood. In a small number of patients with advanced liver disease, swallowed blood may increase risk for hepatic coma.

- Manage bleeding sites with careful packing and suturing techniques.

- **Medication considerations:** Patients preparing to undergo organ or stem cell transplantation may be taking multiple medications. These include anticoagulants, beta blockers, calcium channel blockers, diuretics, and others. Be aware of the side effects of these medications, which range from xerostomia and gingival hyperplasia to orthostatic hypotension and hyperglycemia, and their interactions with drugs that you might prescribe. Likewise, use caution when prescribing medication to patients with end-stage kidney or liver disease. Many medications commonly used in dental practice, including Nonsteroidal anti-inflammatory drugs (NSAIDS), opiates, and some antimicrobials, are metabolized by these organs and are not removed from circulation as quickly in patients with markedly reduced kidney or liver function. Before dental treatment, consult the patient's physician on appropriate drug selection, dosage, and administration intervals.

- **Other medical problems:** Patients with end-stage organ failure may have other major medical conditions. A person with end-stage kidney disease, for example, may have diabetes or significant pulmonary or heart disease. Carefully review your patient's medical history to determine what additional treatment considerations your patient may have.

Dental Treatment before Transplantation

Whenever possible, all active dental disease should be eliminated before transplantation, since post-operative immunosuppression decreases a patient's ability to resist systemic infection.

- Eliminate or stabilize sites of oral infection. Patients with active dental disease who can tolerate treatment should receive indicated dental care. Depending on the patient's condition, temporary restoration may be appropriate until his or her health improves.

- Extract nonrestorable teeth.

- Consider removing orthodontic bands or adjusting prostheses if a patient is expected to receive cyclosporine after transplant because some people taking this drug will develop gingival hyperplasia. The overgrowth can be minimized with good plaque control, and removing orthodontic bands may make it easier to maintain good oral hygiene.

- Conduct dental procedures on days that your patient with end-stage renal disease does not undergo hemodialysis.

- Pay special attention to your patient's anxiety and pain tolerance.

- Counsel the patient about oral health. Explain that effective oral hygiene is crucial before and after transplantation. The patient may experience fewer oral and dental problems after transplantation by reducing the number of oral bacteria and inhibiting their proliferation.

- Instruct patients to bring a current list of their medications, including over-the-counter drugs, to every appointment and note those medications that may be problematic.

Managing Oral Health after Transplantation

Except for emergency dental care, patients who receive organ or stem cell transplants should avoid dental treatment for at least 3 months. Dosage of immunosuppressive drugs is highest in the early post-transplant period, and patients are at greatest risk for serious complications, such as rejection of the transplanted organ, during that time. Once the graft has stabilized (which typically occurs within 3 to 6 months of the transplant procedure) and the medical team clears the patient for dental treatment, patients can be treated in the dental office with proper precautions.

Preparing for Dental Treatment after Transplantation

Treatment after transplantation requires consultation with your patient's physician. The medical consult can help you understand your patient's general health and ability to tolerate treatment. Post-transplant patients vary widely in their ability to endure dental treatment and heal following invasive procedures. Your discussion needs to address whether your patient requires antibiotic prophylaxis and if the physician will need to adjust other medications before treatment.

- **Infection:** Patients who have had a transplant procedure are at increased risk for serious infection. Bacterial, viral, and fungal infections are more common, especially immediately after the procedure. The decision to premedicate for invasive dental procedures and selection of the appropriate regimen should be done in consultation with the patient's physician.

- **Medication considerations:** Your transplant patient may be taking one or more medications that affect dental treatment. Immunosuppressive drugs can cause gingival hyperplasia, poor healing, and infections and may interact with commonly prescribed medications. Anticoagulant medications may contribute to excessive bleeding problems, whereas a patient taking steroids is at risk for acute adrenal crisis. The patient's physician may want to adjust these medications several days before an invasive dental procedure.

Dental Treatment after Transplantation

All new dental disease should be treated after the patient's transplant has stabilized.

- Check your patient's blood pressure before you begin treatment. Know baseline levels for each patient and call his or her physician immediately if blood pressure exceeds accepted thresholds. Do not treat a patient when this problem is present.

- Know your patient's bleeding potential and take appropriate steps to manage excessive bleeding.

- Prescribe an antimicrobial rinse when appropriate.

- Recommend saliva substitutes and fluoride rinses if your patient has dry mouth.

- Advise your patients to follow a conscientious oral hygiene routine and emphasize the importance of oral health.

- Examine the patient's mouth thoroughly for dental infection, since immunosuppressive drugs can hide signs of a problem.

As a result, infections are often more advanced than they appear when detected. Treat all infections aggressively.

• Watch for signs of adrenal insufficiency with surgical stress in patients taking steroids. These patients may require hydrocortisone replacement therapy at the time of extensive dental procedures to avoid adrenal insufficiency syndrome. A person experiencing this condition may become hypertensive, weak, feverish, and nauseated and should be transported immediately to a hospital for treatment.

• Exercise care in prescribing medications to avoid potentiating the renal and hepatic toxicities of immunosuppressant drugs. Consult the patient's physician to ensure proper drug selection and dosing.

Some Dental Complications after Transplantation

Chronic Graft-Versus Host Disease

In patients who receive a stem cell transplant from a donor, an autoimmune like disease called chronic graft-versus host disease (cGVHD) may develop, usually within two years of transplantation. cGVHD may affect multiple organ systems, including the mouth, and you should screen stem cell transplant patients at every dental visit because treatment and supportive care for pain, sensitivity, and dry mouth are important.

Oral cGVHD has three components: mucosal involvement, sclerotic involvement of the mouth and surrounding tissues, and salivary gland involvement:

Mucosa: The oral mucosa presents with the classic findings in cGVHD, including lichenoid changes, erythema, ulcerations, hyperkeratotic patches, and mucosal atrophy.

Musculoskeletal tissue: Limited mouth opening and limited tongue mobility may be caused by involvement of the temporomandibular joints or by sclerotic changes in the perioral tissues.

Salivary glands: Salivary gland dysfunction may result from medication, inflammation, and fibrosis of the major and minor salivary glands.

Treatment and supportive care for the oral effects of cGVHD should be coordinated with the patient's medical team. Patients may need artificial saliva for dry mouth; topical immunosuppressive agents, such as steroid rinses, to manage their oral disease; and palliative agents, such as lidobenalox rinse or viscous lidocaine, to manage oral pain.

Oral Cancer

The long-term use of immunosuppressive drugs and other treatments puts transplant patients at risk of developing cancers, including cancers of the oral cavity. Squamous cell carcinoma, especially of the tongue, salivary gland, lip, or throat; oral Kaposi's sarcoma; and lymphoma are among the malignancies that sometimes occur in transplant patients. Because early detection of oral cancer is essential for effective treatment, screen patients at every appointment, and biopsy new oral lesions that lack a clear etiology.

Organ Rejection

If a patient's body begins to reject a transplanted organ, only emergency dental care may be provided. Before dental treatment, talk with the patient's physician about antibiotic prophylaxis or other special needs.

Tips for Dental Management of the Organ Transplant or Stem Cell Transplant Patient

See Your Dentist before Transplant

Before an organ or stem cell transplant, have a dental checkup. Your mouth should be as healthy as possible before your transplant procedure. Treating cavities, periodontal (gum) disease, and any other mouth problems ahead of time can help prevent or reduce the side effects of transplant drugs. Also, keeping your mouth clean and free of dental disease is important for your general health too.

See Your Dentist after Transplant

Make sure your dentist knows that you are a transplant patient. Give your dentist the contact information for your transplant doctor. Your dentist should speak with your transplant team before dental treatment. Together, they will work out a dental care plan that safely meets your needs. For example, they may decide that you need to take antibiotics before dental treatment, or your doctor may adjust the dosage of your transplant drugs.

Bring a list of all your drugs, including over-the-counter drugs, to every dental appointment. Remember to tell your dentist if your drugs have changed.

Talk to your dentist about your general health. If you have diabetes or other health conditions, make sure your dentist knows. In the same way, tell your transplant doctor if you have mouth problems.

Tell Your Dentist about Mouth Problems

Transplant drugs suppress your immune system so that the donated organ or cells are less likely to be rejected by your body. Unfortunately, the side effects of these drugs make you more likely to develop problems in your mouth.

Tell your dentist about any problems that develop in your mouth. Transplant drugs can cause many different kinds of mouth problems. Your dentist can help you manage the mouth problems caused by transplant drugs:

Infections: When your immune system is suppressed, you are at much greater risk of developing infections, such as yeast (thrush) or herpes simplex infections, and tooth decay. Get treatment if you experience redness, painful or sensitive areas, swelling, pus, white patches, fever, or other problems.

Dry mouth: Not having enough saliva to keep your mouth moist can lead to tooth decay.

Mouth ulcers: Sores in the soft lining of the mouth can make chewing, speaking, or swallowing painful.

Enlarged gums: Gums can grow so large that they cover part of the teeth, making brushing and flossing difficult and increasing the chance of bleeding and infection.

Mouth cancers: Some people, especially those who used tobacco, develop mouth cancer after an organ or stem cell transplant.

Keep Your Mouth Healthy

You can do a lot to keep your mouth healthy after your transplant procedure. Brush and floss every day. Good daily oral hygiene is vital to keeping your mouth healthy by reducing levels of harmful germs. If you have any questions about brushing and flossing, particularly if your mouth is sore after transplant, ask your dentist or dental hygienist.

Look inside your mouth every day. Check how it feels with your tongue. Side effects from transplant drugs may show up as white or red patches, sores, or ulcers. You may notice dryness in your mouth, bleeding gums when you brush, or a growth. Call your dentist if you notice any changes or problems.

Chapter 55

Osteoporosis Affects Bones and Teeth

Chapter Contents

Section 55.1

Oral Health and Bone Disease

This section includes text excerpted from "Oral Health and Bone
Disease," National Institute of Arthritis and Musculoskeletal and
Skin Diseases (NIAMS), May 2016.

Health Concerns

Osteoporosis and tooth loss are health concerns that affect many
older men and women. Osteoporosis is a condition in which the bones
become less dense and more likely to fracture. This disease can affect
any bone in the body, although the bones in the hip, spine, and wrist
are affected most often. In the United States, more than 53 million
people either already have osteoporosis or are at high risk due to low
bone mass. Research suggests a link between osteoporosis and bone
loss in the jaw. The bone in the jaw supports and anchors the teeth.
When the jawbone becomes less dense, tooth loss can occur, a common
occurrence in older adults.

Skeletal Bone Density and Dental Concerns

The portion of the jawbone that supports our teeth is known as the
alveolar process. Several studies have found a link between the loss
of alveolar bone and an increase in loose teeth (tooth mobility) and
tooth loss. Women with osteoporosis are three times more likely to
experience tooth loss than those who do not have the disease.

Low bone density in the jaw can result in other dental problems as
well. For example, older women with osteoporosis may be more likely
to have difficulty with loose or ill-fitting dentures and may have less
optimal outcomes from oral surgical procedures.

Periodontal Disease and Bone Health

Periodontitis is a chronic infection that affects the gums and the
bones that support the teeth. Bacteria and the body's own immune system break down the bone and connective tissue that hold teeth in place.
Teeth may eventually become loose, fall out, or have to be removed.

Although tooth loss is a well-documented consequence of periodontitis, the relationship between periodontitis and skeletal bone density is less clear. Some studies have found a strong and direct relationship among bone loss, periodontitis, and tooth loss. It is possible that the loss of alveolar bone mineral density leaves bone more susceptible to periodontal bacteria, increasing the risk for periodontitis and tooth loss.

Role of the Dentist and Dental X-Rays

Research supported by the National Institute of Arthritis and Musculoskeletal and Skin Diseases (NIAMS) suggests that dental X-rays may be used as a screening tool for osteoporosis. Researchers found that dental X-rays were highly effective in distinguishing people with osteoporosis from those with normal bone density.

Because many people see their dentist more regularly than their doctor, dentists are in a unique position to help identify people with low bone density and to encourage them to talk to their doctors about their bone health. Dental concerns that may indicate low bone density include loose teeth, gums detaching from the teeth or receding gums, and ill-fitting or loose dentures.

Effects of Osteoporosis Treatments on Oral Health

It is not known whether osteoporosis treatments have the same beneficial effect on oral health as they do on other bones in the skeleton. Additional research is needed to fully clarify the relationship between osteoporosis and oral bone loss; however, scientists are hopeful that efforts to optimize skeletal bone density will have a favorable impact on dental health.

Bisphosphonates, a group of medications available for the treatment of osteoporosis, have been linked to the development of osteonecrosis of the jaw (ONJ), which is cause for concern. The risk of ONJ has been greatest in patients receiving large doses of intravenous bisphosphonates, a therapy used to treat cancer. The occurrence of ONJ is rare in individuals taking oral forms of the medication for osteoporosis treatment.

Taking Steps for Healthy Bones

A healthy lifestyle can be critically important for keeping bones strong. You can take many important steps to optimize your bone health:

- Eat a well-balanced diet rich in calcium and vitamin D.

- Engage in regular physical activity or exercise. Weight-bearing activities—such as walking, jogging, dancing, and weight training—are the best for keeping bones strong.

- Don't smoke, and limit alcohol intake.

- Report any problems with loose teeth, detached or receding gums, and loose or ill-fitting dentures to your dentist and your doctor.

Section 55.2

Osteogenesis Imperfecta (OI)

This section contains text excerpted from "Osteogenesis Imperfecta (OI)," Eunice Kennedy Shriver National Institute of Child Health and Human Development (NICHD), December 16, 2013.

Osteogenesis imperfecta means "imperfect bone formation" and is commonly known as "brittle bone disease" or OI. It is a rare genetic disorder that affects the protein collagen, which is found in bone, teeth, skin, tendons, and parts of the eye. People with osteogenesis imperfecta have bones that can break easily, sometimes with no obvious cause. *Eunice Kennedy Shriver* National Institute of Child Health and Human Development (NICHD) research has been instrumental in discovering the genes that cause some types of OI. The Institute continues to conduct and support research on many aspects of OI, including genetics and treatment.

What Is Osteogenesis Imperfecta (OI)?

OI, or "brittle bone disease," is a condition causing fragile bones that break easily, sometimes for no obvious reason. Some people with OI have only a few fractures in their lifetimes. Others have hundreds. People who have severe forms of OI have fragile bones that are also deformed. Most people with OI experience physical disability. OI also can cause weak muscles, brittle teeth, a curved spine, and hearing loss. Most forms of OI are caused by abnormal genes that are passed down from one or both parents to their children.

There are currently 11 types of OI. Types I through IV are the most common. They are autosomal dominant forms of the disease. Autosomal dominance is a pattern of inheritance common to some genetic diseases. "Autosomal" means that the abnormal gene is located on one of the numbered, or non-sex, chromosomes. "Dominant" means that a single copy of the abnormal gene is enough to cause the disease; in other words, a person only needs to get the abnormal gene from one parent in order to inherit the disease, even though the matching gene from the other parent is normal. This is in contrast to an autosomal recessive disorder, where two copies of the mutation are needed to cause the disease; in other words, a person must inherit the abnormal gene from both parents in order to inherit the disease. Types VI through XI are autosomal recessive.

What Causes Osteogenesis Imperfecta?

OI is caused by defects in or related to a protein called type 1 collagen. Collagen is an essential building block of the body. The body uses type 1 collagen to make bones strong and to build tendons, ligaments, teeth, and the whites of the eyes.

Certain gene changes, or mutations, cause the collagen defects. Mutations in several genes can lead to OI. About 80%–90% of OI cases are caused by autosomal dominant mutations in the type 1 collagen genes, COL1A1 and COL1A2. Mutations in one or the other of these genes cause the body to make either abnormally formed collagen or too little collagen. Mutations in these genes cause OI Types I through IV.

The remaining cases of OI (types VI–XI) are caused by autosomal recessive mutations in any of six genes (SERPINF1, CRTAP, LEPRE1, PPIB, SERPINH1, and FKBP10) that code for proteins that help make collagen. These mutations also cause the body to make too little collagen or abnormally formed collagen.

These gene changes are inherited, or passed down from parents to their children; people who have OI are born with it. However, in some cases, the gene mutation is not inherited and occurs after conception.

How Many People Are Affected by or at Risk of Osteogenesis Imperfecta?

Infants who have recognizable OI at birth make up about 1 in every 16,000 to 20,000 births. The incidence rate is similar in people with milder forms of OI that become apparent later in life. OI affects all genders, races and ethnic groups equally.

What Are the Symptoms of Osteogenesis Imperfecta?

All types of OI have some degree of bone fragility and fracturing, and many have some degree of bone deformity.

The symptoms of OI vary by type:

Type I

- Most common and mildest form of OI. It can be so mild that healthcare providers do not diagnose it in some people until they are adults.
- Bone fractures occur mostly in years before puberty and decrease in frequency after puberty.
- Normal height; a few inches shorter than same gender relatives
- Little or no bone deformity
- Brittle teeth in rare cases
- Hearing loss in some cases
- Blue sclera (whites of the eyes)
- Easy bruising
- Mild delay in motor skills

Type II

- Severe; usually results in stillborn birth or death in the first months of life
- Severe bone deformity

Type III

- Most severe, nonlethal form
- Hundreds of fractures starting very early in life
- Severe bone deformities and physical disability that worsen over time
- Sclera may be blue or grey
- Triangular face and prominent forehead
- Scoliosis (abnormal curving of the spine)
- Sunken or protruding chest wall

- Brittle teeth
- Hearing loss
- Very short height
- Motor skill delays
- Usually need wheelchairs

Type IV

- Similar to type I but with mild to moderate bone deformity
- Dozens of fractures on average, most of which occur before puberty or after middle age
- Motor skill delays
- People with type IV often need braces or crutches to walk
- Short height
- Brittle teeth
- Hearing loss in some cases
- White or blue sclera
- Scoliosis
- Large head
- Easy bruising

Type V

- Identical symptoms to Type IV except:
- Normal sclera
- Normal teeth
- Severely limited ability to twist forearms clockwise or counterclockwise
- Distinguished from Type IV by differing bone features at microscopic level

Type VI

- Identical symptoms to Type IV except:
- Normal teeth

- Greater frequency of fractures
- Distinguished from Type IV by differing bone features at microscopic level

Type VII and VIII

- Similar to Types II and III
- Severe or lethal bone deformity
- Type VII can also involve small head, blue sclera, bulging eyes
- Some people with Type VIII have lived into their second or third decade

Type IX

- Moderate to severe bone deformity and similar to Types III and IV
- White sclera
- Short height

Type X

- Severe and often leads to death.

Type XI

- Bone deformities worsen over time

The bone deformities and collagen defects common to OI can affect various internal organs, leading to secondary problems. These include:

Lung Problems

People with OI are more vulnerable to lung problems, including asthma and pneumonia. Viral and bacterial infections can become severe. In fact, respiratory failure is the most common cause of death in people with OI.

Lung problems result from a combination of factors. If the ribs and spine do not develop normally, there may be less space for the lungs to expand. Collagen also is an important building block of connective tissue in the lungs. If the body does not make enough collagen, or makes abnormal collagen, the lungs do not work properly. This makes it difficult for people with OI to get enough oxygen through their bodies. In addition, they may have problems coughing effectively to clear away mucus.

Heart Problems

Heart problems, such as incorrectly working valves and arteries, sometimes occur in people with OI.

Neurological Problems

People with OI often have enlarged heads, called macrocephaly. They can also have a condition called hydrocephalus, in which fluid builds up inside the skull, causing the brain to swell.

People with severe OI often have basilar invagination, a malformation of the spinal column that puts pressure on the spinal cord and brainstem. It worsens over time and can cause severe headaches, changes in facial sensation, lack of control over muscle movements, and difficulty swallowing. If untreated, basilar invagination can lead to rapid neurological decline and inability to breathe.

How Do Healthcare Providers Diagnose Osteogenesis Imperfecta?

If OI is moderate or severe, healthcare providers usually diagnose it during prenatal ultrasound at 18 to 24 weeks of pregnancy.

If a parent or sibling has OI, a healthcare provider can test the DNA of the fetus for the presence of an OI mutation. In this case, a healthcare provider obtains a sample of fetal cells by chorionic villus sampling (CVS) or amniocentesis. The fetal cells can also be tested for the presence of abnormal collagen.

For amniocentesis, a healthcare provider takes a small amount of fluid from the sac surrounding the fetus for testing. He or she takes the sample by inserting a thin needle into the uterus through the abdomen. For CVS, a healthcare provider uses a similar procedure to take a sample of tissue from the placenta for testing.

If OI is not detected prenatally, parents or a healthcare provider may notice symptoms in an infant or child. The healthcare provider may perform the following:

- Physical exam, which includes:

  - Measuring the length of limbs

  - Measuring the head circumference

- Examining the eyes and teeth
- Examining the spine and rib cage
- Personal and family medical history, which include questions about:
  - Broken bones
  - Hearing loss
  - Brittle teeth
  - Adult height
  - Racial background
  - Whether close relatives have had children together
- X-ray
- Bone density test
- Bone biopsy, in some cases

Healthcare providers may send blood or skin samples to a lab for collagen or genetic testing. These tests usually confirm whether a person has OI.

What Are the Treatments for Osteogenesis Imperfecta?

OI treatments are designed to prevent or control symptoms and vary from person to person. Early intervention is important to ensure optimal quality of life and outcomes. Treatment for OI and its related symptoms may include:

Fracture Care

Casting, splinting, and bracing fractured bones can help them heal properly. However, bones may weaken if they are held in one place for long periods. Healthcare providers try to strike a balance between healing fractures and maintaining bone strength.

Physical Therapy

Physical therapy aims to maintain functioning in as many aspects of life as possible. A usual program combines muscle strengthening with aerobic conditioning. Many children with OI have delayed motor skills because their muscles are weak. A physical rehabilitation program can include strengthening of deltoids, biceps, and important lower muscles, such as the gluteus maximus, gluteus medius, and trunk extensors. When these muscles are strong, children can lift their arms and legs against the pull of gravity and get around independently.

Bracing

For some people with OI, wearing braces on the legs can provide support for weak muscles, decrease pain, and keep joints properly aligned. Braces can allow people to get around and function more easily.

Surgical Procedures

Some people with OI undergo surgery to correct bone deformities, including scoliosis and basilar invagination. A common surgical procedure for OI patients, "rodding," is the placement of metal rods in the long bones of the legs. This strengthens them and helps prevent fractures. Some rods get longer as the legs grow. But they also can work their way out of the bone. Surgery can also be performed to improve hearing loss.

Medication

Bisphosphonates are drugs used to treat osteoporosis. They also are useful for OI, especially in children. These drugs do not build new bone, but they slow the loss of existing bone. They have been shown to reduce vertebral compressions and some long bone fractures. However, controlled trials show no improvement in motor skill or decrease in bone pain.

Treatments for Related Conditions

Although these treatments are not specifically for OI, individuals with OI might rely on the following to address conditions related to OI

- Hearing aids for hearing loss
- Crowns and similar dental devices for brittle teeth
- Oxygen administration for people with lung problems

Chapter 56

Periodontal Disease Associated with Chronic Diseases

Potential Impact of Maternal Periodontitis on Reproductive Outcomes

Recent United States studies indicate that periodontal disease during pregnancy may be a newly identified obstetric risk factor for preterm delivery and fetal growth restriction. Mothers with periodontal disease early in pregnancy or with worsening periodontal status during pregnancy appear to have 2–8 times the risk for preterm delivery as other mothers. Maternal periodontitis confers risk that is particularly high at the earlier gestational ages, rather than late in pregnancy. As a result, the impact on neonatal morbidity and mortality is dramatic. Babies of mothers with periodontal infections that disseminate to the fetus are twice as likely as other babies to be admitted to the neonatal intensive care unit and three times more likely to require extended hospital stay beyond 7 days. Other studies conducted on Bangladeshi patients in London, however, failed to find an association between maternal clinical signs of periodontitis and prematurity.

This chapter includes text excerpted from "Public Health Implications of Chronic Periodontal Infections in Adults," Centers for Disease Control and Prevention (CDC), July 10, 2013.

These findings suggest that there may be significant ethno-racial or geographical differences in attributable risk.

Early findings from antepartum periodontal treatment intervention trials point to a potentially dramatic 5-fold reduction in the rate of prematurity. This trial, conducted by Lopez and colleagues, divided almost 400 women into a treatment and a delayed treatment group. They reported that periodontal treatment during pregnancy not only is safe but may improve pregnancy outcomes. Other new findings suggest that approximately 25% of pregnant women demonstrate increased periodontal pocketing during pregnancy and that this condition raises the risk for prematurity. The research suggests that preventing periodontal disease initiation and progression, even in relatively healthy individuals, may improve pregnancy outcomes. The transfer of maternal oral organisms or microbial components to the fetus has been documented, suggesting that there may be translocation of specific oral organisms, such as *Campylobacter rectus*, contributing to prematurity and growth restriction. Thus, there is emerging evidence that this linkage with prematurity may represent a specific infection of the fetus by oral organisms of maternal origin. The identification of specific infectious etiological organisms in this pathology will have diagnostic and therapeutic implications. To prove that periodontal therapy has potential protective benefits against obstetric complications, however, researchers must conduct multi-centered, randomized clinical trials.

Periodontal care will become an integral as part of obstetric care if maternal periodontal disease interventions and/or elimination of specific periodontal pathogens are shown to improve pregnancy outcomes. Further studies are needed to define the key pathogens and pathology mechanisms to optimize potential for diagnostic and therapeutic strategies will enable characterization of appropriate at-risk populations for demonstration projects to determine the effectiveness of reducing the burden of oral infection on obstetric and neonatal morbidity and mortality. In addition, education and outreach programs are needed to help coordinate and integrate obstetric and dental services.

Diabetes and Periodontal Disease

Diabetes mellitus appears to be the best studied disease related to periodontal disease. Extensive studies show that individuals with diabetes are more susceptible to periodontal disease than those without diabetes. For example, diabetes mellitus, types 1 and 2, are well established as increasing the risk for severe periodontal disease, with earlier onset among people with diabetes than among others.

Recently, the concept has developed that people with both diabetes and periodontal disease suffer from more severe diabetes over time as a result of the systemic effects of periodontal infection. For example, Taylor and colleagues found that people with diabetes who also had periodontal disease suffered from worsened glycated hemoglobin over time than did those diabetics who did not have periodontal disease. This and similar observations led to a series of clinical trials in which periodontal therapy, especially therapy involving adjunctive systemic and/or local antibiotics, was found to be effective in treating periodontal disease in people with diabetes and also resulted in reduction of glycated hemoglobin levels. Further studies, especially randomized controlled clinical trials, are required to determine whether the reduction of glycated hemoglobin brought about by resolving periodontal infections in patients with diabetes will result in reducing complications such as retinopathy, nephropathy, and other clinical complications of diabetes.

Other studies have assessed why patients with diabetes respond to periodontal infection with aggravated host destructive responses. One theory suggests that there is a general hyperinflammatory response associated with advanced glycation end products (AGE). This response triggers inflammatory cells through AGE receptors with a release of proinflammatory mediators leading to excessive tissue destruction. This hyperinflammatory response is manifest at the monocyte and neutrophil (cellular) levels. Other mechanisms that explain the increased pathology seen in diabetes patients as a result of periodontal infection include altered vascular physiology, reduced immune response, particularly protective response by neutrophils, and reduced ability for tissues to heal.

Many possible theories explain why glycated hemoglobin is reduced when periodontal infections are resolved in diabetes patients. There is some evidence that systemic overflow of tumor necrosis factor-alpha (TNF-alpha) and other inflammatory cytokines from periodontal lesions may act in concert with TNF-alpha from other sources, such as adipocytes, to increase insulin resistance. In addition to insulin resistance, it is thought that impaired beta cell function leads to reduced insulin secretion resulting in sustained elevated glucose concentrations and elevated glycated hemoglobin with associated increase in complication rates in diabetes patients. However, the role of periodontal infection in beta cell dysfunction is not known, however.

Clinical consequences of reduced glycated hemoglobin in response to treating periodontal infection are yet to be determined. It is possible, however, that treating periodontal infection in patients with diabetes will reduce systemic TNF-alpha and other mediators derived from infected periodontal tissues and, thus, reduce the systemic effects of periodontal infections. Hence, treating periodontal disease may modulate, in some part, factors associated with increased insulin resistance. Studies are needed to assess the mechanisms involved in this two-way relationship with diabetes mellitus increasing the risk for periodontal disease, and periodontal infections increasing or resulting in poor glycemic control. In addition, large prospective, randomized controlled trials are warranted to determine the effects of periodontal therapy on glycemic control and important complications of diabetes including cardiovascular disease, nephropathy, and retinopathy. The public health implications of these studies are potentially important because periodontal disease and diabetes mellitus are common chronic diseases.

Potential Public Health Implications of Periodontal Disease and Cardiovascular Disease Relationships

Periodontitis is a destructive disease that affects the supporting structures of the teeth including the periodontal ligament, cementum, and alveolar bone. Periodontitis represents a chronic, mixed infection by gram-negative bacteria, such as *Porphyromonas gingivalis*, *Prevotella intermedia*, *Bacteroides forsythus*, *Actinobacillus actinomycetemcomitans*, and gram positive organisms, such as *Peptostreptococcus micros* and *Streptococcus intermedius*. Due to periodic changes in concepts of periodontal disease pathogenesis and restructuring and renaming periodontal disease types, actual prevalence and incidence estimates for periodontal disease have been debated for decades. It is generally thought that in developed countries, 44% to 57% of adults have moderate periodontitis, and about 7% to 15% have advanced periodontitis. Partly because of uncertainty about the public health importance of this disease and partly because primary prevention depends on personal oral hygiene behavior and professional services, public health programs to prevent periodontal disease are underdeveloped.

Since 1989, a number of cross-sectional, case-control, and longitudinal studies have reported that the clinical signs of periodontitis may be associated with cardiovascular events; other studies have reported no significant association. Several basic science and animal studies also have reported systemic effects of periodontal infection. Cardiovascular disease is the top cause of death in the United States for men and women and carries with it considerable morbidity. In addition, total costs for cardiovascular disease in 2003 were estimated to reach almost

$352 billion. This presentation assumes that periodontal disease will be shown to be a risk factor for cardiovascular disease. Because periodontal and cardiovascular diseases are highly prevalent in the U.S. population, periodontal disease also becomes a public health problem worthy of attention, even though the strength of the association may be only moderate.

As a result of this link with cardiovascular disease, interest in periodontal disease prevention and treatment is likely to intensify in the private and public health sectors and in the general public. One consequence of this link is that dentists and physicians may need to focus more on primary prevention of infection by periodontal pathogens and, in patients with disease, they may need to focus more on secondary prevention. End-points for secondary prevention will involve eliminating periodontal pathogens and reducing inflammation, while pocket reduction, tooth retention, and regenerative procedures may become less important. Controlling inflammation and infection may create an increased need for anti-infective and anti-inflammatory pharmacological strategies for high-risk patients.

Chapter 57

Pregnancy and Oral Health

As a Woman, Why Do I Have to Worry about Oral Health?

Everyone needs to take care of their oral health. But female hormones can lead to an increase in some problems, such as:

- Cold sores and canker sores

- Dry mouth

- Changes in taste

- Higher risk of gum disease

Taking good care of your teeth and gums can help you avoid or lessen oral health problems.

I'm Pregnant. Do I Need to Take Special Care of My Mouth?

Yes! If you are pregnant, you have special oral health needs.

Before you become pregnant, it is best to have regular dental checkups. You want to keep your mouth in good health before your pregnancy.

This chapter includes text excerpted from "Oral Health Fact Sheet," Office on Women's Health (OWH), U.S. Department of Health and Human Services (HHS), July 16, 2012. Reviewed September 2016.

Also, remember that what you eat affects the development of your unborn child—including teeth. Your baby's teeth begin to grow during the third and sixth months of pregnancy, so it is important that you eat a balanced diet that includes calcium, protein, phosphorous, and vitamins A, C, and D.

If you are pregnant:

- Have a complete oral exam early in your pregnancy. Because you are pregnant, your dentist might not take routine X-rays. But if you need X-rays, the health risk to your unborn baby is small.

- Remember dental work during pregnancy is safe. The best time for treatment is between the 14th and 20th weeks. In the last months, you might be uncomfortable sitting in a dental chair.

- Have all needed dental treatments. If you avoid treatment, you may risk your own and your baby's health.

- Use good oral hygiene to control your risk of gum diseases. Pregnant women may have changes in taste and develop red, swollen gums that bleed easily. This condition is called pregnancy gingivitis. Both poor oral hygiene and higher hormone levels can cause pregnancy gingivitis. Until now, it was thought that having gum disease could raise your risk of having a low-birth-weight baby. Researchers have not been able to confirm this link, but studies are still under way to learn more.

I'm a New Mother. What Can I Do for My Baby's Oral Health?

You can do a lot! Below are some things you need to know about your baby's oral health.

- The same germs that cause tooth decay in your mouth can be passed to your baby. Do not put your baby's items, such as toys, spoons, bottles, or pacifiers in your mouth.

- Wipe your baby's teeth and gums with a clean gauze pad or baby toothbrush after each nursing and feeding. This can help remove sugars found in milk that can cause tooth decay and also get your baby used to having her teeth cleaned on a regular basis.

- If you bottle-feed your baby, try to finish bottle weaning by age 1.

- Avoid giving your baby bottles or pacifiers at naps and bedtime. Sucking on a bottle when lying down can cause cavities and lead to "baby bottle tooth decay."

- All babies should visit a dentist by age 1. The dentist will screen for problems in your baby's mouth. You will also be shown how to care for your child's teeth and mouth.

- Talk with your doctor about the best water choices for infants. Fluoride is good for teeth. But too much fluoride can harm development of tooth enamel in infants.

Chapter 58

Tobacco Use Associated Oral Changes

Chapter Contents

Section 58.1

Betel Quid Use and Its Impact on Oral Health

This section contains text excerpted from "Betel Quid
with Tobacco (Gutka)," Centers for Disease Control and
Prevention (CDC), February 18, 2016.

Betel quid is a combination of betel leaf, areca nut, and slaked
lime.

- In many countries, tobacco is also added, and the product is
  known as *gutka, ghutka,* or *gutkha.*

- Other ingredients and flavorants are also added according to
  local preferences and customs (e.g., sweeteners, catechu, or
  spices such as cardamom, saffron, cloves, anise seeds, turmeric,
  and mustard).

Gutka is commercially available in foil packets and tins and is
consumed by placing a pinch of the mixture in the mouth between the
gum and cheek and gently sucking and chewing. The excess saliva
produced by chewing may be swallowed or spit out.

Use

- Betel quid and gutka use is reported to have stimulant and
  relaxation effects.

- Global estimates report that up to 600 million men and women
  use some variety of betel quid.

- Betel quid with or without tobacco is widely used in the Indian
  subcontinent (i.e., Bangladesh, India, Pakistan) as well as
  throughout Asia and the Pacific region (e.g., Cambodia, China,
  Indonesia, Malaysia, Philippines, Taiwan, Thailand).

Health Effects

The following conditions have been associated with betel quid/gutka
use:

Precancerous Conditions

- Oral precancerous lesions, including erythroplakia (a reddened patch in the mouth) and leukoplakia (a white patch on the mucous membranes in the mouth that cannot be wiped off).

- Oral submucous fibrosis (OSF), a precancerous lesion that stiffens the soft pink tissue that lines the inside of the mouth (i.e., oral mucosa).

Cancer

- Oral cancers—predominantly carcinomas of the lip, mouth, tongue, and pharynx

- Cancer of the esophagus

Other Health Effects

- Reproductive health outcomes such as increased risk of having a low birth-weight infant

- Nicotine addiction

Section 58.2

Smoking, Gum Disease, and Tooth Loss

This section contains text excerpted from "Smoking, Gum Disease, and Tooth Loss," Centers for Disease Control and Prevention (CDC), September 1, 2015.

What Is Gum Disease?

Gum (periodontal) disease is an infection of the gums and can affect the bone structure that supports your teeth. In severe cases, it can make your teeth fall out. Smoking is an important cause of severe gum disease in the United States.

Gum disease starts with bacteria (germs) on your teeth that get under your gums. If the germs stay on your teeth for too long, layers of plaque (film) and tartar (hardened plaque) develop. This buildup leads to early gum disease, called gingivitis. When gum disease gets worse, your gums can pull away from your teeth and form spaces that get infected. This is severe gum disease, also called periodontitis. The bone and tissue that hold your teeth in place can break down, and your teeth may loosen and need to be pulled out.

Warning Signs and Symptoms of Gum Disease

* Red or swollen gums
* Tender or bleeding gums
* Painful chewing
* Loose teeth
* Sensitive teeth
* Gums that have pulled away from your teeth

How Is Smoking Related to Gum Disease?

Smoking weakens your body's infection fighters (your immune system). This makes it harder to fight off a gum infection. Once you have gum damage, smoking also makes it harder for your gums to heal.

What Does This Mean for Me If I Am a Smoker?

* You have twice the risk for gum disease compared with a nonsmoker.
* The more cigarettes you smoke, the greater your risk for gum disease.
* The longer you smoke, the greater your risk for gum disease.
* Treatments for gum disease may not work as well for people who smoke.

Tobacco use in any form—cigarettes, pipes, and smokeless (spit) tobacco—raises your risk for gum disease.

How Can Gum Disease Be Prevented?

You can help avoid gum disease with good dental habits.

* Brush your teeth twice a day.

- Floss often to remove plaque.

- See a dentist regularly for checkups and professional cleanings.

- Don't smoke. If you smoke, quit.

How Is Gum Disease Treated?

Regular cleanings at your dentist's office and daily brushing and flossing can help treat early gum disease (gingivitis). More severe gum disease may require:

- Deep cleaning below the gum line.

- Prescription mouth rinse or medicine.

- Surgery to remove tartar deep under the gums.

- Surgery to help heal bone or gums lost to periodontitis. Your dentist may use small bits of bone to fill places where bone has been lost. Or your dentist may move tissue from one place in your mouth to cover exposed tooth roots.

If you smoke or use spit tobacco, quitting will help your gums heal after treatment.

Part Seven

Finding and Financing Oral Health in the United States

Chapter 59

Access to Oral Healthcare

Chapter Contents

Section 59.1

Oral Health Status

This section includes text excerpted from "Oral Health
in America: A Report of the Surgeon General (Executive
Summary)," National Institute of Dental and Craniofacial
Research (NIDCR), March 7, 2014.

The Burden of Oral Diseases and Disorders

Oral diseases are progressive and cumulative and become more
complex over time. They can affect our ability to eat, the foods we
choose, how we look, and the way we communicate. These diseases
can affect economic productivity and compromise our ability to work
at home, at school, or on the job. Health disparities exist across population groups at all ages. Over one third of the U.S. population (100
million people) has no access to community water fluoridation. Over
108 million children and adults lack dental insurance, which is over
2.5 times the number who lack medical insurance. The following are
highlights of oral health data for children, adults, and the elderly.

Children

- Cleft lip/palate, one of the most common birth defects, is estimated to affect 1 out of 600 live births for whites and 1 out of
  1,850 live births for African Americans.

- Other birth defects such as hereditary ectodermal dysplasias,
  where all or most teeth are missing or misshapen, cause lifetime
  problems that can be devastating to children and adults.

  - Dental caries (tooth decay) is the single most common
    chronic childhood disease—5 times more common than
    asthma and 7 times more common than hay fever.

- Over 50 percent of 5- to 9-year-old children have at least one cavity or filling, and that proportion increases to 78 percent among
  17-year-olds. Nevertheless, these figures represent improvements
  in the oral health of children compared to a generation ago.

- There are striking disparities in dental disease by income. Poor children suffer twice as much dental caries as their more affluent peers, and their disease is more likely to be untreated. These poor-non poor differences continue into adolescence. One out of four children in America is born into poverty, and children living below the poverty line (annual income of $17,000 for a family of four) have more severe and untreated decay.

- Unintentional injuries, many of which include head, mouth, and neck injuries, are common in children.

- Intentional injuries commonly affect the craniofacial tissues.

- Tobacco-related oral lesions are prevalent in adolescents who currently use smokeless (spit) tobacco.

- Professional care is necessary for maintaining oral health, yet 25 percent of poor children have not seen a dentist before entering kindergarten.

- Medical insurance is a strong predictor of access to dental care. Uninsured children are 2.5 times less likely than insured children to receive dental care. Children from families without dental insurance are 3 times more likely to have dental needs than children with either public or private insurance. For each child without medical insurance, there are at least 2.6 children without dental insurance.

- Medicaid has not been able to fill the gap in providing dental care to poor children. Fewer than one in five Medicaid-covered children received a single dental visit in a recent year-long study period. Although new programs such as the State Children's Health Insurance Program (SCHIP) may increase the number of insured children, many will still be left without effective dental coverage.

- The social impact of oral diseases in children is substantial. More than 51 million school hours are lost each year to dental-related illness. Poor children suffer nearly 12 times more restricted-activity days than children from higher-income families. Pain and suffering due to untreated diseases can lead to problems in eating, speaking, and attending to learning.

Although this measure has not been fully implemented, the results have been dramatic. Dental caries began to decline in the 1950s among children who grew up in fluoridated cities, and by the late 1970s, decline in decay was evident for many Americans. The application of science to improve diagnostic, treatment, and prevention strategies has saved billions of dollars per year in the nation's annual health bill. Even more significant, the result is that far fewer people are edentulous (toothless) today than a generation ago.

The theme of prevention gained momentum as pioneering investigators and practitioners in the 1950s and 1960s showed that not only dental caries but also periodontal diseases are bacterial infections. The researchers demonstrated that the infections could be prevented by increasing host resistance to disease and reducing or eliminating the suspected microbial pathogens in the oral cavity. The applications of research discoveries have resulted in continuing improvements in the oral health of Americans, new approaches to the prevention and treatment of dental diseases, and the growth of the science.

Adults

- Most adults show signs of periodontal or gingival diseases. Severe periodontal disease (measured as 6 millimeters of periodontal attachment loss) affects about 14 percent of adults aged 45 to 54.

- Clinical symptoms of viral infections, such as herpes labialis (cold sores), and oral ulcers (canker sores) are common in adulthood, affecting about 19 percent of adults 25 to 44 years of age.

- Chronic disabling diseases such as temporomandibular disorders, Sjögren's syndrome, diabetes, and osteoporosis affect millions of Americans and compromise oral health and functioning.

- Pain is a common symptom of craniofacial disorders and is accompanied by interference with vital functions such as eating, swallowing, and speech. Twenty-two percent of adults reported some form of oral-facial pain in the past 6 months. Pain is a major component of trigeminal neuralgia, facial shingles (post-herpetic neuralgia), temporomandibular disorders, fibromyalgia, and Bell's palsy.

- Population growth as well as diagnostics that are enabling earlier detection of cancer means that more patients than ever before are undergoing cancer treatments. More than 400,000 of these patients will develop oral complications annually.

- Immunocompromised patients, such as those with HIV infection and those undergoing organ transplantation, are at higher risk for oral problems such as candidiasis.

- Employed adults lose more than 164 million hours of work each year due to dental disease or dental visits.

- For every adult 19 years or older without medical insurance, there are three without dental insurance.

- A little less than two thirds of adults report having visited a dentist in the past 12 months. Those with incomes at or above the poverty level are twice as likely to report a dental visit in the past 12 months as those who are below the poverty level.

Older Adults

- Twenty-three percent of 65- to 74-year-olds have severe periodontal disease (measured as 6 millimeters of periodontal attachment loss). (Also, at all ages men are more likely than women to have more severe disease, and at all ages people at the lowest socioeconomic levels have more severe periodontal disease.)

- About 30 percent of adults 65 years and older are edentulous, compared to 46 percent 20 years ago. These figures are higher for those living in poverty.

- Oral and pharyngeal cancers are diagnosed in about 30,000 Americans annually; 8,000 die from these diseases each year. These cancers are primarily diagnosed in the elderly. Prognosis is poor. The 5-year survival rate for white patients is 56 percent; for blacks, it is only 34 percent.

- Most older Americans take both prescription and over-the-counter drugs. In all probability, at least one of the medications used will have an oral side effect—usually dry mouth. The inhibition of salivary flow increases the risk for oral disease because saliva contains antimicrobial components as well as minerals that can help rebuild tooth enamel after attack by acid-producing, decay-causing bacteria. Individuals in long-term care facilities are prescribed an average of eight drugs.

- At any given time, 5 percent of Americans aged 65 and older (currently some 1.65 million people) are living in a long-term care facility where dental care is problematic.

- Many elderly individuals lose their dental insurance when they retire. The situation may be worse for older women, who generally have lower incomes and may never have had dental insurance. Medicaid funds dental care for the low-income and disabled elderly in some states, but reimbursements are low. Medicare is not designed to reimburse for routine dental care.

At the same time, more needs to be done to ensure that messages of health promotion and disease prevention are brought home to all Americans. In this regard, a fourth theme of the report is that general health risk factors, such as tobacco use and poor dietary practices, also affect oral and craniofacial health. The evidence for an association between tobacco use and oral diseases has been clearly delineated in almost every Surgeon General's report on tobacco since 1964, and the oral effects of nutrition and diet are presented in the Surgeon General's report on nutrition (1988). All the health professions can play a role in reducing the burden of disease in America by calling attention to these and other risk factors and suggesting appropriate actions.

Clearly, promoting health and preventing disease are concepts the American people have taken to heart. For the third decade the nation has developed a plan for the prevention of disease and the promotion of health, embodied in the U.S. Department of Health and Human Services (2000) document, Healthy People 2010. As a nation, we hope to eliminate disparities in health and eradicate cancer, birth defects, AIDS and other devastating infections, mental illness and suicide, and the chronic diseases of aging. To live well into old age free of pain and infirmity, and with a high quality of life, is the American dream.

Scientists today take that dream seriously in researching the intricacies of the craniofacial complex. They are using an ever-growing array of sophisticated analytic tools and imaging systems to study normal function and diagnose disease. They are completing the mapping and sequencing of human, animal, microbial, and plant genomes, the better to understand the complexities of human development, aging, and pathological processes. They are growing cell lines, synthesizing molecules, and using a new generation of biomaterials to revolutionize tissue repair and regeneration. More than ever before, they are working in multidisciplinary teams to bring new knowledge and expertise to the goal of understanding complex human diseases and disorders.

The Status of Oral Health in America

- Microbial infections, including those caused by bacteria, viruses, and fungi, are the primary cause of the most prevalent oral diseases. Examples include dental caries, periodontal diseases, herpes labialis, and candidiasis.

- The etiology and pathogenesis of diseases and disorders affecting the craniofacial structures are multifactorial and complex, involving an interplay among genetic, environmental, and behavioral factors.

- Many inherited and congenital conditions affect the craniofacial complex, often resulting in disfigurement and impairments that may involve many body organs and systems and affect millions of children worldwide.

- Tobacco use, excessive alcohol use, and inappropriate dietary practices contribute to many diseases and disorders. In particular, tobacco use is a risk factor for oral cavity and pharyngeal cancers, periodontal diseases, candidiasis, and dental caries, among other diseases.

- Some chronic diseases, such as Sjögren's syndrome, present with primary oral symptoms.

- Oral-facial pain conditions are common and often have complex etiologies.

- Over the past five decades, major improvements in oral health have been seen nationally for most Americans.

- Despite improvements in oral health status, profound disparities remain in some population groups as classified by sex, income, age, and race/ethnicity. For some diseases and conditions, the magnitude of the differences in oral health status among population groups is striking.

- Oral diseases and conditions affect people throughout their lifespan. Nearly every American has experienced the most common oral disease, dental caries.

- Conditions that severely affect the face and facial expression, such as birth defects, craniofacial injuries, and neoplastic diseases, are more common in the very young and in the elderly.

- Oral-facial pain can greatly reduce quality of life and restrict major functions. Pain is a common symptom for many of the conditions affecting oral-facial structures.

- National and state data for many oral and craniofacial diseases and conditions and for population groups are limited or nonexistent. Available state data reveal variations within and among states in patterns of health and disease among population groups.

- Research is needed to develop better measures of disease and health, to explain the differences among population groups, and to develop interventions targeted at eliminating disparities.

Section 59.2

Disparities in Oral Health

This section includes text excerpted from "Disparities in Oral Health," Centers for Disease Control and Prevention (CDC), May 17, 2016.

A Worrying Factor

Oral health disparities are profound in the United States. Despite major improvements in oral health for the population as a whole, oral health disparities exist for many racial and ethnic groups, by socioeconomic status, gender, age, and geographic location.

Some social factors that can contribute to these differences are lifestyle behaviors such as tobacco use, frequency of alcohol use, and poor dietary choices. Just like they affect general health, these behaviors can affect oral health. The economic factors that often relate to poor oral health include access to health services and an individual's ability to get and keep dental insurance.

Disparities in Oral Health

Some of the oral health disparities that exist include the following:

- **Overall.** Non-Hispanic blacks, Hispanics, and American Indians and Alaska Natives generally have the poorest oral health of any racial and ethnic groups in the United States.

- **Children and Tooth Decay.** The greatest racial and ethnic disparity among children aged 2–4 years and aged 6–8 years is seen in Mexican American and black, non-Hispanic children.

- **Adults and Untreated Tooth Decay.** Blacks, non-Hispanics, and Mexican Americans aged 35–44 years experience untreated tooth decay nearly twice as much as white, non-Hispanics.

- **Tooth Decay and Education.** Adults aged 35–44 years with less than a high school education experience untreated tooth decay nearly three times that of adults with at least some college education.

- In addition, adults aged 35–44 years with less than a high school education experience destructive periodontal (gum) disease nearly three times that of adults with a least some college education.

- **Adults and Oral Cancer.** The 5–year survival rate is lower for oral pharyngeal (throat) cancers among black men than whites (36% versus 61%).

- **Adults and Periodontitis.** 47.2% of U.S. adults have some form of periodontal disease. In adults aged 65 and older, 70.1% have periodontal disease.

- Periodontal Disease is higher in men than women, and greatest among Mexican Americans and Non-Hispanic blacks, and those with less than a high school education.

Healthy People 2020 Works to Eliminate Oral Health Disparities

Healthy People 2020 is the nation's framework to improve the health of all Americans. The overarching goals of Healthy People 2020 are to increase quality and years of healthy life and eliminate health disparities. Interventions such as community water fluoridation and school-based dental sealant programs can help achieve this goal.

Reduces and aids in preventing tooth decay among different socio-economic, racial, and ethnic groups. Currently, this Healthy People 2020 objective is moving toward its target of 79.6% of community water having fluoride.

School-based dental sealant programs provide sealants to children who may not receive routine dental care. This includes children at highest risk for tooth decay: those from low-income families and certain racial and ethnic groups. Sealants are thin plastic coatings applied to the tiny grooves on the chewing surfaces of the teeth.

Chapter 60

Expenditures and Financing of Oral Healthcare

Chapter Contents

Section 60.1

Overview of Expenditures

This section includes text excerpted from "National Health
Expenditures 2014 Highlights," Centers for Medicare and
Medicaid Services (CMS), December 3, 2015.

In 2014, U.S. healthcare spending increased 5.3 percent following
growth of 2.9 percent in 2013 to reach $3.0 trillion, or $9,523 per person. The faster growth experienced in 2014 was primarily due to the
major coverage expansions under the Affordable Care Act, particularly
for Medicaid and private health insurance. The share of the economy
devoted to healthcare spending was 17.5 percent, up from 17.3 percent
in 2013.

Health Spending by Type of Service or Product: Personal Healthcare

- **Hospital Care:** Spending for hospital care increased 4.1 percent to $971.8 billion in 2014 compared to 3.5 percent growth in
  2013. The faster growth in 2014 was influenced by a resurgence
  in growth of non-price factors, such as the use and intensity of
  services. In addition, hospital services experienced faster growth
  in Medicaid, private health insurance, and Medicare spending
  compared to 2013. Lastly, ACA-related coverage expansion contributed to increased hospital spending for both Medicaid and
  private health insurance.

- **Physician and Clinical Services:** Spending on physician and
  clinical services increased 4.6 percent in 2014 to $603.7 billion
  from 2.5 percent growth in 2013 when spending was at a historical
  low. Faster growth in both price and non-price factors contributed
  to the acceleration in overall spending for physician and clinical
  services. Medicaid, private health insurance, and Medicare spending for physician and clinical services all accelerated in 2014.

- **Other Professional Services:** Spending for other professional
  services reached $84.4 billion in 2014, an increase of 5.2 percent,

which is an acceleration from 3.5 percent in 2013. Spending in this category includes establishments of independent health practitioners (except physicians and dentists) that primarily provide services such as physical therapy, optometry, podiatry, or chiropractic medicine.

- **Dental Services:** Spending for dental services increased 2.8 percent in 2014 to $113.5 billion, faster than in 2013 when growth was 1.5 percent. Private health insurance (which accounted for almost half of dental spending in 2014) increased 3.4 percent after growing 1.3 percent in 2013. Out-of-pocket spending for dental services (which accounted for 40 percent of spending in 2014) increased slightly at 0.2 percent in 2014, following growth of 1.0 percent in 2013.

- **Other Health, Residential, and Personal Care Services:** Spending for other health, residential, and personal care services grew 4.1 percent in 2014 to $150.4 billion, which was a slowdown compared to 4.7 percent growth in 2013. This category includes expenditures for medical services that are generally delivered by providers in non-traditional settings such as schools, community centers, and the workplace; as well as by ambulance providers and residential mental health and substance abuse facilities.

- **Home Healthcare:** Spending growth for freestanding home healthcare agencies accelerated in 2014, increasing 4.8 percent to $83.2 billion following growth of 3.3 percent in 2013. The faster growth in 2014 was attributable to increased spending by the two largest payers of home health, Medicare, with growth of 3.3 percent, and Medicaid, with growth of 3.5 percent. Combined, both payers of home healthcare represented 77 percent of total home health spending.

- **Nursing Care Facilities and Continuing Care Retirement Communities:** Spending for freestanding nursing care facilities and continuing care retirement communities increased 3.6 percent in 2014 to $155.6 billion, an acceleration from growth of 1.3 percent in 2013. The faster growth in 2014 was due to the increased spending in Medicare, with 4.1 percent growth, and Medicaid, with 3.1 percent growth.

- **Prescription Drugs:** Retail prescription drug spending accelerated in 2014, growing 12.2 percent to $297.7 billion compared to the 2.4 growth in 2013. The rapid growth in 2014 was due to increased spending for new medications (particularly for specialty drugs such as hepatitis C), a smaller impact from patent expirations, and brand-name drug price increases. Private health insurance, Medicare, and Medicaid spending on prescription drugs all accelerated in 2014.

- **Durable Medical Equipment:** Retail spending for durable medical equipment reached $46.4 billion in 2014 and increased 3.2 percent, faster than the 2.8 percent growth in 2013. Spending in this category includes items such as contact lenses, eyeglasses and hearing aids.

- **Other Non-durable Medical Products:** Retail spending for other non-durable medical products, such as over-the-counter medicines, medical instruments, and surgical dressings, grew 2.4 percent to $56.9 billion in 2014. This was a slower rate of growth than in 2013, when spending grew 3.5 percent.

Health Spending by Major Sources of Funds

- **Medicare:** Medicare spending grew 5.5 percent to $618.7 billion in 2014, an acceleration from 3.0 percent growth in 2013. This increase was primarily attributable to faster growth in spending for prescription drugs, physician and clinical services, and government administration and the net cost of insurance. Medicare accounted for 20 percent of total healthcare spending.

- **Medicaid:** Total Medicaid spending, which accounted for 16 percent of total national health expenditures, increased 11.0 percent in 2014 after growing 5.9 percent in 2013. State and local Medicaid expenditures only grew 0.9 percent, while federal Medicaid expenditures increased 18.4 percent in 2014. The increased spending by the federal government was largely driven by the newly eligible enrollees under the ACA, which were fully financed by the federal government.

- **Private Health Insurance:** Total private health insurance expenditures increased 4.4 percent (33 percent of total healthcare spending) to $991.0 billion in 2014, faster than the 1.6 percent growth in 2013 which was the slowest rate since 1967. The faster rate of growth reflected the impacts of the ACA, including the introduction of Marketplace plans, health insurance premium tax credits, health insurance industry fees, and mandated benefit design changes. Average monthly marketplace enrollment was 5.4 million in 2014.

- **Out-of-Pocket:** Out-of-pocket spending grew 1.3 percent in 2014 to $329.8 billion which was slightly slower than annual growth of 2.1 percent in 2013. The slowdown in 2014 was influenced by the expansion of insurance coverage and the corresponding drop in the number of individuals without health insurance.

Section 60.2

Finding Low-Cost Dental Care

This section includes text excerpted from "Finding Low-Cost Dental Care," National Institute of Dental and Craniofacial Research (NIDCR), June 7, 2016.

Role of National Institute of Dental and Craniofacial Research (NIDCR) towards Dental Care

The National Institute of Dental and Craniofacial Research (NIDCR), one of the federal government's National Institutes of Health (NIH), leads the nation in conducting and supporting research to improve oral health. As a research organization, NIDCR does not provide financial assistance for dental treatment. The resources listed below, however, may help you find the dental care you need. You also can contact the NIDCR's National Oral Health Information Clearinghouse at 1-866-232-4528 or nidcrinfo@mail.nih.gov if you have questions or need additional information.

Some of the resources offer an internet address but no phone number. If you do not have internet access, you may wish to call the NIDCR toll-free number (listed above), visit your local library, or ask a friend or family member for help.

Clinical Trials

NIDCR sometimes seeks volunteers with specific dental, oral, and craniofacial conditions to participate in research studies, also known as clinical trials. Researchers may provide study participants with limited free or low-cost dental treatment for the particular condition they are studying. To learn more about clinical trials, visit the NIDCR website and click on "Clinical Trials." To find a clinical trial, contact:

- ClinicalTrials.gov—a database of government and private clinical trials in the United States and around the world.

- NIH Clinical Research Studies—a database of clinical trials at the NIH Clinical Center in Bethesda, Maryland; to talk with someone about studies at the Clinical Center, call: 1–800–411–1222.

Dental Schools and Dental Hygiene Schools

Dental schools can be a good source of quality, reduced-cost dental treatment. Most of these teaching facilities have clinics that allow dental students to gain experience treating patients while providing care at a reduced cost. Experienced, licensed dentists closely supervise the students. At most schools, there are also clinics where graduate students and faculty members provide care.

Dental hygiene schools may offer supervised, low-cost preventive dental care as part of the training experience for dental hygiene students. To find a dental or dental hygiene school in your area, contact:

- Dental Schools—American Dental Association.

- Dental Hygiene Schools—American Dental Hygienists' Association.

Community Health Centers

The federal government's Health Resources and Services Administration (HRSA), runs federally funded community health centers across the country that provide free or reduced-cost health services, including dental care. To find a health center in your area, visit:

- HRSA.gov and type your location in the "Find a Health Center" box.

Medicaid and CHIP

- Medicaid is a state-run program that provides medical benefits—and in some cases dental benefits—to eligible individuals and families. States are required to provide dental benefits for children covered by Medicaid, but states can choose whether to provide dental benefits for adults. Most states provide only limited dental services for adults, while some offer extensive services. Visit the Medicaid website and click on "Learn How to Apply for Coverage" or contact your state Medicaid program.

- CHIP is a state-run program for children whose families earn too much to qualify for Medicaid but can't afford private insurance. CHIP provides dental services to children up to age 19. Dental services covered under this program vary from state to state. To find children's dental care programs in your state, visit Insure Kids Now or call 1–877–KIDS–NOW (1–877–543–7669).

Medicare

Medicare is a federal health insurance program for people 65 and older and for people under 65 with specific disabilities. Medicare only covers dental services related to certain medical conditions or treatments. It does not cover dentures or most routine care like checkups, cleanings, or fillings. Visit Medicare Dental Services or call 1–800–MEDICARE (1–800–633–4227). Have your Medicare number handy when you call.

State and Local Resources

Your state or local health department may know of programs in your area that offer free or reduced-cost dental care. To find state and local resources:

- Call your local or state health department to learn more about their financial assistance programs.
- Call 2–1–1 to find services in your area.

Section 60.3

Dental Coverage in the Market Place

This section includes text excerpted from "Dental coverage in the Marketplace," HealthCare.gov, Centers for Medicare and Medicaid Services (CMS), April 18, 2015.

Dental Coverage Is Available Two Ways

In the Health Insurance Marketplace, you can get dental coverage two ways: as part of a health plan, or by itself through a separate, stand-alone dental plan. You can buy a dental plan through the federal Marketplace only when you enroll in a health plan at the same time.

1. **Health plans that include dental coverage.** In the Marketplace, dental coverage is included in some health plans. You can see which plans include dental coverage when you compare them. If a health plan includes dental coverage, you'll pay one monthly premium for both. The premium shown for the plan includes both health and dental coverage.

2. **Separate, stand-alone dental plans.** In some cases separate, stand-alone plans are offered. You may want this if the health coverage you choose doesn't include dental coverage, or if you want different dental coverage. If you choose a separate dental plan, you'll pay a separate, additional premium.

How to Get Marketplace Dental Coverage

When you complete your Marketplace application and get your results, you can select a health plan that include dental coverage. If you decide you want a stand-alone dental plan, you can choose one after you select your health plan. You can't buy a dental plan from the Marketplace unless you're enrolling in a Marketplace health plan at the same time.

Dental Plan Categories: High and Low

There are two categories of Marketplace dental plans: High and low coverage levels.

1. The high coverage level has higher premiums but lower copayments and deductibles. So you'll pay more every month, but you'll pay less when you use dental services.

2. The low coverage level has lower premiums but higher copayments and deductibles. So you'll pay less every month, but you'll pay more when you use dental services.

When you compare dental plans in the Marketplace, you'll find details about each plan's costs, copayments, deductibles, and services covered.

Adult and Child Dental Insurance in the Marketplace

Under the healthcare law, dental insurance is treated differently for adults and children 18 and under.

Dental coverage for children is an essential health benefit. This means if you're getting health coverage for someone 18 or younger, dental coverage **must be available** for your child either as part of a health plan or as a stand-alone plan. **Note:** While dental coverage for children must be **available** to you, you **don't** have to buy it.

Dental coverage isn't an essential health benefit for adults. Insurers don't have to offer adult dental coverage.

Under the healthcare law, most people must have health coverage or pay a fee. Dental coverage is optional, even for children. So you don't need it to avoid the penalty.

Can I Cancel My Marketplace Dental Coverage and Still Keep My Health Coverage?

It depends.

- **If you have a separate, stand-alone dental plan**, you can cancel any time during the year by contacting your plan directly, or by contacting the Marketplace call center.

  - **Important:** Don't cancel your **dental** plan on Health-Care.gov if you want to keep your **health** plan. Selecting **"Remove"** in **"My Plans and Programs"** under your dental plan will cancel both your dental and health plans.

- **If you have a health plan that includes dental benefits** and want to modify that plan, you can change to another health plan that doesn't include dental benefits only during Open Enrollment. The 2016 Open Enrollment Period started November 1, 2015.

Outside Open Enrollment, you can change health plans only if you have a qualifying life event that gives you a Special Enrollment Period (SEP). Learn more about how you qualify for a Special Enrollment Period. If you qualify for an SEP, you can choose a new health plan with or without dental coverage. But you can't get dental coverage by itself.

Chapter 61

Fluoride and Sealants at School-Based Services

What Are Dental Sealants?

Sealants are thin plastic coatings applied to the tiny grooves on the chewing surfaces of the back teeth. This is where most tooth decay in children and teens occurs. Sealants protect the chewing surfaces from decay by keeping germs and pieces of food out.

What Are School-Based Sealant Programs?

School-based dental sealant delivery programs provide sealants to children unlikely to receive them otherwise. Such programs:

- Define a target population within a school district

- Verify unmet need for sealants

- Get financial, material, and policy support

This chapter contains text excerpted from the following sources: Text beginning with the heading "What Are Dental Sealants?" is excerpted from "School-Based Dental Sealant Programs," Centers for Disease Control and Prevention (CDC), July 10, 2013; Text under the heading "Implementation of Evidence-Based Preventive Interventions: School-Based and School-Linked Dental Sealant Programs" is excerpted from "Implementation of Evidence-Based Preventive Interventions: School-Based and School-Linked Dental Sealant Programs," Centers for Disease Control and Prevention (CDC), July 10, 2013.

- Apply rules for selecting schools and students

- Apply sealants at school or offsite in clinics

School-based sealant programs are especially important for reaching children from low-income families who are less likely to receive private dental care. Programs generally target schools by using the percentage of children eligible for federal free or reduced-cost lunch programs Tooth decay may result in pain and other problems that affect learning in school-age children.

CDC-Sponsored Expert Work Group Publishes Updated Recommendations for School-Based Sealant Programs

The recommendations were developed by a work group of experts in the fields of caries prevention and treatment, oral epidemiology, and evidence-based reviews. The work group also included representatives from professional dental organizations.

The expert work group examined new evidence on:

- The effectiveness of sealants in preventing new decay and progression of early decay

- Methods to assess decay

- Sealant placement techniques

- Scientific reviews of program practices

Based on this evidence, the following recommendations are provided for practitioners in school-based programs:

- Seal pit-and-fissure tooth surfaces that are sound or have early decay, prioritizing first and second permanent molars.

- Use visual assessment to differentiate surfaces with the earliest signs of tooth decay from more advanced lesions.

- X-rays are not needed solely for sealant placement.

- A toothbrush can be used to help clean the tooth surface before acid etching.

- When resources allow, have an assistant help the dental professional place sealants.

- Provide sealants to children even if follow-up examinations for every child cannot be guaranteed. These recommendations are designed to guide practices of state and community public health programs for planning, implementing, and evaluating school-based sealant programs, as well as to complement the American Dental Association Council on Scientific Affairs' evidence-based clinical recommendations for sealant use published in 2008.

Implementation of Evidence-Based Preventive Interventions: School-Based and School-Linked Dental Sealant Programs

School-based and school-linked dental sealant programs (SBSP) are highly effective strategies for preventing tooth decay in children. School-based sealant programs provide pit and fissure sealants to children in a school setting, and school-linked programs screen the children in school and refer them to private dental practices or public dental clinics that place the sealants.

School-based and school-linked programs generally target vulnerable populations that may be at greater risk for developing decay and less likely to receive dental care. When developing, coordinating, and implementing a SBSP, state oral health program strategies should:

- Promote policies that allow the use of dental personnel to the top of their licensure. State health departments may educate decision makers on the potential cost savings and increased utilization of school-based sealant programs when dentists are not required to be on site when the sealants are placed.

- Develop referral networks. School-based and school-linked programs are encouraged to work with dental practitioners in their communities so they can provide referrals to dental homes for children who currently do not have one.

- Increase efficiency. School-based and school-linked sealant programs are encouraged to collaborate with targeted schools to increase the number of children that can be seen in schools. Programs should work with school staff to identify children with dental needs and to ensure that parental consent forms are returned in order to increase the cost-effectiveness and efficiency of these programs.

Data collection and analysis. State health departments are encouraged to work with all school sealant programs in their state to systematically collect and analyze data in order to document program impact and efficiency. Centers for Disease Control and Prevention

(CDC) has developed software (SEALS) that can assist sealant programs in their data efforts.

CDC grantee states are required to report the following measures related to SBSP coverage annually:

- Percentage of eligible schools with a school-based/linked sealant program.

- Percentage and number of children attending these schools receiving at least one permanent molar sealant from SBSP stratified by grade and age.

CDC grantee states are required to report the following measures related to SBSP effectiveness annually:

- Percentage of children with caries experience.

- Percentage of children with untreated decay.

- Percentage of children without sealants at screening.

- Number of molar sealants placed.

- Percentage of children referred for dental treatment.

- Percentage of children with referrals for urgent dental treatment.

CDC grantee states should conduct an analysis documenting the effectiveness of their SBSP. This analysis should include baseline measures of sealant prevalence and first molar caries prevalence and severity.

CDC grantee states with advanced capacity should conduct an in-depth cost analysis of their school-based or school-linked dental sealant program. A sealant cost calculator tool will be available to the states in 2015.

Demonstrate progress and leadership. Over funding period, states should demonstrate significant progress toward increasing the proportion of eligible schools participating in a sealant program and the proportion of children in funded schools receiving at least one sealant. Additional elements of leadership include:

- Providing training and technical assistance to community sealant programs, providers, and other types of sealant programs.

- Submission of sealant best practice approaches to Association of State and Territorial Dental Directors (ASTDD) for sharing with other programs.

- Reporting progress toward sustainability and institutionalization of sealant programs through leveraging of funding, partnership participation, billing Medicaid and/or SCHIP or other sources of support.

Reporting analysis of program quality assurance measures, such as sealant retention data.

Chapter 62

Integration of Oral Health and Primary Care Practice

Critical for Implementation of Core Competencies

Discussions about the strategies for implementing Integration of Oral Health and Primary Care Practice (IOHPCP) were framed around the importance of communication and the three systems described below.

Healthcare Professions

A transformation of the current healthcare profession paradigm will require profound multi- faceted change. Stakeholders and advocates agree that interprofessional education and collaboration is key for this change to occur. Healthcare providers and their respective professional organizations are the essential vehicles for health service delivery. The current context of the professions of dentistry, medicine, nursing, and physician assistant are historically rooted in sociological and academic differences in roles which have resulted in isolation of the fields and lack of communication. There is a growing need to have Communication Healthcare professions Finance Healthcare

This chapter includes text excerpted from "Integration of Oral Health and Primary Care Practice," U.S. Department of Health and Human Services (HHS), February 2014.

systems Critical for implementation of core competencies systematic change that includes policy, payment, education, practice, licensure and accreditation to break down the barriers to integrating oral health and overall health.

Healthcare Systems

Healthcare systems are complex operational structures that include access to care, provision of clinical services, and the underlying foundation that supports implementation of the oral health core clinical competencies. An organized and multi-faceted infrastructure needs to be in place for the efficient and effective implementation of the oral health competencies. Infrastructure includes interoperable information technologies (e.g., electronic health records), communication pathways, and business processes. The infrastructure could enable systems to optimize care coordination across medical and dental care environments to improve patient outcomes.

Financing

Financial issues have been shown to be significant barriers to accessing dental care. Medicaid coverage and payment policies vary greatly from state to state. Furthermore, most state Medicaid programs do not provide direct payment for dental services for adults. As a result of these policy decisions, the current system drives the use of more costly alternatives such as emergency department visits. Severe cases often lead to hospitalization, which could have otherwise been managed less expensively in an outpatient setting. In addition, increased reimbursement payment rates would incentivize more dental providers to treat Medicaid patients resulting in increased availability/access to services. Addressing the public and private sectors for payment options will significantly impact access to oral health services.

The above-identified systems are essential to successful implementation of the core clinical competencies within the context of overarching and central communication.

Component III

Identify strategies to implement the core competencies with emphasis on the three identified systems: healthcare professions, healthcare systems, and financial aspects, by employing outcomes of prior meeting recommendations.

Prior meeting topics were used as the conceptual framework to dialogue with a group of nationally recognized participants who have knowledge and expertise in the areas of professional education and practice, interprofessional collaboration, finance and health system change. Health Resources and Services Administration (HRSA) arranged expert panel presentations that focused on these areas. HRSA facilitated group discussions to provide a forum for discussion of implementation strategies for the oral health competencies.

The charge for the discussions was defined by the following assumptions based on the three recurring systems for consideration: healthcare professions, healthcare systems, and finance.

- **Healthcare professions:** The inclusion of the clinical competencies would be within the existing scopes of practice for the health professionals, while explicitly using collaborative practice.

- **Healthcare system:** The participants represent a variety of interdependent resources and systems necessary for the proposed implementation strategy.

- **Finance:** No additional funds would be available for implementation of the core clinical competencies, therefore encouraging the use of innovative concepts.

These three critical systems were individually described to create a model that facilitates understanding. It is important to recognize that in reality, these systems overlap and are interdependent and do not exist in isolation from one another. In planning programs to incorporate oral health clinical competencies, full consideration of these interdependent systems can have a positive impact on the overall goal to improve access to oral healthcare.

Communication among all involved parties is a key element underlying successful engagement and implementation.

Within the parameters of the above assumptions, with focus on the healthcare safety net setting, the approach allowed the participants to identify aspects of health systems that may be included in order to execute a plan. Several themes emerged that informed the basis of the HRSA recommendations for implementing the core competencies. These themes include: a readiness for action, impatience with the status quo, and the critical timing afforded by multiple changes in the healthcare system. Another theme is the emergence of interprofessional education and practice among professions and professional organizations in order to reap benefits from each profession and create a more seamless approach to healthcare. Access to care, particularly for the underserved, has surfaced as a priority that needs to be addressed in order to assure better healthcare outcomes. Finally, sustainability is a consideration that underlies all of the implementation strategies and is dependent on financial viability.

Risks and challenges involved in the implementation of the oral health core clinical competencies were considered. Examples of overarching implementation issues include: time constraints, organizational leadership support, cross-cutting communication and relationships, and turning knowledge into practice. HRSA developed recommendations that provide a foundation for reproducible strategies to improve health. Progress in implementing the competencies will likely be an incremental process that addresses a number of aspects simultaneously, with a vision and goal of improving our population's overall health. This approach emphasizes interrelated care, with competencies not as an "add-on" but seamlessly incorporated into existing practice supported by educational efforts.

The IOHPCP effort highlights the need for a unified approach to address oral health conditions and implement appropriate interventions to improve health outcomes for the most vulnerable populations. The effort will be used to stimulate ongoing communication and collaborations among primary healthcare and dental providers within the health and financial systems to achieve the goal of improving access to oral healthcare for vulnerable and underserved populations in the United States.

The IOHPCP implementation strategies may be applicable to any population where the need is identified. Clinicians applying the competencies should consider both the clinical standards of their profession and the communities they serve.

HRSA synthesized recommendations and considered expert and professional opinions expressed during the IOHPCP meetings. The following recommendations serve as guiding principles and provide a framework for the design of a competency-based, interprofessional practice model to integrate oral health and primary care.

Part Eight

Additional Help and Information

Chapter 63

Glossary of Terms Related to Dental Care and Oral Health

abnormal dental development: Altered tooth development, craniofacial growth, or skeletal development in children secondary to radiotherapy and/or high doses of chemotherapy before age 9.

aerosol: Particles of respirable size (<10 μm) generated by both humans and environmental sources that can remain viable and airborne for extended periods in the indoor environment; commonly generated in dentistry during use of hand pieces, ultrasonic scalers, and air/water syringes.

alcohol-based hand rub: An alcohol-containing preparation designed for application to the hands for reducing the number of viable microorganisms on the hands.

allergen: An antigen capable of inducing allergy or specific hypersensitivity.

allergic contact dermatitis: A type IV or delayed-hypersensitivity reaction resulting from contact with a chemical allergen.

anaphylaxis (immediate anaphylactic hypersensitivity): A severe and sometimes fatal Type 1 reaction in a susceptible person after a second exposure to a specific antigen (e.g., food, pollen, proteins in latex gloves, or penicillin) after previous sensitization.

This glossary contains terms excerpted from documents produced by several sources deemed reliable.

antibody: A protein found in the blood that is produced in response to foreign substances (e.g., bacteria or viruses) invading the body.

antiseptic: A germicide that is used on skin or living tissue for the purpose of inhibiting or destroying microorganisms.

bacterial endocarditis: A bacterial induced inflammation of the lining of the heart and its valves.

bioburden: The microbiological load (i.e., number of viable organisms in or on the object or surface) or organic material on a surface or object prior to decontamination, or sterilization, also known as "bioload" or "microbial load."

biological indicator: A device to monitor the sterilization process that consists of a standardized population bacterial spores known to be resistant to the mode of sterilization being monitored.

bloodborne pathogens: Disease-producing microorganisms spread by contact with blood or other body fluids contaminated with blood from an infected person.

candidiasis (oral): Yeast or fungal infection that occurs in the oral cavity or pharynx or both.

cleft lip or palate: A congenital opening or fissure occurring in the lip or palate.

contaminated: State of having been in contact with microorganisms.

dental caries (dental decay or cavities): An infectious disease that results in de-mineralization and ultimately cavitation of the tooth surface if not controlled or remineralized. Dental decay may be either treated (filled) or untreated (unfilled).

dental implant: A metal device that is surgically placed in the jawbone. It acts as an anchor for an artificial tooth or teeth.

dental plaque: A sticky film of bacteria can build up on teeth. Plaque produces acids that, over time, eat away at the tooth's hard outer surface and create a cavity.

dental sealants: Are thin plastic coatings that protect the chewing surfaces of children's back teeth from tooth decay.

dental visits: Regular use of the oral healthcare delivery system leads to better oral health by providing an opportunity for clinical preventive services and early detection of oral diseases.

dentures: Are false teeth made to replace teeth you have lost. Dentures can be complete or partial. Complete dentures cover your entire upper or lower jaw. Partials replace one or a few teeth.

detergents: Compounds that possess a cleaning action and have hydrophilic and lipophilic parts.

disinfectant: A chemical agent used on inanimate objects (i.e., non-living) (e.g., floors, walls, sinks) to destroy virtually all recognized pathogenic microorganisms, but not necessarily all microbial forms (e.g., bacterial endospores).

disinfection: The destruction of pathogenic and other kinds of micro-organisms by physical or chemical means.

distilled water: Water heated to the boiling point, vaporized, cooled, condensed, and collected so that no impurities are reintroduced.

edentulism/edentulous: A condition characterized by not having any natural teeth.

erythroplakia: An abnormal patch of red tissue that forms on mucous membranes in the mouth and may become cancer.

fluoridation status: Status of a community water system in regards to water fluoridation level. Most water contains some amount of natural fluoride. Fluoridation involves adjusting fluoride in the water to the level optimal for the prevention of dental caries.

functional disabilities: Impaired ability to eat, taste, swallow, or speak because of mucositis, xerostomia, trismus, or infection.

gingivitis: An inflammatory condition of the gum tissue, which can appear reddened and swollen and frequently bleeds easily.

glycocalyx: A gelatinous polysaccharide and/or polypeptide outer covering. The glycocalyx can be identified by negative staining techniques.

hand hygiene: A general term that applies to handwashing, antiseptic handwash, antiseptic hand rub, and surgical hand antisepsis.

hypersensitivity: An immune reaction (allergy) in which the body has an exaggerated response to a specific antigen (e.g., food, pet dander, wasp venom).

immunity: Protection against a disease. Immunity is indicated by the presence of antibodies in the blood and can usually be determined with a laboratory test.

immunization: The process by which a person becomes immune, or protected, against a disease.

irritant contact dermatitis: The development of dry, itchy, irritated areas on the skin, which can result from frequent handwashing and gloving as well as exposure to chemicals.

latex allergy: A type I or immediate anaphylactic hypersensitivity reaction to the proteins found in natural rubber latex.

latex: A milky white fluid extracted from the rubber tree Hevea brasiliensis that contains the rubber material cis-1,4 polyisoprene.

leukoplakia: An abnormal patch of white tissue that forms on mucous membranes in the mouth and other areas of the body.

medical waste (Regulated): Waste sufficiently capable of causing infection during handling and disposal to merit special handling and disposal.

neurotoxicity: Persistent, deep aching and burning pain that mimics a toothache, but for which no dental or mucosal source can be found.

opportunistic infection: An infection caused by a microorganism that does not ordinarily cause disease but is capable of doing so, under certain host conditions.

oral mucositis/stomatitis: Inflammation and ulceration of the mucous membranes; can increase the risk for pain, oral and systemic infection, and nutritional compromise.

oral prophylaxis: Thorough dental cleaning.

oropharynx: The part of the throat at the back of the mouth behind the oral cavity. It includes the back third of the tongue, the soft palate, the side and back walls of the throat, and the tonsils.

orthodontic devices: *See* dentures.

osteonecrosis: Blood vessel compromise and necrosis of bone exposed to high-dose radiation therapy, resulting in decreased ability to heal if traumatized and extreme susceptibility to infection.

parts per million (PPM): A measure of concentration in solution.

periodontal diseases: Periodontal diseases include gingivitis and periodontitis. Both are inflammatory conditions of the gingival tissues.

prevalence: The number of disease cases (new and existing) within a population at a given time.

public water supply system (PWS): A public water system provides water for human consumption to the public through piped or other constructed conveyances.

radiation caries: Lifelong risk of rampant dental decay that may begin within 3 months of completing radiation treatment if changes in either the quality or quantity of saliva persist.

retraction: The entry of oral fluids and microorganisms into waterlines through negative water pressure.

root caries: Dental decay that occurs on the root portion of a tooth. (In younger persons, root surfaces are usually covered by gum [gingival] tissue.)

sterilant: A liquid chemical germicide that destroys all forms of microbiological life, including high numbers of resistant bacterial spores.

sterile/sterility: State of being free from all living microorganisms.

tooth decay: A commonly known term for dental caries, an infectious, transmissible, disease caused by bacteria.

trismus tissue fibrosis: Loss of elasticity of masticatory muscles that restricts normal ability to open the mouth.

ventilation: The process of supplying and removing air by natural or mechanical means to and from any space.

X-ray: A type of radiation used in the diagnosis and treatment of cancer and other diseases. In low doses, X-rays are used to diagnose diseases by making pictures of the inside of the body. In high doses, X-rays are used to treat cancer.

xerostomia/salivary gland dysfunction: Dryness of the mouth because of thickened, reduced, or absent salivary flow; increases the risk for infection and compromises speaking, chewing, and swallowing.

Chapter 64

Directory of Local Dental Schools

Alabama

University of Alabama at Birmingham (UAB)
School of Dentistry
1919 7th Ave. S.
Ste. 406
Birmingham, AL 35294
Phone: 205-934-3000
Website: www.dental.uab.edu

Arizona

ASDOH Dental Care West
20325 N. 51st Ave.
Unit 156
Glendale, AZ 85308
Phone: 623-251-4700
Website: www.atsu.edu/asdoh

Arizona School of Dentistry and Oral Health (ASDOH)
ASDOH Dental Clinic
5855 E. Still Cir.
Mesa, AZ 85206
Phone: 480-248-8100
Toll-Free: 866-626-2878
Website: www.atsu.edu/asdoh

Midwestern University
College of Dental Medicine
19555 N.
59th Ave.
Glendale, AZ 85308
Phone: 623-572-3215
Website: www.midwestern.edu

Excerpted from "Local Dental Schools," National Institute of Dental and Craniofacial Research (NIDCR), February 26, 2014. All contact information was verified and updated in September 2016.

California

University of California at Los Angeles (UCLA)
Center for Children's Health Media
10833 Le Conte Ave.
CHS-Box 951668
Los Angeles, CA 90095
Phone: 310-206-3904
Toll-Free: 800-825-2631
Fax: 310-825-2951
Website: www.dentistry.ucla.edu/patient-care

University of California at San Francisco (UCSF)
Student Dental Clinic
707 Parnassus Ave.
San Francisco, CA 94143
Phone: 415-502-5800
Toll-Free: 866-678-8399
Website: dentistry.ucsf.edu/patient-services

Loma Linda University (LLU)
School of Dentistry
11092 Anderson St.
Loma Linda, CA 92350
Phone: 909-558-4222
Website: dentistry.llu.edu

University of the Pacific Arthur A. Dugoni
School of Dentistry
155 Fifth St.
San Francisco, CA 94103
Phone: 415-929-6400
Fax: 415-929-6654
Website: dental.pacific.edu/Dental_Services.html

University of Southern California (USC)
Herman Ostrow School of Dentistry
925 W. 34th St.
Los Angeles, CA 90089
Phone: 213-740-2800
Website: dentistry.usc.edu/patient-care/contact
E-mail: patientfeedback@usc.edu

Colorado

University of Colorado School of Dental Medicine
Anschutz Medical Campus
13065 E. 17th Ave.
Aurora, CO 80045
Phone: 303-724-6900
Website: www.ucdenver.edu/academics/colleges/dentalmedicine/PatientCare/Pages/BecomeaPatient.aspx

Connecticut

University of Connecticut
School of Dental Medicine
263 Farmington Ave.
Farmington, CT 06030
Phone: 860-679-3415
Website: sdm.uchc.edu

District of Columbia

Howard University (HU)
College of Dentistry
600 W. St. N.W.
Washington, DC 20059
Phone: 202-806-0456;
202-806-0008
Website: www.dentistry.howard.edu/patientcare.htm

Florida

University of Florida (UF)
College of Dentistry
1395 Center Dr.
P.O. Box 100405
Gainesville, FL 32610
Phone: 352-273-5800
Toll-Free: 800-633-3953
Fax: 352-392-3070
Website: www.dental.ufl.edu/
Patients

*Nova Southeastern
University (NSU)*
College of Dental Medicine
3301 College Ave.
Fort Lauderdale, FL 33314
Phone: 954-262-7500
Toll-Free: 800-541-6682
Website: dental.nova.edu/clinics/
index.html

Georgia

*The Dental College of
Georgia at Augusta
University*
1430 John Wesley Gilbert Dr.
Augusta, GA 30912
Phone: 706-721-7019
Toll-Free: 877-44-AFLAC
(1-877-442-3522)
Fax: 706-721-6276
Website: www.georgiahealth.
edu/dentalmedicine/
patientservices/
becomingapatient.html

Illinois

*University of Illinois at
Chicago (UIC)*
College of Dentistry
801 S. Paulina St.
Chicago, IL 60612
Phone: 312-996-7555
Toll-Free: 855-260-0996
Website: dentistry.uic.edu/depts/
patientservices/index.cfm
E-mail: gradcoll@uic.edu

*Southern Illinois University
(SIU)*
School of Dental Medicine
2800 College Ave.
Alton, IL 62002
Phone: 618-474-7000
Toll-Free: 800-447-SIUE
(800-447-7483)
Website: www.siue.edu/dental

Indiana

Indiana University (IU)
School of Dentistry
1121 W. Michigan St.
Indianapolis, IN 46202
Phone: 317-274-7433
Toll-Free: 888-373-IUSD
(888-373-4873)
Website: www.dentistry.iu.edu/
index.php/patient-services
E-mail: ds-ps@iupui.edu

Iowa

University of Iowa
College of Dentistry
801 Newton Rd.
Dental Sciences Bldg.
Iowa City, IA 52242
Phone: 319-335-7499
Toll-Free: 888-857-7038
Website: www.dentistry.uiowa.
edu/missions/patientcare/
becoming_a_patient.shtml

Kentucky

*University of Louisville
(UofL)*
School of Dentistry
501 S. Preston St.
Louisville, KY 40202
Phone: 502-852-5096
Toll-Free: 800-334-UofL
(800-334-8635)
Website: louisville.edu/dental/
patients
E-mail: DENTALCA@louisville.
edu

University of Kentucky (UK)
College of Dentistry
800 Rose St.
Lexington, KY 40536
Phone: 859-323-3368
Toll-Free: 800-333-8874
Website: dentistry.uky.edu

Louisiana

*Louisiana State University
(LSU)*
School of Dentistry
1100 Florida Ave.
New Orleans, LA 70119
Phone: 504-619-8700
Toll-Free: 888-769-8841
Website: www.lsusd.lsuhsc.edu/
patients.html

Maryland

University of Maryland
Baltimore College of Dental
Surgery
650 W. Baltimore St.
Baltimore, MD 21201
Phone: 410-706-7101
Toll-Free: 866-787-8637
Website: www.dental.
umaryland.edu

Massachusetts

Tufts University
School of Dental Medicine
1 Kneeland St.
Boston, MA 02111
Phone: 617-636-6828
Toll-Free: 866-351-5184
Website: dental.tufts.edu

Boston University
Goldman School of Dental
Medicine
100 E. Newton St.
Boston, MA 02118
Phone: 617-638-4700
Website: www.bu.edu/dental/
patients

Harvard School of Dental Medicine
188 Longwood Ave.
Boston, MA 02115
Phone: 617-432-1434
Website: www.
harvarddentalcenter.harvard.
edu/asp-html

Michigan

University of Detroit Mercy (UDM)
School of Dentistry
2700 Martin Luther King Jr.
Blvd.
Detroit, MI 48208
Phone: 313-494-6700
Website: dental.udmercy.edu/
patient

University of Michigan
School of Dentistry
1011 N. University Ave.
Ann Arbor, MI 48109
Phone: 734-763-6933
Toll-Free: 888-707-2500
Website: dent.umich.edu/
patientservices

Minnesota

University of Minnesota
School of Dentistry
515 Delaware St. S.E. 7th Fl.
Minneapolis, MN 55455
Phone: 612-625-2495
Website: www.dentistry.umn.
edu/patients/index.htm
E-mail: umdentcl@umn.edu

Mississippi

University of Mississippi
School of Dentistry
2500 N. State St.
Jackson, MS 39216
Phone: 601-984-6080
Toll-Free: 888-815-2005
Website: dentistry.umc.edu/
patients/becoming_a_patient.
html

Missouri

University of Missouri–Kansas City
School of Dentistry
650 E. 25th St.
Kansas City, MO 64108
Phone: 816-235-2100
Toll-Free: 800-776-8652
Website: dentistry.umkc.edu/
Patient_Information/index.shtml

Nebraska

Creighton University
School of Dentistry
2500 California Plaza
Omaha, NE 68178
Phone: 402-280-2700
Fax: 402-280-5013
Website: www.creighton.edu/
dentalschool/informationfor
patients/index.php

University of Nebraska Medical Center (UNMC)
College of Dentistry
4000 E. Campus Loop S.
Box 830740
Lincoln, NE 68583-0740
Phone: 402-472-1333
Toll-Free: 800-922-0000
Website: www.unmc.edu/dentistry

Nevada

University of Nevada, Las Vegas (UNLV)
School of Dental Medicine
1700 W. Charleston Blvd.
P.O. Box 7410
Las Vegas, NV 89106
Phone: 702-774-2400
Toll-Free: 877-895-2794
Website: dentalschool.unlv.edu/clinics.html

New Jersey

University of Medicine and Dentistry of New Jersey (UMDNJ)
New Jersey Dental School
110 Bergen St.
Newark, NJ 07103
Phone: 973-972-7370
Website: www.unmc.edu/dentistry

New York

Columbia University
School of Dental and Oral Surgery
630 W. 168th St.
New York, NY 10032
Phone: 212-305-6100
Website: dental.columbia.edu/patients/index.html

New York University
College of Dentistry
345 E. 24th St.
New York, NY 10010
Phone: 212-998-9800
Website: www.nyu.edu/dental/patientinfo/index.html

State University of New York at Stony Brook (SUNY)
School of Dental Medicine
Health Sciences Center
S. Dr.
Stony Brook, NY 11794
Phone: 631-632-8989
Website: dentistry.stonybrookmedicine.edu

State University of New York at Buffalo
School of Dental Medicine
325 Squire Hall
3435 Main St.
Buffalo, NY 14214
Phone: 716-829-2836
Website: dental.buffalo.edu/Patients.aspx

North Carolina

University of North Carolina at Chapel Hill
UNC School of Dentistry
CB #7450
Chapel Hill, NC 27599-7450
Phone: 919-537-3942
Website: www.dentistry.unc.edu/patient
E-mail: underwoj@dentistry.unc.edu

Ohio

Case Western Reserve University
CWRU School of Dental Medicine
10900 Euclid Ave.
Cleveland, OH 44106
Phone: 216-368-2000
Website: dental.case.edu

Ohio State University College of Dentistry
305 W. 12th Ave.
Columbus, OH 43210
Phone: 614-292-2751
Website: dent.osu.edu/patients/index.php

Oklahoma

University of Oklahoma (OU)
College of Dentistry
1201 N. Stonewall Ave,
Oklahoma City, OK 73117-1214
Phone: 405-271-6326
Website: dentistry.ouhsc.edu/patients.php
E-mail: OUCOD-CommCtr@ouhsc.edu

Oregon

Oregon Health and Science University (OHSU)
School of Dentistry
3181 S.W. Sam Jackson Park Rd.
Portland, OR 97239-3098
Phone: 503-494-8311
Website: www.ohsu.edu/xd/health/ohsu-near-you/portland/south-waterfront/school-of-dentistry.cfm

Pennsylvania

University of Pittsburgh
School of Dental Medicine
3501 Terr. St.
Pittsburgh, PA 15261
Phone: 412-648-8616
Website: www.dental.pitt.edu/patients/index.php

Temple University
School of Dentistry
3223 N. Broad St.
Philadelphia, PA 19140
Phone: 215-707-2880
Website: dentistry.temple.edu

University of Pennsylvania
School of Dental Medicine
240 S. 40th St.
Philadelphia, PA 19104
Phone: 215-898-8965
Website: www.dental.upenn.edu/patient_care/dental_school_clinics/patient_information

Puerto Rico

University of Puerto Rico
School of Dentistry
Medical Sciences Campus
P.O. Box 365067
San Juan, PR 00936
Phone: 787-758-2525
Website: dental.rcm.upr.edu/

Medical University of South Carolina (MUSC)
College of Dental Medicine
173 Ashley Ave.
P.O. Box 250507
Charleston, SC 29425
Phone: 843-792-2101
Website: academicdepartments. musc.edu/dentistry/patient_care/ walk_in_care.htm

Tennessee

Meharry Medical College
School of Dentistry
1005 D.B. Todd Jr. Blvd.
Nashville, TN 37208
Phone: 615-327-6348
Website: www.mmc.edu

University of Tennessee
College of Dentistry
875 Union Ave.
Memphis, TN 38163
Phone: 901-448-6468
Website: www.uthsc.edu/ dentistry

Texas

University of Texas (UT)
School of Dentistry
7500 Cambridge St.
Houston, TX 77054
Phone: 713-500-4000
Website: www.uth.edu/index/ maps/inside/sd.htm

University of Texas
San Antonio Dental School
8210 Floyd Curl Dr.
San Antonio, TX 78229
Phone: 210-567-3700
Website: dental.uthscsa.edu/ becomeapatient.php

Texas A&M College of Dentistry
3302 Gaston Ave.
Dallas, TX 75246
Phone: 214-828-8100
Website: dentistry.tamhsc.edu

Virginia

Virginia Commonwealth University (VCU)
School of Dentistry
520 N. 12th St.
P.O. Box 980566
Richmond, VA 23298
Phone: 804-828-9190
Website: vcudentalcare.com
E-mail: dentalcare@vcu.edu

Washington

University of Washington (UW)
School of Dentistry
Health Sciences Bldg.
1959 N.E. Pacific St. D322
Seattle, WA 98119-6365
Phone: 206-616-6996;
206-685-1022
Toll-Free: 866-791-1278
Website: www.dental.
washington.edu/patient/patient-
care-guide.html-0

West Virginia

West Virginia University
School of Dentistry
Robert C. Byrd Health Sciences
Center.
P.O. Box 9400
Morgantown, WV 26506-9400
Phone: 304-293-2521
Toll-Free: 800-982-8242
Website: dentistry.hsc.wvu.edu/
Patient-Services

Wisconsin

Marquette University
School of Dentistry
1801 W. Wisconsin Ave.
Milwaukee, WI 53233
Phone: 414-288-6790
Toll-Free: 800-222-6544
Website: www.marquette.edu/
dentistry

Directory of Organizations That Provide Information about Dental Care and Oral Health Resources

Government Agencies That Provide Information about Dental and Oral Health

Administration for Children and Families (ACF)
Office of Head Start (OHS)
330 C St. S.W. 4th Fl.
Washington, DC 20201
Toll-Free: 866-763-6481
Fax: 202-205-9721
Website: www.acf.hhs.gov/office-of-head-start

Agency for Healthcare Research and Quality (AHRQ)
5600 Fishers Ln.
Rockville, MD 20850
Toll-Free: 800-358-9295
Phone: 301-427-1364
Website: www.ahrq.gov

Resources in this chapter were compiled from several sources deemed reliable; all contact information was verified and updated in September 2016.

Celiac Disease Awareness Campaign (CDAC)
National Digestive Diseases
Information Clearinghouse
(NDDIC)
2 Information Way
Bethesda, MD 20892
Toll-Free: 800-891-5389
Toll-Free TTY: 866-569-1162
Website: www.celiac.nih.gov
E-mail: celiac@info.niddk.nih.
gov

Centers for Disease Control and Prevention (CDC)
1600 Clifton Rd.
Atlanta, GA 30329-4027
Toll-Free: 800-CDC-INFO
(800-232-4636)
Toll-Free TTY: 888-232-6348
Website: www.cdc.gov
E-mail: OADS@cdc.gov

Centers for Medicare and Medicaid Services (CMS)
7500 Security Blvd.
Baltimore, MD 21244
Toll-Free: 800-633-4227
Toll-Free TTY: 877-486-2048
Website: www.cms.hhs.gov

Clinical Trials Center (CTC)
10 Cloister Ct. Bldg. 61
Bethesda, MD 20892
Toll-Free: 800-411-1222
Toll-Free TTY: 866-411-1010
Website: clinicalcenter.nih.gov
E-mail: prpl@mail.cc.nih.gov

Eunice Kennedy Shriver National Institute of Child Health and Human Development (NICHD)
31 Center Dr.
Bldg. 31 Rm. 2A32
Bethesda, MD 20892
Toll-Free: 800-370-2943
Toll-Free TTY: 888-320-6942
Fax: 866-760-5947
Website: www.nichd.nih.gov
E-mail:
NICHDInformationResource
Center@mail.nih.gov

Head Start
Administration for Children and Families (ACF)
370 L'Enfant Promenade S.W.
Washington, DC 20447
Toll-Free: 866-763-6481
Website: eclkc.ohs.acf.hhs.gov/
hslc/hs
E-mail: HeadStart@eclkc.info

Health Resources and Services Administration (HRSA)
5600 Fishers Ln.
Rockville, MD 20857
Toll-Free: 888-275-4772
Toll-Free TTY: 877-489-4772
Website: www.hrsa.gov

Medicaid-CHIP State Dental Association (MSDA)
4411 Connecticut Ave. N.W.
#401
Washington, DC 20008
Phone: 202-248-3993
Fax: 202-248-2315
Website: www.medicaiddental.
org

National Cancer Institute (NCI)
NCI Public Inquiries Office
9609 Medical Center Dr.
BG 9609 MSC 9760
Bethesda, MD 20892-9760
Toll-Free: 800-4-CANCER
(800-422-6237)
Website: www.cancer.gov

National Diabetes Education Program (NDEP)
1 Diabetes Way
Bethesda, MD 20814
Toll-Free: 888-693-NDEP
(888-693-6337)
Toll-Free TTY: 866-569-1162
Fax: 703-738-4929
Website: www.ndep.nih.gov
E-mail: ndep@mail.nih.gov

National Diabetes Information Clearinghouse (NDIC)
1 Information Way
Bethesda, MD 20892
Toll-Free: 800-860-8747
Toll-Free TTY: 866-569-1162
Fax: 703-738-4929
Website: www.diabetes.niddk.nih.gov
E-mail: healthinfo@niddk.nih.gov

National Digestive Diseases Information Clearinghouse (NDDIC)
2 Information Way
Bethesda, MD 20892
Toll-Free: 800-891-5389
Phone: 301-654-3810
Toll-Free TTY: 866-569-1162
Website: digestive.niddk.nih.gov
E-mail: nddic@info.niddk.nih.gov

National Institute of Dental and Craniofacial Research (NIDCR)
National Oral Health Information Clearinghouse (NOHIC)
1 NOHIC Way
Bethesda, MD 20892
Toll-Free: 866-232-4528
Fax: 301-480-4098
Website: www.nidcr.nih.gov
E-mail: nidcrinfo@mail.nih.gov

National Institute of Diabetes and Digestive and Kidney Diseases (NIDDK)
31 Center Dr. MSC 2560
Bldg. 31 Rm. 9A06
Bethesda, MD 20892
Phone: 301-496-3583
Website: www2.niddk.nih.gov

National Institute of Neurological Disorders and Stroke (NINDS)
NIH Neurological Institute
P.O. Box 5801
Bethesda, MD 20824
Toll-Free: 800-352-9424
Phone: 301-496-5751
TTY: 301-468-598
Website: www.ninds.nih.gov

National Institute on Aging (NIA)
31 Center Dr. MSC 2292
Bldg. 31 Rm. 5C27
Bethesda, MD 20892
Toll-Free: 800-222-2225
Phone: 301-496-1752
Toll-Free TTY: 800-222-4225
Fax: 301-496-1072
Website: www.nia.nih.gov
E-mail: niaic@nia.nih.gov

National Institute on Deafness and Other Communication Disorders (NIDCD)
31 Center Dr.
MSC 2320
Bethesda, MD USA 20892-2320
Toll-Free: 800-241-1044
Toll-Free TTY: 800-241-1055
Fax: 301-770-8977
Website: www.nidcd.nih.gov
E-mail: nidcdinfo@nidcd.nih.gov

National Institutes of Health (NIH)
9000 Rockville Pike
Bethesda, MD 20892
Phone: 301-496-4000
TTY: 301-402-9612
Website: www.nih.gov
E-mail: NIHinfo@od.nih.gov

National Oral Health Information Clearinghouse (NOHIC)
Bethesda, MD 20892-2190
Toll-Free: 866-232-4528
Phone: 301-496-4261
Website: www.nidcr.nih.gov
E-mail: nidcrinfo@mail.nih.gov

NIH Osteoporosis and Related Bone Diseases
National Resource Center (NRC)
2 AMS Cir.
Bethesda, MD 20892
Toll Free: 800-624-BONE
(800-624-2663)
Phone: 202-223-0344
TTY: 202-466-4315
Fax: 202-293-2356
Website: www.bones.nih.gov
E-mail: NIHBoneInfo@mail.nih.gov

U.S. Department of Health and Human Services (HHS)
200 Independence Ave. S.W.
Washington, DC 20201
Toll-Free: 877-696-6775
Website: www.hhs.gov

U.S. Environmental Protection Agency (EPA)
1200 Pennsylvania Ave. N.W.
Ariel Rios Bldg.
Washington, DC 20460
Phone: 202-272-0167
TTY: 202-272-0165
Website: www.epa.gov

U.S. Food and Drug Administration (FDA)
10903 New Hampshire Ave.
Silver Spring, MD 20993
Toll-Free: 888-INFO-FDA
(888-463-6332)
Website: www.fda.gov

Private Agencies That Provide Information about Dental and Oral Health

*Academy of General
Dentistry (AGD)*
560 W. Lake St., 6th Fl.
Chicago, IL 60661
Toll-Free: 888-243-3368 ext.
5300
Fax: 312-335-3443
Website: www.agd.org
E-mail: membership@agd.org

*American Academy of
Cosmetic Dentistry (AACD)*
402 W. Wilson St.
Madison, WI 53703
Toll-Free: 800-543-9220
Phone: 608-222-8583
Fax: 608-222-9540
Website: www.aacd.com

*American Academy of
Implant Dentistry (AAID)*
211 E. Chicago Ave., Ste. 750
Chicago, IL 60611
Toll-Free: 888-929-9298
Phone: 312-335-1550
Fax: 312-335-9090
Website: www.aaid-implant.org
E-mail: info@aaid.com

*American Academy of Oral
Medicine (AAOM)*
2150 N 107th St.
Ste. 205
Seattle, WA 98133
Phone: 206-209-5279
Fax: 425-771-9588
Website: www.aaom.com/
patients
E-mail: info@aaom.com

*American Academy of
Pediatric Dentistry (AAPD)*
211 E. Chicago Ave., Ste. 1600
Chicago, IL 60611-2637
Phone: 312-337-2169
Fax: 312-337-6329
Website: www.aapd.org

*American Academy of
Periodontology (AAP)*
737 N. Michigan Ave.
Ste. 800
Chicago, IL 60611
Phone: 312-787-5518
Fax: 312-787-3670
Website: www.perio.org

*American Association of
Endodontists (AAE)*
211 E. Chicago Ave.
Ste. 1100
Chicago, IL 60611
Toll-Free: 800-872-3636
Phone: 312-266-7255
Fax: 866-451-9020
Website: www.aae.org
E-mail: info@aae.org

*American Association of Oral
and Maxillofacial Surgeons
(AAOMS)*
9700 W. Bryn Mawr Ave.
Rosemont, IL 60018-5701
Toll-Free: 800-822-6637
Phone: 847-678-6200
Fax: 847-678-6286
Website: www.aaoms.org

American Association of Orthodontists (AAO)
401 N. Lindbergh Blvd.
St. Louis, MO 63141
Toll-Free: 800-424-2841
Phone: 314-993-1700
Fax: 314-997-1745
Website: www.aaomembers.org
E-mail: info@aaortho.org

American Dental Assistants Association (ADAA)
140 N. Bloomingdale Rd.
Bloomingdale, IL 60108
Toll-Free: 877-874-3785
Phone: 312-541-1550
Fax: 630-351-8490
Website: www.dentalassistant. org

American Dental Association (ADA)
211 E. Chicago Ave.
Chicago, IL 60611
Toll-Free: 800-621-8099
Website: www.ada.org

American Dental Hygienists Association (ADHA)
444 N. Michigan Ave., Ste. 3400
Chicago, IL 60611
Phone: 312-449-8900
Website: www.adha.org

American Diabetes Association (ADA)
1701 N. Beauregard St.
Alexandria, VA 22311
Toll-Free: 800-DIABETES
(800-342-2383)
Website: www.diabetes.org

American Head and Neck Society (AHNS)
11300 W. Olympic Blvd.
Ste. 600
Los Angeles, CA 90064
Phone: 310-437-0559
Fax: 310-437-0585
Website: www.ahns.info

Children's Dental Health Project (CDHP)
1020 19th St. N.W., Ste. 400
Washington, DC 20036
Phone: 202-833-8288
Fax: 202-833-8288
Website: www.cdhp.org
E-mail: info@cdhp.org

Cleft Palate Foundation (CPF)
1504 E. Franklin St., Ste. 102
Chapel Hill, NC 27514
Toll-Free: 800-242-5338
Phone: 919-933-9044
Fax: 919-933-9604
Website: www.cleftline.org

Cleveland Clinic
9500 Euclid Ave.
Cleveland, OH 44195
Toll-Free: 800-223-2273
TTY: 216-444-0261
Website: www.clevelandclinic. org

FACES: The National Craniofacial Association
P.O. Box 11082
Chattanooga, TN 37401
Toll-Free: 800-332-2373
Phone: 423-266-1632
Website: www.faces-cranio.org

Health Physics Society (HPS)
1313 Dolley Madison Blvd., Ste. 402
McLean, VA 22101
Phone: 703-790-1745
Fax: 703-790-2672
Website: www.hps.org
E-mail: HPS@BurkInc.com

Juvenile Diabetes Research
Foundation International
(JDRF)
26 Broadway 14th Fl.
New York, NY 10004
Toll-Free: 800-533-CURE
(800-533-2873)
Website: www.jdrf.org
E-mail: faces@faces-cranio.org

National Academy of
Sciences (NAS)
500 5th St. N.W.
Washington, DC 20001
Phone: 202-334-2000
Website: www.
nationalacademies.org

National Dental Association
(NDA)
3517 16th St. N.W.
Washington, DC 20010
Phone: 202-588-1697
Fax: 202-588-1244
Website: www.ndaonline.org

National Eating Disorders
Association (NEDA)
165 W. 46th St.
New York, NY 10036
Toll-Free: 800-931-2237
Phone: 212-575-6200
Fax: 212-575-1650
Website: www.
nationaleatingdisorders.org

Hispanic Dental Association
(HDA)
3085 Stevenson Dr.
Ste. 200
Springfield, IL 62703
Phone: 217-529-6517
Fax: 217-529-9120
Website: www.hdassoc.org
E-mail: gchda@hdassoc.org

National Maternal and
Child Oral Health Resource
Center (OHRC)
Georgetown University
2115 Wisconsin Ave. N.W.
Ste. 601
Washington, DC 20007
Phone: 202-784-9771
Fax: 202-784-9777
Website: www.mchoralhealth.
org
E-mail: OHRCinfo@georgetown.
edu

The Nemours Foundation
1600 Rockland Rd.
Wilmington, DE 19803
Phone: 302-651-4000
Website: www.kidshealth.org
E-mail: AskCompliance@
nemours.org

Oral Health America (OHA)
180 N. Michigan Ave.
Ste. 1150
Chicago, IL 60601
Phone: 312-836-9900
Fax: 312-836-9986
Website: www.
oralhealthamerica.org
E-mail: info@oralhealthamerica.
org

Sjögren's Syndrome Foundation (SSF)
6707 Democracy Blvd., Ste. 325
Bethesda, MD 20817
Toll-Free: 800-475-6473
Phone: 301-530-4420
Fax: 301-530-4415
Website: www.sjogrens.org

Special Care Dentistry Association (SCDA)
401 N. Michigan Ave., Ste. 2000
Chicago, IL 60611
Phone: 312-527-6764
Fax: 312-673-6663
Website: scdaonline.org
E-mail: SCDA@SCDAOnline.org

Support for People with Head and Neck Cancer (SPOHNC)
P.O. Box 53
Locust Valley, NY 11560
Toll-Free: 800-377-0928
Fax: 516-671-8794
Website: www.spohnc.org
E-mail: info@spohnc.org

TNA Facial Pain Association
408 W. University Ave., Ste. 602
Gainesville, FL 32601
Toll-Free: 800-923-3608
Phone: 352-384-3600
Fax: 352-384-3600
Website: www.fpa-support.org

Index

Index

Y

yogurt
  calcium rich foods 155
  healthy diet 25
  soft foods 53
  teeth sensitivity 84

Z

zaleplon (Sonata), non-
  benzodiazepines 99
zinc
  denture adhesives 130
  dental amalgam filling 109
zolpidem (Ambien), oral sedatives 99